THE ORIGINS OF MODERN PSYCHIATRY

£29.50

✓

THE ORIGINS OF MODERN PSYCHIATRY

Edited by

C. Thompson

Charing Cross and Westminster Medical School
London UK

A Wiley Medical Publication

JOHN WILEY & SONS
Chichester · New York · Brisbane · Toronto · Singapore

Library of Congress Cataloging-in-Publication Data

The origins of modern psychiatry.
  (A Wiley medical publication)
  Includes index.
  1. Psychiatry—History—Sources. I. Thompson,
Chris. II. Series. [DNLM: 1. Mental Disorders.
2. Psychiatry—history.   WM 11.1 069]
RC438.075   1987   616.89′009   87–8163

ISBN 0 471 91581 5

British Library Cataloguing in Publication Data:

The origins of modern psychiatry.
  1. Psychiatry—History
  I. Thompson, Chris
  616.89′009′034   RC438

  ISBN 0 471 91581 5

Typeset by Photo·graphics, Honiton, Devon
Printed by Anchor Brendon Ltd, Tiptree, Colchester

List of Contributors

P.E .Bebbington, MA PhD MRCP MRCPsych, *Honorary Senior Lecturer, MRC Social Psychiatry Unit, Institute of Psychiatry, London, UK*

G.E. Berrios, MA (Oxon) MD FRCPsych, *Consultant and University Lecturer in Psychiatry, University of Cambridge; Librarian, Royal College of Psychiatrists, London, UK*

Dorothy Joan Bicknell, MD FRCPsych, *Professor of the Psychiatry of Mental Handicap, St George's Hospital Medical School, London, UK*

Felicity De Zulueta, MA BSc MB ChB MRCPsych, *Consultant Psychotherapist, Charing Cross Hospital, London, UK*

R.D.T. Farmer, MB BS MRCGP, *Professor of Community Medicine, Charing Cross and Westminster Medical School, London, UK*

C.P.L. Freeman, MB ChB MRCPsych, *Consultant Psychotherapist, Royal Edinburgh Hospital, Edinburgh, Scotland*

E.H. Hare, FRCP FRCPsych MD, *Physician Emeritus, Maudsley Hospital, London, UK*

D. Leigh, MD FRCP, *Physician Emeritus, Maudsley Hospital, London, UK*

H.G.Morgan, MD (Cantab) FRCP FRCPsych DPM (Lond), *Professor of Mental Health, University of Bristol, UK*

H.R. Rollin, MD MRCP FRCPsych, *Emeritus Consultant Psychiatrist, Horton Hospital, Surrey, UK*

C. Thompson, MB BSc MPhil MD MRCPsych, *Charing Cross and Westminster Medical School, London, UK*

T.H. Turner, BA MB BS MRCPsych DHMSA, *Consultant Psychiatrist, St Bartholomew's & Hackney Hospitals, London, UK*

G. Wilkinson, BSc MPhil MB ChB MRCP MRCPsych, *Honorary Senior Lecturer, General Practice Research Unit, Institute of Psychiatry, London, UK*

Contents

Introduction: The Origins of Modern Psychiatry
C.Thompson   1

1. 1856: JOHN CONNOLLY
    THE TREATMENT OF THE INSANE WITHOUT MECHANICAL
    RESTRAINTS
    London, Smith, Elder and Co, Reprinted 1973, Dawsons, Folkestone,
    In Psychiatric Monograph series
    P.E. Bebbington   7

2. 1866: J. LANGDON H. DOWN MD LOND
    OBSERVATIONS ON AN ETHNIC CLASSIFICATION OF IDIOTS
    Lectures and reports from the London Hospital for 1866, 259–262
    D.J. Bicknell   15

3. SIR WILLIAM WITHEY GULL MD BART
    ANOREXIA NERVOSA
    Transcripts of the Clinical Society of London, 1874, 7, 22–28; British
    Medical Journal, 1873, 527–528; Lancet, 1888, 516–517
    H.G. Morgan   25

4. 1878: D. HACK TUKE MD
    INSANITY IN ANCIENT AND MODERN LIFE WITH CHAPTERS ON
    ITS PREVENTION.
    Chapter VII Facts and Figures in Regard to the Increase of Insanity.
    London, Macmillan & Co
    E.H. Hare   49

5. 1888: HUGHLINGS JACKSON
    ON A PARTICULAR VARIETY OF EPILEPSY ('INTELLECTUAL AURA'):
    ONE CASE WITH SYMPTOMS OF ORGANIC BRAIN DISEASE. Brain
    II, 179–207
    T.H. Turner   59

6. 1893: J. BREUER AND S. FREUD
    ON THE PSYCHICAL MECHANISM OF HYSTERICAL PHENOMENA:
    PRELIMINARY COMMUNICATION.
    In Studies of Hysteria, Standard Edition, 2, 3.
    F. de Zulueta   87

7. 1897: E. DURKHEIM
    SUICIDE
    (Translation) London, Routledge and Kegan Paul, 1952.
    Book 1 Chapter 1 Suicide and Psychopathic States
    Book 3 Chapter 1 The Social Element of Suicide
    R.D.T. Farmer   105

8. 1899: HENRY MAUDSLEY MD
    THE CAUSATION AND PREVENTION OF INSANITY
    In Pathology of the Mind. Appleton and Co., New York, Chapter 3
    H.R. Rollin   139

9. 1911: EUGEN BLEULER
    THE FUNDAMENTAL SYMPTOMS IN DEMENTIA PRAECOX OR THE
    GROUP OF SCHIZOPHRENIAS
    (Trans J. Zinkin 1950) International Universities Press, New York,
    The Fundamental Symptoms
    G.E.Berrios   165

10. 1913: HIDEYO NOGUCHI MD AND J. W. MOORE MD
    DEMONSTRATION OF *TREPONEMA PALLIDUM* IN THE BRAIN IN
    CASES OF GENERAL PARALYSIS
    Journal of Experimental Medicine 17, 232-238
    D. Leigh   211

11.   E. KRAEPELIN
      DEMENTIA PRAECOX AND PARAPHRENIA (1919)
      (Translated by R. M. Barclay from the 8th edition Psychiatrie, Barth,
      Leipzig) Livingstone, Edinburgh.
      INTRODUCTORY LECTURES ON CLINICAL PSYCHIATRY
      (1906 Second edition, translated by T. Johnstone) Baillière, Tindall and
      Cox, London, Lecture III, Dementia Praecox
      G. Wilkinson   225

12.   E. KRAEPELIN
      MANIC DEPRESSIVE INSANITY AND PARANOIA (1921)
      (Translated by R M Barclay, from 8th edition Psychiatrie, Barth Leipzig)
      Livingstone, Edinburgh.
      INTRODUCTORY LECTURES ON CLINICAL PSYCHIATRY
      (1906 Second edition, translated by T. Johnstone) Bailliere, Tindall and
      Cox, London, Lecture I, Melancholia
      C. Thompson   245

13.   1938: U. CERLETTI AND L. BINI
      A NEW METHOD OF SHOCK THERAPY: 'ELECTROCONVULSIVE
      TREATMENT' (SUMMARY)
      Boll Acad Med Roma, 64, 136–138
      C.P.L. Freeman   259

Index   273

Introduction: The Origins of Modern Psychiatry

In the last few years the history of Psychiatry has undergone a transformation, with increases in activity and popularity. What used to be the preserve of a few retired psychiatrists has become a growth point of psychiatric research. At a Royal Society of Medicine Symposium in London entitled *Research with a Future* the paper on History of Psychiatry at first appeared out of place. This impression was thoroughly dispelled by the speaker who gave a reasoned account of the importance of research into the history of psychiatry. As with all fields of research which cross professional boundaries there is still, however, a place for the interested psychiatrist to make a valuable contribution. This has been recognized by the inauguration of the history of psychiatry group of the Royal College of Psychiatrists. All of the contributors to this book are psychiatrists (with the exception of one community physician) who have had an interest in the history of psychiatry over a number of years, most having already written extensively on the subject.

A study of the history of ideas in any subject is important not only as an abstract field of enquiry, but also as a method of retaining an appropriate perspective on the current status of the subject and proposed developments. In most cases 'new' ideas have been thought of before. It is easy to distort the history of a subject like psychiatry, which has always had contentious areas within it. Indeed, almost without exception, the papers chosen for this anthology are concerned with controversies. While many of them are purely scientific controversies, in psychiatry it is impossible to ignore the ethical and social dilemmas often contained therein. In that respect psychiatry, far more than the technical subjects of medicine, is closer to the mainstream of the history of ideas. Examples of distortions have been the views of the antipsychiatrists in which all progress in psychiatry has been forced upon a reluctant and reactionary profession by enlightened outside influences. The data to hand do not support this interpretation of history. Connolly and Gardiner-Hill were psychiatrists who worked against tremendous pressure from the 'community' to liberalize the hospitals and institutions to which the 'mad' were committed, and there are many other examples of the liberalizing influence of psychiatrists themselves upon the treatment of patients in this and earlier centuries.

Psychiatry is a subject which is still developing and in order to understand present controversies and assess the adequacy of proposed changes an historical perspective is essential. For example, a knowledge of the treatment before the advent of the victorian asylum of those who were poor and mad is both a warning to those planning community services without adequate fiscal provision, and a lesson in the historical inadequacy of the view that asylums were simply machines for social control.

The motivation for this book came from a realization of the difficulty of obtaining access to the historical material itself. A case in point is the volume on suicide by Durkheim. This is a reference known by every self-respecting psychiatric trainee and most medical students, but very few will have read even the most relevant parts of the translation, gaining all of their knowledge of it from textbooks and reviews. It is difficult to find a copy in even the most well-stocked medical libraries. Thus there seemed to be a need for an anthology of original works covering the formative years of psychiatry as practised today.

This book deals with the years between 1856, when Connolly was experimenting with non-restraint, and 1938, when the first successful treatment for acute psychiatric disorder was introduced—electroconvulsive therapy (ECT). It would be impossible to cover all the major contributions during this period, and there are many important developments which have been missed by setting these two landmarks as the limits. However this was a period of extraordinary change in which the foundations of our present practice were laid down. Before this period there were great contributions such as Prichard's monograph on *Moral Insanity* or Burton's *Anatomy of Melancholy*. Since the discovery of ECT there have of course been further enormous changes in the treatment of acute psychiatric illness which have transformed the specialty still further. These developments were thought to be too recent for inclusion here.

Each of the original works are accompanied by a commentary written by a modern expert in the field, aiming to set the work in historical context and to bring out the points which are still most relevant today.

We start then in 1856, the year in which John Connolly published *The Treatment of the Insane Without Mechanical Restraints*. In fact the extracts chosen are from his Hanwell reports for the years 1845 and 1846 because these best convey the impact and excitement of his 'great experiment'. Argument still persists over the roles of Gardiner-Hill and Charlesworth in

Lincoln versus Connolly at Hanwell in this advance and the interested reader can find more about the former in the paper by Walk (1970). Dr Paul Bebbington, a senior lecturer in today's social psychiatry, sets the scene by describing the status of the mentally ill immediately before and during Connolly's era.

Ten years later one of the first attempts to subdivide the class of 'idiots' appeared. Greatly flawed as the paper is, Professor Joan Bicknell points out that Down's approach to the mentally handicapped was unusual for it's humanity. His ideas about the significance of this group of 'Down's syndrome' cases were rooted in the incorrect notions of race prevalent at the time and were not an expression of any personal race hatred. Further subdivision of mental handicap followed, leading eventually to discrete aetiologies and in some cases therapies.

Three related items on anorexia nervosa have been included. The 1874 paper from the *Transcripts of the Clinical Society of London* is the substantive first paper. However, the *British Medical Journal* reported the discussion of that paper in 1873, before publication of the transcript. A further report in the *Lancet* 1888 carried woodcuts of one of the first recognized cases and has value as a detailed description. Professor Morgan points to the courage of Gull in attributing this sometimes fatal illness to psychological causes.

Daniel Hack Tuke was the third in a family of famous psychiatrists and a prolific writer on psychiatry. It was difficult to choose a single example of his work. The chapter on the increase in insanity is valuable today because current theories of the causes of schizophrenia (for example, the viral hypothesis) have demanded a re-examination of the emergence of insanity during the 19th century. Doctor Edward Hare has been a distinguished contributor to this literature in recent times and has reappraised this rather statistical work. After extensive research he has also given us the first brief biography of D. H. Tuke.

The gradual delineation of the diseases of the brain towards the end of the 19th century brought the alienists and the neurologists ever closer together and the description in 1888 by Hughlings Jackson of the intellectual aura associated with what we now call temporal lobe epilepsy led to a gradual recognition of the importance of this area of the brain for investigations of psychiatric illnesses. Today the relationship between the temporal lobe and symptoms of the major psychoses remains a major theme of research in biological psychiatry. Doctor Trevor Turner discusses the relationship between neurology and psychiatry at that time.

Less than ten years later a new strand in the story emerged: psychoanalysis. The formulation of the psychical mechanism of hysteria presented in this preliminary communication has had an influence far greater than might have been expected at the time. The ideological gap between the psychoanalytic and the biological views of psychiatric disorder persists to this day, while the pendulum continues to swing first in favour of one then the other approach. The influence of this and succeeding psychoanalytic papers on the mainstream of intellectual life has been profound. Indeed it was a reaction to the claim that the analytic approach to the mind was scientific that led Karl Popper to formulate his view of science, which has become dominant in the philosophy of science and which has largely destroyed the scientific credibility of psychoanalysis. However, non-science is not necessarily nonsense and psychoanalysis still boasts a large number of adherents within psychiatry.

Durkheim's book on suicide is one of the first empirical studies of a social phenomenon and hence is as important for sociologists as for psychiatrists. Two chapters in the book are particularly relevant to psychiatry, those on psychopathic states and on the social element of suicide. Dr Farmer, as a community physician and an editor of a book on suicide, is able to direct appropriate criticism of this otherwise seminal work towards Durkheim's uncritical use of data.

Maudsley was a towering figure in 19th century English psychiatry, using both his intellect and his wealth to promote the study of mental illness. As shown by Dr Rollin he represents another connection with the mainstream of thought, being a correspondent of Charles Darwin. The contribution chosen here has a particularly modern ring to it in many respects, standing as it does for the multiple causation theory of psychiatric illness, but putting genetic influences well to the fore. In common with many victorian writers however he spreads ideas across many pages and hence is somewhat inaccessible for most present day readers. He has therefore been heavily edited, I hope without losing the important elements of his argument.

Modern as he seems in many respects Maudsley still used what is now an outdated nosology. The beginnings of our modern classification appear with the contributions by Bleuler and Kraepelin. There were many editions of Kraepelin's books and dementia praecox was first put forward as an idea in 1893. Thus Bleuler's contribution comes later in strict chronology, but here, because I have taken the descriptions of dementia praecox and manic depression from 1919 and 1921, respectively, Bleuler appears to come first. Dr Berrios is an influential writer on the history of psychiatric concepts and is thorough in his dissection of schizophrenia and it's origins.

The Kraepelin chapters are each taken from two sources: one a theoretical work to elucidate the concept and the other one of the lectures on clinical psychiatry. These latter have great impact, bringing alive the atmosphere of the clinical lecture theatre of the day and each case demonstrating more about Kraepelin's method than would more detail from the theoretical works.

The Bleuler and Kraepelin contributions are separated by possibly one of the greatest discoveries of the time: the proof that *Treponema pallidum* caused general paralysis of the insane by the demonstration of the microorganisms in the brain. This discovery bolstered the case for a biological psychiatry and for the exploration of other physical causes of psychiatric illness. It helped to classify the psychoses and led to the search for a specific treatment. Dr Leigh puts all this in detailed context in a lively account, including descriptions of the lives and personalities of the main protagonists.

Finally we come to 1938 and the discovery of the therapeutic effects of ECT. This paper is an obviously hurried account given by Cerletti and Bini and the subsequent confusion over the attribution of the first description is clearly described by Dr Chris Freeman. With this contribution we enter the modern era and so come to the end of the gestation period which we have identified as taking roughly 83 years from 1856 to 1938. However such historical divisions are arbitrary and any anthology such as this one inevitably leaves out more than it can encompass.

CHRIS THOMPSON

REFERENCE

Walk, A. (1970). Lincoln and Non-restraint, *British Journal of Psychiatry,* **117**, 481–496.

1

The Treatment of the Insane without Mechanical Restraints
John Connolly, 1856

FROM MY SEVENTH REPORT (1845)

"Of the patients admitted during the year, several have come to the asylum in restraints, which have of course always and immediately been removed. In no case has this removal been productive of any accident, or of any inconvenience or difficulty which the officers and attendants of a well-ordered asylum should not be expected to meet, and to overcome. Thirteen of the cases admitted were reported suicidal. The imposition of restraint in some of the cases alluded to appeared inexplicable; as the subjects of them were remarkable for their tranquillity.

"Two female patients among those who had been subjected to severe restraints before coming to the county asylum, had become insane in the puerperal state; and both began to recover almost as soon as admitted. One was an irritable patient, easily excited; the other a delicate and timid woman, easily alarmed. These were among the few cases received at an early stage of the malady; and both patients left the asylum within a few months after admission. (M. B. admitted December, 1844, and discharged March, 1845; and H. L. admitted February, 1845, and discharged March 28th.)

"Without making further allusion to the subject of restraint, I shall on this occasion merely observe that the sixth year, during which the great experiment of managing every kind of case without having recourse to it by day or by night, has been completed without the occurrence of any accident which restraint could have effectually prevented, and without the occurrence of any suicide; and that the non-restraint system appears to be becoming gradually adopted in the greater number of asylums, public and private."

FROM MY EIGHTH REPORT (1846)

"On the 21st day of September last, seven years were completed during which no strait-waistcoat, muff, leg-lock, handcuff, coercion-chair, or other means of mechanical restraint have been resorted to in the Hanwell Asylum, by night or by day. In those seven years, 1,100 cases have been admitted, and treated entirely on the non-restraint system; and the number of patients in the asylum has, during a great part of the same period, amounted to nearly 1,000.

"There are still some asylums in England, Ireland, and Scotland, in which such means of restraint are employed and defended; and travellers from various parts of the Continent, and from the United States of America, apparently prepossessed in favour of such ancient and forcible methods of control, continue to pay hasty visits to Hanwell, and to publish opinions condemnatory of the non-restraint system. In the annual reports of past years, when the experiment was but in an early stage of its progress, and when it was embarrassed by many difficulties, I refrained from engaging in any controversy on the subject; being satisfied that the results would furnish the best test of its being rational and judicious, as well as humane. If such results had not appeared, it would have been my duty to modify or abandon the system, as, in similar circumstances, it would have been my duty to alter or relinquish any other particular in the treatment of the patients. Now, after seven years' patient trial, during which the non-restraint system has been introduced into many other asylums, without the occurrence of any accident against which mechanical restraint would have afforded security, I do not think it desirable more particularly to notice the opinions of writers who have sometimes appeared to visit Hanwell more prepared to argue than disposed to observe; nor should I deem it necessary to refer to this part of the treatment, if it were not that I consider it still requisite to remind those who are most anxious to adopt it, that certain conditions are essential to its being successfully maintained.

"One of the first of these is, a properly constructed building, in which the patients enjoy the advantages of light and air, and a cheerful prospect, and ample space for exercise, and for classification, and means of occupation and recreation. The next is the constant and watchful superintendence of humane and intelligent officers, exercising full but considerate and just control over an efficient body of attendants. Other conditions are connected with such attention to the diet, clothing, lodging, and general cleanliness of the patients, as may exclude all avoidable sources of physical and mental uneasiness. Various employments, a certain extent of instruction, judicious religious attentions, and frequent opportunities of recreation, are indispensable and powerful auxiliaries. The whole treatment, management, and government of the patients and of the asylum, must, in short, be primarily adapted to the cure or improvement of infirm and disordered minds and bodies; and as far removed, on the one hand, from the economy and organization of a workhouse, as, on the other, from the restrictions of a prison.

"In any public asylum constructed and conducted on these principles, and provided with proper resources against accidents incidental to all houses in which a number of insane persons are collected, the practicability and safety of the non-restraint system have now been satisfactorily proved by trials made in some of the largest of such institutions, and continued for several years. Every year in such asylums shows the possibility of removing more restrictions, and of dispensing with some of the precautions for which severe measures constituted the real necessity; so that in every year the comfort and freedom of the patients admits of some further augmentation, and their condition becomes more assimilated to that of the sane, except in points for which their malady intrinsically disqualifies them; and for which an eventual remedy is sought by the indirect operation of a treatment calculated to relieve the feeble from responsibilities they are unequal to bear, from duties they are unable to perform, and all the unavoidable excitements of social life, which the morbidly irritable brain cannot endure.

"The wards of the Hanwell Asylum afford many illustrations of these principles. From some of them, the massive and immoveable tables and other furniture, once supposed to be necessary for safety, have been removed, and more convenient and moveable tables and seats of lighter construction put in their places; many of the window-guards have been found unnecessary; and various additional comforts, including coir-matting on the stone floor by the side of each bed, and a better kind of pillow, have been introduced into the sleeping rooms. The over-crowded state of the larger dormitories has been remedied by lessening the number of beds in them as far as practicable; whilst the admission of light and air has been greatly increased in those apartments by removing the earth or the walls which formerly obstructed the windows, so as to form gentle slopes covered with grass. A great addition to the winter comfort of many of the patients, and to the health of some of the older and feebler among them has been made by the formation of open fire-places in several of the day-rooms. Lavatories, or washing-rooms, have been added to many of the wards, and contribute much to the cleanliness and personal comfort of many of the patients. The substitution of cocoa for gruel, at breakfast, has given universal satisfaction; and the occasional substitution of a currant dumpling for soup, on the only soup-day in the week, has removed almost the only cause of discontent with the general dietary. Allowing white delf plates, and nickel forks, shaped like an ordinary dinner fork, to be used instead of the iron plates and very unsightly as well as more dangerous forks formerly used, has given an air of neatness to the dinner-table in several of the wards, which will, in all probability, be gradually extended to the rest. The tranquil and orderly patients have had the first benefit of some of these changes; and subsequently, the infirm, whose hands are often nearly helpless, and to whom the former forks, especially, were very inconvenient; but the other alterations have been more general. The extreme order with which the patients sit down to dinner, particularly on the male side of the asylum, and even in what are called the refractory wards, leaves no room for doubting that all the patients may in time participate in the benefit of every one of these improvements."

Time has treated John Connolly (1794–1866) kindly. He is seen as he appears in his lithograph portrait in the Wellcome Institute, a pleasant, gentle and humane man. It is true that not all his contemporaries had quite this view of him, and Dr Wycherley in Charles Reade's novel *Hard Cash* is a thinly veiled and not wholly complimentary representation. However, the extracts from his Hanwell reports show the fervour of his commitment to the abolition of physical methods of control. Mere kindliness is insufficient to explain this commitment, in which Connolly clearly exemplifies the attitudes of the moral treatment tradition.

In Britain, this tradition had a number of intellectual roots. Grange (1962) has traced the changes in the 18th century towards a more positive evaluation of emotion. Throughout most of this period, psychology had been very much the study of intellectual processes, but by 1804 the romantic view of emotion as the catalyst of action had gained support. In Paris at this time, Philippe Pinel (1745–1826) was concerned not with the intellect but with emotions, with what was then called the 'moral' aspects of man. He was particularly interested in an insanity of the emotions, later demarcated by Prichard (1833) as moral insanity and by Maudsley (1867) as affective insanity. For Pinel, the care of insanity had to be approached by a balancing of the passions. Liberty was an important part of this approach because it permitted a 'non-dangerous effervescence' of passions that would, in other circumstances, be destructive of sanity. It was this that led to his dramatic gesture in freeing the patients at the Salpêtrière and Bicêtre of their chains.

Another source of the moral treatment movement grew from the actions of William Tuke (1732–1822), a layman, who founded the Retreat in York in 1792 for the care of Quaker lunatics. As Lewis (1955) points out, the ideological basis of practice in the Retreat was established without knowledge of Pinel's work, whose *Traité Medicophilosophique sur l'Aliénation* was not translated into English until 1806. Tuke was motivated by the pacific Quaker concerns with humanitarian philanthropy, and the spiritual value of the individual. Management of the insane without physical restraint was almost a necessary outcome of such views, which in turn informed concepts of mental illness. This is seen clearly in the work of Tuke's grandson Samuel (1784–1857) who published his description of the Retreat in 1813. He clearly regards insanity as a *mental* illness, which is thus likely to respond to treatments that appeal to the mind. This led logically to a policy of using mental assets to overcome the deleterious effets of illness. Tuke describes three components of treatment: 'We shall therefore enquire, 1. By what means the power of the patient to control the disorder, is strengthened and assisted. 2. What modes of coercion are employed, when restraint is absolutely necessary. 3. By what means the general comfort of the insane is promoted' (p. 133).

Tuke specifically rejects the use of fear. Skultans (1979) points out that underlying these principles was an emphasis on self-control. The moral treatment movement made the cruel handling of the insane unacceptable for two reasons. It went hand in hand with a belief in the persisting human status of the mentally ill, and it undermined the ideological basis that permitted men who would regard themselves as kindly and well intentioned to carry out the acts of cruelty detailed by Connolly among others.

William Tuke also had empirical doubts about the 'medical' treatments for insanity of the time. He persuaded his medical colleague Dr Fowler to carry out clinical trials of the prevalent medical remedies. With the possible exception of warm baths for melancholics, none had any effect.

The advent of the moral treatment ideology and the rebuttal of traditional medical remedies had two effects readily apparent from that first testing of the waters, the 1815 Parliamentary Commission. Many physicians, notably James Monro, physician to the Bethlem, revealed great pessimism about the value of a medical approach to the insane. At the same time, there was considerable evidence of a medical backlash.

Scull (1979) is probably wrong in arguing that mental illness was only separated from other forms of deviance during the 19th century. The writings of earlier physicians show clearly that they regarded mental illness as a suitable subject for study (Hunter and MacAlpine, 1963; Jeste *et al.*, 1985). Doctors already regarded insanity as falling within their province, and they were very suspicious of what was essentially a secular development. Scull (1979) suggests that moral treatment was an inadequate ideology for the emergent discipline of psychiatry, as it lent itself too little to the conspiratorial requirements of a profession.

However, the movement's modesty rendered it vulnerable to hijacking. It was taken over by the medical profession in the next 20 years through two processes. Firstly, it was assimilated: extreme positions were avoided and it became a recognized part of overall medical management. Secondly, physicians were able to claim a special expertise once more by their attention to a description and classification built upon the intellectual foundations of the moral treatment movement. This is clear from the writings of Prichard (1833). After 42 years of existence, the Retreat got its first medical superintendant and this was the climate in which Robert Gardiner Hill (1811–78) and John Connolly made their innovations in the management of the insane in the new County Asylums. Hill was Superintendant of the Lincoln Asylum from 1835 to 1840 during which period he abolished all restraints.

> 'But, it may be demanded, What mode of treatment do you adopt in place of restraint? How do you guard against accidents? How do you provide for the safety of attendants? In short what is the substitute for coercion? The answer may be summed up in a few words, viz – classification – watchfulness – vigilant and unceasing attendance by day and by night – kindness, occupation and attention to health, cleanliness and comfort and the total absence of every description of other occupation by the attendants (Hill, 1839).

Connolly's very similar practice at the Middlesex County Asylum in Hanwell dated from 1839 and culminated in the volume from which the extracts reprinted here are taken.

However, even as Connolly and Hill were lending their humanitarianism and benign optimism to the institutions they served, other developments, less benign, were already under way that would undermine their practice.

The most salient demographic feature of 19th century Britain was the speed of urbanization. Scull (1979) argues that this increased the cost and the difficulty of caring for the insane. The 1834 Poor Law Act with its principle of 'less eligibility' set the scene for an overall growth in institutionalism, documented by Skultans (1979). Increasing numbers of paupers were housed in the new Workshouses, and with them many pauper lunatics. An Act of Parliament passed in 1808 enabled the counties to set up asylums for pauper lunatics. Few did so, and in 1845 Shaftesbury's Lunacy Act gave the government power to compel the establishment of asylums in each county. As it was considerably more expensive to house lunatics in the new asylums than in the Workhouse, this was seen by its progenitors as an act of philanthropy. Scull (1979) argues that it was only possible because the medical profession had established itself as the definitive agent for the control of mental illness. Moreover, the Act was passed during a prevailing atmosphere of therapeutic optimism arising from the writings of Hill and Connolly. The moral treatment movement had always been located in asylums, and the idea of cure had become entwined in that of the benign institution. Shaftesbury certainly saw his 1845 Act as a mechanism for providing the mentally ill with the early treatment thought necessary for cure.

The reality almost immediately betrayed the hope. As Scull (1979, p. 219) says, 'The asylum's early association with social reform gave a humanitarian gloss to these huge, cheap, more or less overtly custodial, dumps. . .'. He also argues that the opening of asylums immediately reduced tolerance of deviant behaviour. Once the process had been started, the County Authorities repeatedly increased the size of the institutions. Between 1867 and 1877 the numbers of incarcerated lunatics increased by nearly 2000 a year. The ambivalence of the asylums became apparent: while ostensibly about cure, they were also clearly related to social control. 'With the swelling numbers of incurables, pretensions to moral management of patients were abandoned and institutions became increasingly custodial' (Skultans, 1979, p. 122).

There was resistance to these developments. Without avail, the Lunacy Commissioners fought plans by the County for the expansion of Hanwell throughout the 1850s, at a time when it already contained 1000 inmates. In a letter to Sir James Clark, Connolly wrote despairingly 'the magistrates go on adding wing to wing, and story to story, contrary to the opinion of the profession and to commonsense, rendering the institutions most unfavourable to the treatment of patients, and their management most harassing and unsatisfactory to the medical superintendant (quoted in Scull, 1979, p. 117).

By 1877, after Connolly's death, the pretensions of the asylum to curing inmates had gone (Granville, 1877). Scull (1979) documents the decline of recoveries over the century as the asylum became larger. The writings of Henry Maudsley (1874) incorporate this pessimism: the ideologies of the moral managers are in abeyance and the dominant paradigm is a new biologism replete with implications of immutability.

However, ideas never really die: despite the evanescence of his hopes, the beliefs of Connolly and his associates still inform current attitudes in psychiatry and psychology. They can be seen in the ideology of community care, in which the provision of a benign environment helps the mental patient overcome the specific deficits occasioned by his illness; in techniques of rehabilitation; in the conceptual basis of cognitive therapy; and in the practice of occupational therapy. The struggle between the therapeutic and the custodial continues, but we have the advantage of a due wariness of the institution.

P. E. Bebbington

REFERENCES

Grange, K. (1962). The ship symbol as a key to former theories of the emotions. *Bulletin of the History of Medicine*, **36**, 512–523.

Granville, J. M. (1877). *The Care and Cure of the Insane*, Hardwicke and Bogue, London.

Hill, R. G. (1839). *Total Abolition of Personal Restraint in the Treatment of the Insane*, Simpkin and Marshall, London.

Hunter, R. and MacAlpine, I. (1963). *Three Hundred Years of Psychiatry, 1535–1860: A History Presented in Selected English Texts*, Oxford University Press, London.

Jeste, D. V., del Carmen, R., Lohr, J. B. and Wyatt, R. J. (1985). Did schizophrenia exist before the eighteenth century? *Comprehensive Psychiatry*, **26**, 493–503.

Lewis, A. (1955). Philippe Pinel and the English. *Proceedings of the Royal Society of Medicine*, **48**, 581–586.

Maudsley, H. (1867). *The Physiology and Pathology of the Mind*, MacMillan & Co., London.

Maudsley, H. (1874). *Responsibility in Mental Disease*, King, London.

Pinel, P. (1806). *A Treatise on Insanity, in which are contained the principles of nosology of manical disorders* (Transl. D. D. Davis), Todd, Sheffield.

Prichard, J. C. (1833). *A Treatise on Insanity*, Marchant, London.

Scull, A. T. (1979). *Museums of Madness: the Social Organisation of Insanity in Nineteenth Century England*, Penguin, Harmondsworth.

Skultans, V. (1979) *English Madness: Ideas on Insanity, 1580–1890*. Routledge and Kegan Paul, London.

Tuke, S. (1813). *A Description of the Retreat—an Institution near York for Insane Persons of the Society of Friends*, revised edn 1964, Dawsons, London.

2

Observations on an Ethnic Classification of Idiots
J. Langdon H Down MD LOND, 1866

Those who have given any attention to congenital mental lesions, must have been frequently puzzled how to arrange, in any satisfactory way, the different classes of this defect which may have come under their observation. Nor will the difficulty be lessened by an appeal to what has been written on the subject. The systems of classification are generally so vague and artificial, that, not only do they assist but feebly, in any mental arrangement of the phenomena which are presented, but they completely fail in exerting any practical influence on the subject.

The medical practitioner who may be consulted in any given case, has, perhaps in a very early condition of the child's life, to give an opinion on points of vital importance as to the present condition and probable future of the little one. Moreover, he may be pressed as to the question, whether the supposed defect dates from any cause subsequent to the birth or not. Has the nurse dosed the child with opium? Has the little one met with any accident? Has the instrumental interference which maternal safety demanded, been the cause of what seems to the anxious parents, a vacant future? Can it be that when away from the family attendant the calomel powders were judiciously prescribed? Can, in fact, the strange anomalies which the child presents, be attributed to the numerous causes which maternal solicitude conjures to the imagination, in order to account for a condition, for which any cause is sought, rather than hereditary taint or parental influence. Will the systems of classification, either all together, or any one of them, assist the medical adviser in the opinion he is to present, or the suggestions which he is to tender to the anxious parent? I think that they will entirely fail him in the matter, and that he will have in many cases to make a *guarded* diagnosis and prognosis, so guarded, in fact, as to be almost valueless, or to venture an authoritative assertion which the future may *perhaps* confirm.

I have for some time had my attention directed to the possibility of making a classification of the feeble-minded, by arranging them around various ethnic standards,—in other words, framing a natural system to supplement the information to be derived by an inquiry into the history of the case.

I have been able to find among the large number of idiots and imbeciles which come under my observation, both at Earlswood and the out-patient department of the Hospital, that a considerable portion can be fairly referred to one of the great divisions of the human family other than the class from which they have sprung. Of course, there are numerous representatives of the great Caucasian family. Several well-marked examples of the Ethiopian variety have come under my notice, presenting the characteristic malar bones, the prominent eyes, the puffy lips, and retreating chin. The woolly hair has also been present, although not always black, nor has the skin acquired pigmentary deposit. They have been specimens of white negroes, although of European descent.

Some arrange themselves around the Malay variety, and present in their soft, black, curly hair, their prominent upper jaws and capacious mouths, types of the family which people the South Sea Islands.

Nor have there been wanting the analogues of the people who with shortened foreheads, prominent cheeks, deep-set eyes, and slightly apish nose, originally inhabited the American Continent.

The great Mongolian family has numerous representatives, and it is to this division, I wish, in this paper, to call special attention. A very large number of congenital idiots are typical Mongols. So marked is this, that when placed side by side, it is difficult to believe that the specimens compared are not children of the same parents. The number of idiots who arrange themselves around the Mongolian type is so great, and they present such a close resemblance to one another in mental power, that I shall describe an idiot member of this racial division, selected from the large number that have fallen under my observation.

The hair is not black, as in the real Mongol, but of a brownish colour, straight and scanty. The face is flat and broad, and destitute of prominence. The cheeks are roundish, and extended laterally. The eyes are obliquely placed, and the internal canthi more than normally distant from one another. The palpebral fissure is very narrow. The forehead is wrinkled transversely from the constant assistance which the levatores palpebrarum derive from the occipo-tofrontalis muscle in the opening of the eyes. The lips are large and thick with transverse fissures. The tongue is long, thick, and is much roughened. The nose is small. The skin has a slight dirty yellowish tinge, and is deficient in elasticity, giving the appearance of being too large for the body.

The boy's aspect is such that it is difficult to realize that he is the child of Europeans, but so frequently are these characters presented, that there can be no doubt that these ethnic features are the result of degeneration.

The Mongolian type of idiocy occurs in more than ten per cent of the cases which are presented to me. They are always congenital idiots, and never result from accidents after uterine life. They are, for the most part, instances of degeneracy arising from tuberculosis in the parents. They are cases which very much repay judicious treatment. They require highly azotised food with a considerable amount of oleaginous material. They have considerable power of imitation, even bordering on being mimics. They are humorous, and a lively sense of the ridiculous often colours their mimicry. This faculty of imitation may be cultivated to a very great extent, and a practical direction given to the results obtained. They are usually able to speak; the speech is thick and indistinct, but may be improved very greatly by a well-directed scheme of tongue gymnastics. The co-ordinating faculty is abnormal, but not so defective that it cannot be greatly strengthened. By systematic training, considerable manipulative power may be obtained.

The circulation is feeble, and whatever advance is made intellec-tually in the summer, some amount of retrogression may be expected in the winter. Their mental and physical capabilities are, in fact, *directly* as the temperatures.

The improvement which training effects in them is greatly in excess of what would be predicated if one did not know the characteristics of the type. The life expectancy, however, is far below the average, and the tendency is to the tuberculosis, which I believe to be the hereditary origin of the degeneracy.

Apart from the practical bearing of this attempt at an ethnic classification, considerable philosophical interest attaches to it. The tendency in the present day is to reject the opinion that the various races are merely varieties of the human family having a common origin, and to insist that climatic, or other influences, are insufficient to account for the different types of man. Here, however, we have examples of retrogression, or at all events, of departure from one type and the assumption of the characteristics of another. If these great racial divisions are fixed and definite, how comes it that disease is able to break down the barrier, and to simulate so closely the features of the members of another division. I cannot but think that the observations which I have recorded, are indications that the differences in the races are not specific but variable.

These examples of the result of degeneracy among mankind, appear to me to furnish some arguments in favour of the unity of the human species.

Dr John Langdon Down (1828–1896), a physician at The London Hospital and Earlswood, then an asylum for idiots, was one of the first medical men to show compassion for those with mental handicap, and concern for their families. In his day little research was done and the subject attracted almost no clinical interest. Idiocy (of Greek origin, not to partake in public life) and imbecility (from the Latin, not straight) were confused with poverty and hereditary taint. Indeed, it was Langdon Down who strived to separate pauperism from imbecility when, with his medically qualified son, he developed Normansfield in South London as an 'asylum for the imbeciles of the rich'.

This tentative paper of 1866, now regarded as largely inaccurate, is seminal in that it contains the first clinical description of the person now described as having Down's syndrome but for years called a 'Mongol' or 'Mongoloid idiot'.

What was known about Down's syndrome before Langdon Down started to study this group? The term 'cretin' (derived from the word Christian) was commonly used to describe all idiots and had no aetiological significance, and there is a reference to earlier literature from Edinburgh that suggests that Down's syndrome had been singled out as a 'softer type' of cretin.

Of great interest is a painting of the Madonna and Child by Andrea Mantegna in Mantua in the 15th century which appears to be that of a Down's syndrome baby and his mother. Much speculation surrounds this picture and the survival of such a baby to be the subject of the painting. The picture reflects one aspect of an affluent culture separated from ours by 500 years when probably such handicap was reversed, as reflected in the term 'Les enfants du bon Dieu' and conditions were right for the child to survive beyond infancy (Stratford, 1982).

At the same time as Langdon Down was discovering this distinct group among the idiots and imbeciles that he suggested were Mongolian in origin, Séguin in Paris was approaching the plight of the same individuals from the educational viewpoint and there was productive collaboration between these two great men. Indeed, the library of the Royal College of Psychiatrists holds a book sent by Séguin to Langdon Down and presented to the College by Normansfield. Séguin writes as a frontispiece, 'To the man who has done so much for idiots in England'.

Other papers published around the time put forward various aetiological theories, such as Shuttleworth who in 1883 described these infants as 'unfinished children', but all writers of the time were happy to give the credit for the discovery of the condition to Langdon Down.

What of the 1866 paper? Down begins by describing the concern of the parents with an abnormal baby with which we can identify today. Was it opium or calomel, an accident or perinatal damage? The dread of heredity was there as well. Down was a man of his time and struggled to find a meaningful ethnic classification. Undoubtedly in this he was influenced by the writings of individuals such as Chambers (1844), who when speaking of the Mongolian race and not the syndrome, said. . . 'The Mongolian is an arrested infant newly born. . . . In the Caucasian or Indo-European family alone has the primitive organisation been improved upon. The Mongolian, Malayan, American and Negro, comprehending perhaps five-sixths of mankind, are degenerate.'

Could this 'race' of idiots and imbeciles represent throwbacks to certain great divisions of the human family? In Down's appreciation of the problem, the Mogolian race took a large share of the blame! However, some groups of idiots were thought to relate to Ethiopia, Malaya or America. The assumption was that the Caucasian races represented the peak of human evolution and that idiots and imbeciles could be classified in terms of their deviation from the Caucasian norm. The so-called Mongolian idiot was an example of a degeneration thought to be due in most part to parental tuberculosis and living proof that the great divisions between the races of the human family can be crossed in the degenerative process.

Down was of course describing Mongols of Caucasian origin and for many years it was assumed that Down's syndrome only occurred within the industrial areas of the world, thus adding weight to this erroneous ethnic theory. He has been called a racist and questions have been asked as to whether he should be honoured with an eponym so little deserved (Pappworth, 1982). However, mistakes continue to be made. In Pappworth's paper, it is stated that curly hair is not seen in Caucasian Mongols and reddish hair is almost unknown. Both of these are incorrect.

In the years that have followed, interest in Down's syndrome has never waned. The aetiology defied understanding until Professor Jérome Lejeune (1959) identified the extra 21 chromosome as the cause of the syndrome.

He has continued to this day, as Professor of Fundamental Genetics at the University of Paris, to try to identify why the chromosome, when present in triplicate, causes so many anatomical, pathological, physiological and psychological defects.

In the interval between Down's original paper and the discovery by Lejeune, many aetiological theories were proposed, based initially on the mistaken idea that Down's syndrome was more prevalent in the industrial countries. The theory of degeneration to a non-Caucasian race was dropped in favour of industrial pollution, for example. More careful studies in developing countries then showed that Down's syndrome was universal with a remarkably even prevalence of 1 per 650 births. It was the high infant death rate, by natural means or otherwise, among these fragile babies which led to their absence in child and adult populations in the non-industrial parts of the world.

The discovery of the trisomic abnormality led to a new realm of chromosomal and later genetic research. There is now a clear understanding of the difference between non-disjunction or regular trisomy which accounts for 95 per cent of Down's syndrome and is associated with rising maternal age, translocation which accounts for a small number, many of which are familial, and mosaicism where not all cells are affected and the clinical features may be diluted. Epidemiological studies have now resulted in reliable risk tables for Down's syndrome (non-disjunction) for various maternal ages, but serial studies show that the prevalence is changing and the factors cannot always be identified (Owen et al., 1983).

Down, in his paper, drew attention to the characteristic facial appearance which still remains a major feature in the diagnostic process, the poor circulation, the tendency to infection and short life expectancy. Down's description of the personality as lively, humorous and capable of mimicry is still the quoted stereotype, although this is not universal. The facial features have remained of great interest, much studied by ethnologists and there has been speculation as to whether these features lead to certain low expectations on the part of the careers and to stigma within our society. Surgery to correct the epicanthic folds and to reduce the size of the tongue, if enlarged, has fortunately never become popular in this country.

In terms of expectation, the much more important work has been in the field of early intervention and the development of educational techniques that maximize learning and develop self-help, communication, play and eventually academic skills. Literature and support groups are available for parents and a wide range of health, education and social services is available from the time of diagnosis, together with the much needed counselling that the parent may require to accept the child as a full member of the family. Much of this work centres on the research and service development by workers at the Hester Adrian Centre in Manchester* and

---

* Hester Adrian Research Centre, University of Manchester, Manchester M13 9P.

of the parents' and professional's group, The Down's Children's Association . It is now common place for some Down's children to read and write to at least a six year level and to enjoy integrated education in the junior school years. The Warnock report (1978) on special education needs and the Education Act of 1981 have enabled such integration to become part of the expected educational scene in this country.

The vast majority of Down's syndrome children live with their families and many are able to make a contribution to family life, a few reach open employment and fewer make substantial heterosexual relationships, although male infertility is the rule. There are however a few records of Down's syndrome women bearing children by non-Down's men. Down's original statement on the capacity of these children to respond to training 'greatly in excess of what would be predicted' has been fully vindicated.

The lifespan is now rarely shortened by infections, remediable cardiac or intestinal disease or poor medical care, but the natural lifespan seems to be shorter than for non-Down's people because of the apparently universal development of Alzheimer's disease. However, throughout life there is a range of disorders to which Down's people are prone thus increasing morbidity and mortality: cot deaths, leukaemia and other cancers, infections, hypothyroidism, diabetes, cataracts, hearing loss, thymus abnormalities, malabsorption and adult onset epilepsy are all more likely in Down's syndrome, many having an autoimmune origin. Exposure of these energetic youngsters to gymnastics, horse riding and swimming has also revealed a tendency to atlanto-axial dislocation. Psychiatric disorders may also occur: depression, schizophreniform psychoses and anorexia nervosa have all been recognized. To begin to balance this imposing list it is perhaps worth noting that the blood pressure is often low and atheroma is unusual in someone with Down's syndrome.

The wide range of intellect among people with Down's syndrome has at present defeated explanation and it is important that intellectual stereotypes are dropped. In some Down's children with profound intellectual handicap there are additional problems such as perinatal damage or epilepsy but in many there is no explanation and this warrants further investigation. Although Down in his paper mentions both idiots and imbeciles with 'Mongolism', he does not enlarge further; presumably the other unknowns of this syndrome were surely sufficient to occupy him at that time.

Terminology is all important and Down used the phrases of his day, idiocy, imbecility, and mistakenly linked the facial appearance of this syndrome to that of the Mongolian race. Since the theory of ethnic regression was disproved long ago, the term 'Mongol' and its many derivations should now never be used. The term Down's syndrome recognizes the work of the author of the 1866 paper but current emphasis is on people first and handicap second. As the poster recently produced by the Down's Childrens

---

* Downs Children's Association, The Old Rectory, Honeywood Walk, Carshalton, Surrey.

Association reads, 'you call him a Mongol, we call him Down's syndrome, his friends call him David'. A person with Down's syndrome would seem to be an appropriately respectful description.

Langdon Down was also a man with vision beyond his generation. A story, possibly apocryphal, is told of the time when Langdon Down was a medical student and was sheltering from a storm in a West Country farmhouse. In the kitchen was the farmer's wife lovingly caring for her profoundly handicapped daughter. This scene was said to have moved him so much that he was determined to direct his career to understanding and helping such handicapped people. He left the more respectable areas of medicine and was ridiculed when he turned his attention to the idiots and imbeciles. Down was more than a syndrome hunter; he really cared for those he studied. His clinical notes in painstaking copperplate handwriting can still be seen in the bookcases at Normansfield today. Surely he would have approved of the quotation referring to the Mantuan painting of the Madonna and Child with which I end this paper.

> Perhaps Mantegna saw in this child something beyond the deficiencies which now so occupy our attention and perhaps then, the qualities of love, forgiveness, gentleness and innocence were more readily recognized. Has our present age lost access to these qualities and now preoccupies itself with economic considerations of human worth, of profits and losses, of sexuality and intellect? Qualities which are most certainly deficient in Down's syndrome.

> Perhaps we need the Down's syndrome child to help us regain access to the better side of man's nature. (Stratford, 1982).

D. J. Bicknell

REFERENCES

Chambers, R. (1844). *The vestiges of the Natural History of Creation*, Churchill, London.

Lejeune, J., Gauthier, M. and Turpin, R. (1959). Etude des chromosomes somatiques de neuf enfants mongoliens. *Comptes Rendus Hebdomadaires Des Seances de l'Academie des Sciences. D: Sciences Naturelles (Paris),* **248**, 721–1722.

Owen, J. R., Harris, F., Walker, S., McAllister, E. and West, L. (1983). The incidence of Down's syndrome over a 19-year period with special reference to maternal age. *Journal of Medical Genetics,* **20**, 90–93.

Pappworth, M. (1982). Was Down a racist? *World Medicine,* March, 59.

Shuttleworth, G. E. (1883). Physical features of idiocy in relation to classification and prognosis. *Liverpool Medic. Chiv. J.,* **3**, 282.

Stratford, B. (1982). Down's syndrome at the Court of Mantua. *Maternal and Child Health,* June, 250–254.

Warnock Report, The (1978). *Special Education Needs*, Report of the Committee of Enquiry into the education of handicapped people, Cmnd 7212, HMSO, London.

RECOMMENDED FURTHER READING

Lane, D. and Stratford, B. (Eds) (1985). *Current Approahces to Down's Syndrome*, Holt, Rinehart and Winston, London.

3

Anorexia Nervosa
Sir William Withey Gull MD Bart

TRANSCRIPTS OF THE CLINICAL SOCIETY OF
LONDON, 1874

In an address on medicine, delivered at Oxford in the autumn
of 1868, I referred to a peculiar form of disease occurring mostly
in young women, and characterised by extreme emaciation, and
often referred to latent tubercle, and mesenteric disease. I remarked
that at present our diagnosis of this affection is negative, so far as
determining any positive cause from which it springs; that it is
mostly one of inference from our clinical knowledge of the liability
of the pulmonary or abdominal organs to particular lesions, and
by proving the absence of these lesions in the cases in question.
The subjects of this affection are mostly of the female sex, and
chiefly between the ages of 16 and 23. I have occasionally seen it
in males at the same age.

To illustrate the disease I may give the details of two cases, as
fair examples of the whole.

Miss A., æt. 17, under the care of Mr. Kelson Wright, of the
Clapham Road, was brought to me on Jan. 17, 1866. Her emaciation
was very great. (*Vide* Woodcuts Nos. 1 and 2.) It was stated that
she had lost 33 lbs. in weight. She was then 5 st. 12 lbs. Height,
5ft. 5in. Amenorrhœa for nearly a year. No cough. Respirations
throughout chest everywhere normal. Heart-sounds normal. Resps.
12; pulse, 56. No vomiting nor diarrhœa. Slight constipation.
Complete anorexia for animal food, and almost complete anorexia
for everything else. Abdomen shrunk and flat, collapsed. No
abnormal pulsations of aorta. Tongue clean. Urine normal. Slight
deposit of phosphates on boiling. The condition was one of simple
starvation. There was but slight variation in her condition, though
observed at intervals of three or four months. The pulse was noted
on these several occasions as 56 and 60. Resps. 12 to 15. The urine

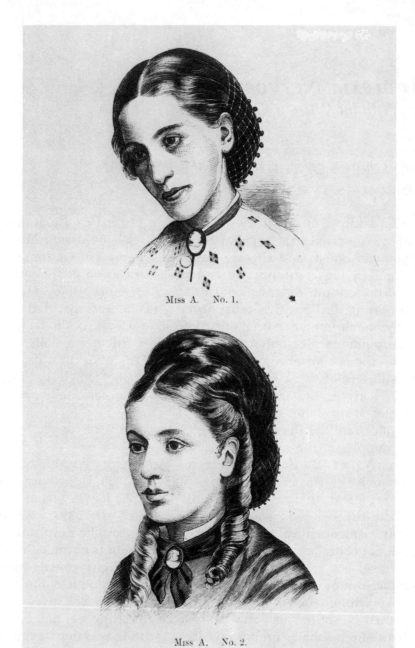

Miss A.   No. 1.

Miss A.   No. 2.

was always normal, but varied in sp. gr., and was sometimes as low as 1005. The case was regarded as one of simple anorexia.

Various remedies were prescribed—the preparations of cinchona, the bichloride of mercury, syrup of the iodide of iron, syrup of the phosphate of iron, citrate of quinine and iron, &c.—but no perceptible effect followed their administration. The diet also was varied, but without any effect upon the appetite. Occasionally for a day or two the appetite was voracious, but this was very rare and exceptional. The patient complained of no pain, but was restless and active. This was in fact a striking expression of the nervous state, for it seemed hardly possible that a body so wasted could undergo the exercise which seemed agreeable. There was some peevishness of temper, and a feeling of jealousy. No account could be gien of the exciting cause.

Miss A. remained under my observation from Jan. 1866 to March 1868, when she had much improved, and gained in weight from 82 to 128 lbs. The improvement from this time continued, and I saw no more of her medically. The Woodcut, Miss A., No. 2, from photograph taken in 1870, shows her condition at that time. It will be noticeable that as she recovered she had a much younger look, corresponding indeed to her age, 21; whilst the photographs, taken when she was 17, give her the appearance of being near 30. Her health has continued good, and I add a fourth photograph taken in 1872.

It will be observed that all the conditions in this case were negative, and may be explained by the anorexia which led to starvation, and a depression of all the vital functions; viz., amenorrhœa, slow pulse, slow breathing. In the stage of greatest emaciation one might have been pardoned for assuming that there was some organic lesion, but from the point of view indicated such an assumption would have been unnecessary.

This view is supported by the satisfactory course of the case to entire recovery, and by the continuance of good health.

Miss B., æt. 18, was brought to me Oct. 8, 1868, as a case of latent tubercle. Her friends had been advised accordingly to take her for the coming winter to the South of Europe.

The extremely emaciated look (*vide* Woodcut, Miss B., No. 1), much greater indeed than occurs for the most part in tubercular cases where patients are still going about, impressed me at once with the probability that I should find no visceral disease. Pulse 50, Resp. 16. Physical examination of the chest and abdomen discovered nothing abnormal. All the viscera were apparently healthy. Notwithstanding the great emaciation and apparent weakness, there was a peculiar restlessness, difficult, I was informed, to control. The mother added, 'She is never tired.' Amenorrhœa since Christmas 1866. The clinical details of this case were in fact almost identical with the preceding one, even to the number of the pulse and respirations.

I find the following memoranda frequently entered in my notebook:—'pulse 56, resp. 12; January 1868, pulse 54, resp. 12; March 1869, pulse 54, resp. 12; March 1870, pulse 50, resp. 12.' But little change occurred in the case until 1872, when the respirations became 18 to 20, pulse 60.

After that date the recovery was progressive, and at length complete. (*Vide* Woodcut, Miss B., No. 2.)

The medical treatment probably need not be considered as contributing much to the recovery. It consisted, as in the former case, of various so-called tonics, and a nourishing diet.

Although the two cases I have given have ended in recovery, my experience supplies one instance at least of a fatal termination to this malady. When the emaciation is at the extremest, œdema may supervene in the lower extremities—the patient may become sleepless—the pulse become quick, and death be approached by symptoms of feeble febrile reaction. In one such case the *post-mortem* revealed no more than thrombosis of the femoral veins, which appeared mto be coincident with the œdema of the lower limbs. Death apparently followed from the starvation alone. This is the clinical point to be borne in mind, and is, I believe, the proper guide to treatment. I have observed that in the extreme emaciation, when the pulse and respiration are slow, the temperature is slightly below the normal standard. This fact, together with the observations made by Chossat on the effect of starvation on animals, and their inability to digest food in the state of inanition, without the aid of external heat, has direct clinical bearings; it being often necessary to supply external heat as well as food to patients. The best means of applying heat is to place an india-rubber tube, having a diameter of 2 inches and a length of 3 or 4 feet, filled with hot water along the spine of the patient, as suggested by Dr. Newington, of Ticehurst.

Food should be administered at intervals varying inversely with the exhaustion and emaciation. The inclination of the patient must be in no way consulted. In the earlier and less severe stages, it is

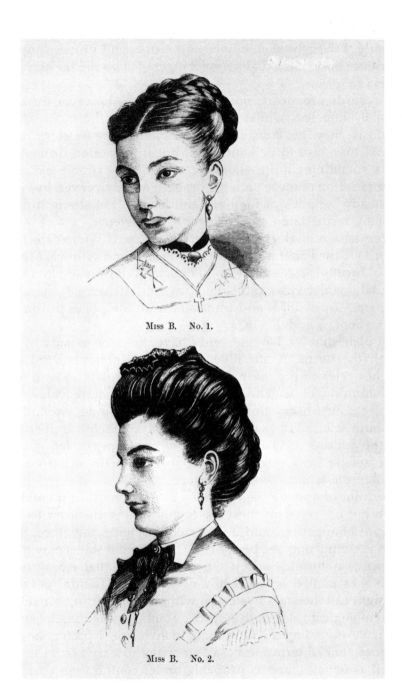

Miss B.   No. 1.

Miss B.   No. 2.

not unusual for the medical attendant to say, in reply to the anxious solicitude of the parents, 'Let her do as she likes. Don't force food.' Formerly, I thought such advice admissible and proper, but larger experience has shown plainly the danger of allowing the starvation-process to go on.

As regards prognosis, none of these cases, however exhausted, are really hopeless whilst life exists; and, for the most part, the prognosis may be considered favourable. The restless activity referred to is also to be controlled, but this is often difficult.

It is sometimes quite shocking to see the extreme exhaustion and emaciation of these patients brought for advice; yet, by warmth and steady supplies of food and stimulants, the strength may be gradually resuscitated, and recovery completed.

After these remarks were penned, Dr. Francis Webb directed my attention to the Paper of Dr. Laségue (Professor of Clinical Medicine in the Faculty of Medicine of Paris, and Physician to La Pitié Hospital), which was published in the 'Archives Générales de Médecine,' April 1873, and translated into the pages of the 'Med. Times,' Sept. 6 and 27, 1873.

It is plain that Dr. Laségue and I have the same malady in mind, though the forms of our illustrations are different. Dr. Laségue does not refer to my address at Oxford, and it is most likely he knew nothing of it. There is, therefore, the more value in his Paper, as our observations have been made independently. We have both selected the same expression to characterise the malady.

In the address at Oxford I used the term *Apepsia hysterica*, but before seeing Dr. Laségue's Paper, it had equally occurred to me that *Anorexia* would be more correct.

The want of appetite is, I believe, due to a morbid mental state. I have not observed in these cases any gastric disorder to which the want of appetite could be referred. I believe, therefore, that its origin is central and not peripheral. That mental states may destroy appetite is notorious, and it will be admitted that young women at the ages named are specially obnoxious to mental perversity. We might call the state hysterical without committing ourselves to the etymological value of the word, or maintaining that the subjects of it have the common symptoms of hysteria. I prefer, however, the more general term 'nervosa,' since the disease occurs in males as well as females, and is probably rather central than peripheral. The importance of discriminating such cases in practice is obvious; otherwise prognosis will be erroneous, and treatment misdirected.

In one of the cases I have named the patient had been set abroad for one or two winters, under the idea that there was a tubercular tendency. I have remarked above that these wilful patients are often allowed to drift their own way into a state of extreme exhaustion, when it might have been prevented by placing them under different moral conditions.

The treatment required is obviously that which is fitted for persons of unsound mind. The patients should be fed at regular intervals, and surrounded by persons who would have moral control over them; relations and friends being generally the worst attendants.

ADDENDUM

As a further ilustration, I may add the following correspondence on one of these cases with Dr. Anderson, of Richmond.

Miss C., æt. 15 years 8 months, was sent to me in April 1873. The clinical history was that she had been ailing for a year, and had become extremely emaciated. (Woodcut, Miss C., No. 1.) The catamenia had never appeared. Pulse 64, resp. 16. Very sleepless for six months past. All the viscera healthy. Urine normal. Lower extremities œdematous. Mind weakened. Temper obstinate. Great restlessness. No family history of disease beyond the fact that the maternal grandmonther had had peculiar nervous symptoms. I wrote the following letter to Dr. Anderson:-

'Dear Dr. Anderson,—I saw Miss C. to-day. The case appears to be an extreme instance of what I have proposed to call "Apepsia hysterica," or "Anorexia nervosa." (*See* "Address on Medicine at Oxford," 1868.) I believe it to be essentially a failure of the powers of the gastric branches of the pneumogastric nerve. It differs from tuberculosis, though that state may subsequently arise, by the pulse, which I found to be 64, by the breathing, 16, the cleanness of the tongue, &c. In fact, the disease will be most correctly interpreted if it is remembered that no symptom more positive than emaciation is presented in and throughout its course.

'I would advise warm clothing, and some form of nourishing food every two hours, as milk, cream, soup, eggs, fish, chicken. I must only urge the necessity of nourishment in some form, otherwise the venous obstruction, which has already begun to show itself by œdema of the legs, will go on to plugging of the

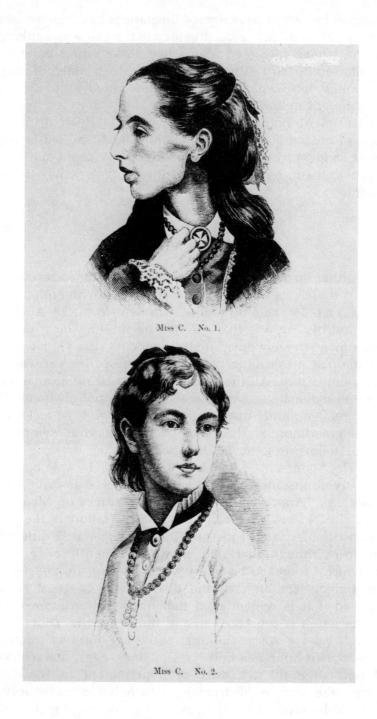

Miss C. No. 1.

Miss C. No. 2.

vessels. With the nourishment I would conjoin a dessert-spoonful of brandy every two or three hours. Whilst the present state of weakness continues, fatigue must be limited, and if the exhaustion increases beyond its present degree the patient should for a time be kept in a warm bed. I do not at present prescribe medicines, because the nursing and the food are more important than anything else. Such cases not unfrequently come before me; but as the morbid state is not yet generally recognised, I should be glad if you would second my wish of having a photograph taken of Miss C. in her present state, that we may compare it with some later one, if, as I hope, our plan of treatment is successful, as in my experience it generally is. I would, as I say, enclose a prescription, but I feel it most necessary to insist on food and stimulants, at least for a time:

'yours truly,

'April 30, 1873.'

On May 24 I received the following note from Dr. Anderson:-
'Dear Sir William,—I enclose photograph of Miss C. . . . There is rather an improvement in one respect, viz. there is less aversion to food. Want of sleep and swelling of the feet are the two great troubles. You have given us all new hope, however, and I trust I may one day sent you a *plump* photograph, like what she was two years ago. With renewed thanks, I am, dear Sir William, yours very truly,'

On Oct. 23, 1873, I received a further report.
'Dear Sir William,—Miss C. is now at Shanklin, but returns very soon. I hear she is much better. She had a bad slough on the leg near the ankle, from persisting in wearing a tight boot.
'The great difficulty was to keep her quiet, and to make her eat and drink. Every step had to be fought. She was most loquacious and obstinate, anxious to overdo herself bodily and mentally. I will give you particulars when they return, but I am told she is much improved. Rest, and food, and stimulants as prescribed, undoubtedly did her a great deal of good. She used to be a nice, plump, good-natured little girl. Believe me, &c.'
The last report I received was on April 15, 1874.
'Dear Sir W.,—I am sure you will be delighted to hear that Miss C, in whose case you were so kindly interested, . . . has now made

a complete recovery, and is getting plump and rosy as of yore. . . .' (*Vide* Woodcut, Miss C., No. 2.)

BRITISH MEDICAL JOURNAL, 1873

Anorexia Hysterica (Apepsia Hysterica).—Sir W. Gull said that in the Address in Medicine delivered at the meeting of the British Medical Association at Oxford in August 1868, and published at the time in the medical journals, he had referred to a form of disease occurring mostly in young women between the ages of fifteen and twenty-three, and characterised by extreme emaciation, and often supposed to be due to latent tubercle, mesenteric disease, or so-called atrophy. This state he proposed at the time to call *apepsia hysterica*, and added in a note appended to that address: "I have ventured to apply this term to the state indicated, in the hope of directing more attention to it." In the paper now brought forward, the word *anorexia* had been preferred to that of *apepsia*, as more fairly expressing the facts, since what food is taken, except in the extreme stages of the disease, is well digested. Dr. Laségue, of La Pitié Hospital, Paris, in April last published remarks on this state (translated into the *Medical Times and Gazette* of September last), which he also called *anorexia hysterica*. Dr. Laségue seems not to have known of the reference to this morbid condition which was made by the author of the paper at the time named; therefore Dr. Laségue's observations are the more confirmatory, having been made from an independent point of view. The author believed that the want of appetite was due to a morbid mental state. He had not observed, in the special cases in question, any gastric disorder to which the want of appetite could be referred. He believed that the origin was central, not peripheral. It was notorious that certain mental states were apt to destroy the appetite, and it would be admitted that young women of the ages named were especially obnoxious to mental perversity. We might call the state hysterical without committing ourselves to the strict etymological value of the word, or maintaining that the subjects of anorexia hysterica had any of the common symptoms of hysteria proper. The author then gave details of two well marked cases of this malady, with photographs of the patients in the stage of extreme atrophy, and after they had recovered their weight and strength. In the starvation stage, when the patients in the stage of extreme atrophy, and after they had recovered their weight and strength. In the starvation stage, when the patients were for the most part brought for advice, all the functions were found to be below the normal standard, but otherwise normal. Temperature half a degree to a degree below normal; respiration 12; pulse 56 to 60. An examination of the viscera of the chest and abdomen discovered nothing texturally abnormal. In fact, the clinical characteristics were those of starvation only, without any signs of visceral disease. It was remarkable how long this condition often continued, and with how little change in the vital functions, the pulsations and respirations remaining at the low standard named for a year or two or more. Such patients, thogh extremely wasted, complained of no pain, nor, indeed, of any *malaise*, but often very singularly restless and wayward, if the prostration had not reached its extremest point. In one case only had a fatal issue occurred, though sometimes the exhaustion was so great as to make possible recovery seem very doubtful. In this fatal case, thrombosis took place in the femoral veins; the patient became feverish, and died. Death followed from the thrombosis and the starvation only. The *post mortem* examination discovered no tubercular or other lesion. The author insisted that the diagnosis of these cases was to be made from the slowness of the pulse and breathing, from the slightly depressed temperature, and the absence of any sign of visceral disease in the chest and abdomen; whilst the emaciation was explicable by the fact of chronic starvation. In reference to treatment, he contended that the patients require moral control; and that, if possible, a change in the domestic relations should be made; that, from the beginning, food should be given at short intervals; and that patients should not be left to their own inclinations in the matter. If the exhaustion had reached an extreme point, then it might be necessary to apply external heat to the body, as well as to administer food; as Chossat had long ago shown that starved animals, when the inanition was extreme, could not digest food without the aid of external heat. One of the best ways of applying heat in such cases was that suggested by Dr. Newington of Ticehurst, by an India-rubber tube, having a diameter of two inches and a half, and a length of about four feet. This tube, filled with hot water, and placed in the bed along the spind of the patient, is often of great value. The author had not observed much advantage from the administration of drugs, whether tonics or alternatives. Believing the disease to be due to a want of mental equilibrium, he would rather trust to moral influences and to feeding than to medicines, though these might still be amongst the *adjuvantia*.

Dr. Quain was very glad Sir William Gull had brought forward this subject, for these were cases with which he (Dr. Quain) had been long familiar, and which he thought of great interest. His experience, however, differed from Sir William Gull's in this respect, that some of the cases he had seen were more severe than those narrated in the paper, and he saw no evidence in some of them to connect them with a merely nervous origin. In fact, the words "anorexia hysterica" were but names. He narrated one case which he regarded as typical. Some years ago, a young lady, who was gradually losing all inclination for food, was sent to him from Lancashire. The disinclination for food progressed, and became so great that at last she altogether ceased to take food. She was an amiable girl, and by no means of a nervous temperament. She became so reduced, that in appearance she resembled nothing so much as one of the mummies in the British Museum. The skin of the front of the abdomen became so sunken that it reached the backbone; the abdomen contained almost nothing; and the bones everywhere seemed covered with skin only, a bedsore exposing the sacrum. She lost all power of voluntary movement, and at length became insensible. Under the persevering use of essence of beef-tea, flavoured with cloves to resemble medicine, with the brandy mixture of the *Pharmacopæia* in the intervals, she rallied and recovered. A few months ago, Dr. Quinn was consulted with regard to her marriage, she being then in perfect health. Now that, which was the worst case of the kind witnessed by Dr. Quinn, for which reason he had narrated the particulars, could not be called "hysterical"; there was simply a loathing of food. Dr. Quain had always looked upon these cases as due to some local condition of congestion of the mucous membrane, and was inclined to consider the real cause as peripheral rather than central.—Dr. Greenhow mentioned two cases in which he had been consulted; and in his treatment always insisted upon the necessity of making an alteration in the moral surroundings of the patient. Called to see a young lady at St. Leonard's, emaciated to the last degree, he had at once arranged for her removal from home to the house of a private family near London, where the whole course of her daily life was changed. She shortly began to eat, and in six weeks was well. She had a relative who was of unsound mind. Dr. Greenhow's second case came of a family in which insanity existed. The girl was greatly emaciated; but, upon being removed to the house of a doctor, she at once improved. She then returned to her family, and had a relapse; but, upon removal from home, again recovered. From the day that the moral surroundings were altered, she became better. The moral management of these cases is to be insisted upon; medical treatment is of little use.—Mr. Brudeneli Carter had, many years ago, witnessed the great success which attended the late Mr. Mackenzie's treatment of these cases by the taking of them from home, and therefore advocated the moral management of the patient. The beginning of the disease is a desire to obtain sympathy from friends; for this purpose, some repulsive idea is conjured up by the fancy when food is presented, so that it is set aside with abhorrence. In one case which had come under Mr. Carter's observation, the patient always thought of putrid cat-pudding when pressed to eat; thus food caused her to vomit, and she gained her own way. At length, however, the vomiting beat her; then she became frightened, and gave in, confessed how she had caused the dislike for food, began to eat, and recovered.—Dr. Poore inquired if any of the symptoms proper to starvation were present in any of the cases. It would be remembered that, in the case of the Welsh fasting girl, when the patient was watched and food was really withheld, she soon became restless, her temperature and pulse rose, and she had fœter of the breath.—Dr. Symes Thompson thought it difficult to draw a line between these cases and certain cases of insanity in which disinclination for food is a prominent symptom. A patient, about whose sanity he had been consulted, was put under restraint and sent to Bethlehem Hospital, as otherwise she would have starved herself to death. She at once improved, and, after six or eight weeks, was sent home. She became worse, and finally succeeded in starving herself to death. Starvation is often, as in such a case, the most manifest sign of insanity. Dr. Thompson considered that there was no symptom of hysteria in the cases they had discussed; the malady was more mental than physical.—Dr. Greenhow stated that, in both the cases attended by him, there was restlessness at night, but the temperature and pulse were not elevated. There was no mental alienation in either case; but simply a disgust for, and inability to take, food.—Dr. Theodore Williams thought Sir William Gull's cases exhibited disease of the mind rather than disease of the body. He asked whether the introduction of food into the patient's stomach against her will would fatten the body? Is fattening of the body possible against the patient's will? He advised recourse to the use of nutrient enemata in extreme cases.—A Member narrated the case of a young lady whose tastes varied; at one time she exhibited a great aversion to bibles; then she passed on to show a strong dislike to food. She had none of the ordinary symptoms of hysteria, and seemed to require no sympathy. Her father had died "out of his mind," as it was said.—Dr. Edis spoke of a young lady who had lost a dear relative, and had disgust for food. She was accounted insane, and was sent to an asylum. Refusing food at the asylum, she was nourished with enemata. At first she seemed apathetic, but soon began to take a little food by the mouth, and quickly recovered. Removal from friends, and perhaps the giving of enemata, are chief points in the treatment.—Dr. Quain begged to mention another case, one of the earliest he had seen, in which this loathing of food existed, and which, after the patient had been reduced to a state of extreme emaciation, was relieved by a copious discharge of fluid by vomiting and diarrhœa. The recovery in that instance dated from that event, and seemed to show that it was due to some relief of congestion by this spontaneous discharge. In some of these cases no special sympathy was sought for by the patients; they greatly desired to get well. It was not that they would not, but they could not, take food.—Sir William Gull would not insist on the etymological meaning of *hysteria*, in applying that term to these cases. The nervous equilibrium of the patient is not quite right. Still, it would be unfair for the doctor to go into the world and say that they are of unsound mind. Some of the patients certainly had other symptoms of hysteria. Sir James Paget had seen one of the cases after her recovery from anorexia, and she was then suffering from hysterical hip-joint. The disinclination to take food seemed to be due to some vagary of the pneumogastric. Many nerves of the trunk may take on hysterical action, without much damage to the individual; but, when the pneumogastric is so affected, the results are serious. It is evident the patient must be prevailed upon to take food by some means or other. There seems to be some hysterical condition of the pneumogastrics, which Sir William Gull considers to be of central origin. There is no congestion of any part; the tongue is clean, urine clear. Then, as to the evidences of starvation, the Welsh fasting girl died not of starvation but of urinæmia, after being deprived of drink for six days. Had only water been allowed her, she would have lived much longer. Without air, an individual lasts about four minutes; with air, but without food or water, he lives about eight days; deprived of food only, he lives for forty or fifty days. The cases which Sir William Vull had described were not strictly insane; there was, however, something wrong in the nervous equilibrium, and usually something queer in the family history.

LANCET, Clinical Notes, 1888

It may interest the readers of The Lancet to look at the accompanying wood engravings, which were made from photographs of a case of extreme starvation (anorexia nervosa) which was brought to me on April 20th of last year by Dr. Leachman, of Petersfield. Dr. Leachman, was good enough subsequently to send me the following notes; and afterwards, at my request, the two photographs, taken by Mr. C. S. Ticehurst, of Petersfield. The case was so extreme that, had it not been photographed and accurately engraved, some assurance would have been necessary that the appearances were not exaggerated, or even caricatured, which they were not.

Miss K. R.—, aged fourteen, the third child in a family of six, one of whom died in infancy. Father died, aged sixty-eight, of pneumonic phthisis. Mother living, and in good health. Has a sister the subject of various nervous symptoms, and a nephew epileptic. With these exceptions, there have been no other neurotic cases on either side in the family, which is a large one. The patient, who was a plump, healthy girl until the beginning of last year (1881) began in early February, without apparent cause, to evince a repugnance to food: and soon afterwards declined to take any whatever, except half cups of tea or coffee. On March 16th she travelled from the North of England, and visited me on April 20th. She was then extremely emaciated, and persisted in walking through the streets to my house, though an object of remark to the passers-by. Extremities blue and cold. Examination showed no organic disease. Respiration 12 to 14; pulse 46; temperature 97. Urine normal. Weight 4 st. 7 lb.; height 5 ft. 4in. Patient expressed herself as quite well. A nurse was obtained from Guy's and light food ordered every few hours. In six weeks Dr. Leachman reported her condition to be fairly good; and on July 27th the mother wrote: "K— is nearly well, I have no trouble now about her eating. Nurse

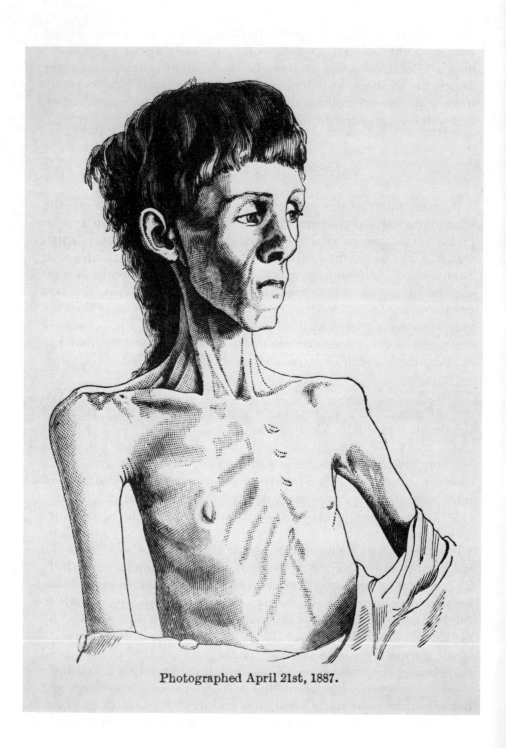

Photographed April 21st, 1887.

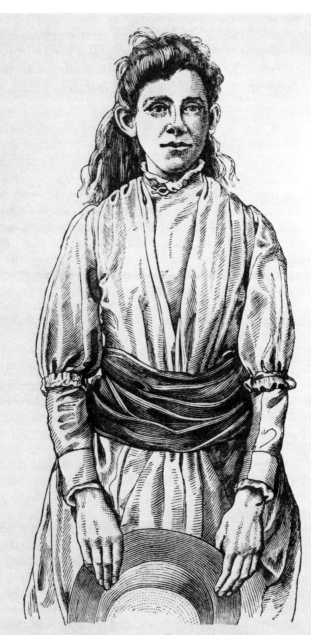

Photographed June 14th, 1887.

has been away three weeks." This story, in fine, is an illustration of most of these cases, perversions of the "ego" being the cause and determining the course of the malady. As part of the pathological history, it is curious to note, as I did in my first paper, the persistent wish to be on the move, though the emaciation was so great and the nutritive functions at an extreme ebb.

To look back at William Gull's papers on anorexia nervosa produces many rewards. Perhaps most important of all is the way in which they remind us that our present day understanding has had a long, painful development and is still far from complete. The present review will consider three aspects of Gull's papers; it begins with an evaluation of his clinical description, followed by examination of the way in which he interpreted his findings, leading to discussion of their impact upon subsequent development of ideas concerning the syndrome of anorexia nervosa.

CLINICAL DESCRIPTION

Gull had sufficient confidence in his clinical skills to be able to exclude organic causes of weight loss in what otherwise was a most perplexing disorder, occurring typically but not exclusively in adolescent and young adult females. At a time when the understanding of psychological factors leading to weight loss was so rudimentary, we cannot but admire Gull's insight in realizing that the clinical findings were inconsistent with organic disease, such as latent tuberculosis, which might only later declare itself fully. It would have been only too easy to fall back onto such a safe diagnostic position at a time when organic illness of this nature was far commoner than it is today.

We should acknowledge too the concern which Gull showed to emphasize the long-term outcome of anorexia nervosa and to be optimistic about it. To do so he used woodcut illustrations and these remain to this day arresting in their impact. In his later communication to the *Lancet* (1888), which also included woodcut illustrations of a fourth patient who suffered from anorexia nervosa, he justified this approach by commenting: 'The case was so extreme that, had it not been photographed and accurately engraved, some assurance would have been necessary that the appearances were not exaggerated, or even caricatured, which they were not.' The woodcuts supported his assertion that 'none of these cases, however exhausted are really hopeless, while life exists, and for the most part, the prognosis may be considered favourable'. He was careful to emphasize however that the outcome may in some be fatal, due to nothing else but simple starvation.

Throughout his paper Gull asserted that the emaciation of anorexia nervosa was due to simple starvation, without any evidence of visceral disease. He commented on how little changed were the 'vital functions' accompanying emaciation of this type even over long periods of time provided that the weight loss was not too excessive, and he was clearly impressed not only by the absence of malaise or pain, but also at the presence of what he called a 'singular restlessness'. His astonishment at this is captured in his comment 'it barely seems possible that a body so wasted could undergo the exercise which seemed agreeable'. He regarded the restlessness itself as a morbid feature, referring to it as a 'peculiar restlessness difficult to control', and in the case of Miss C the great difficulty was to keep her quiet because she was, according to her general practitioner 'loquacious and obstinate, anxious to overdo herself bodily and mentally'. Retention of such physical energy and well-being clearly meant to Gull that organic disease, such as abdominal tuberculosis, was unlikely to have been a primary cause of the weight loss.

Gull was of course a general physician pre-eminent in his time. Whilst we can look back and admire such clinical acumen regarding his physical findings, he was clearly less at ease with the behaviour and mental attitudes of these 'wayward' young women. He identified a 'morbid mental state' noting that 'it is notorious that certain mental states are apt to destroy appetite, and it would be admitted that young women of the ages named are especially obnoxious (liable) to mental perversities'. His other comments refer to peevishness of temper, wilfulness, weakening of the mind, and obstinate temper. All this conjures up a vivid picture of perplexity and consternation on the part of Gull at the intense resistance which such patients develop when exhorted to eat even small amounts of food.

Having identified the causal importance of a disordered mental state, Gull emphasized that treatment should be primarily moral (psychological) in nature. The recommended regular administration of food, away from the attention of over-anxious relatives, with firm control—'the patients should not be left to their own inclinations on the matter'—is remarkably similar to the approach commonly advocated today in trying to persuade the anorexic patient to eat.

Gull's advice that heat should be applied through the use of a long rubber tube applied to the patient's spine in order to stimulate digestion of food is probably the only aspect of his paper that seems dated. This contrasts with his firm stand against polypharmacy, in which he dismisses with careful, measured judgement the use of a whole variety of fashionable medicines which included bichloride of mercury, syrup of the phosphate of iron, and citrate of quinine and iron. Today when iatrogenic complications are still a matter of concern in anorexia nervosa, we should be grateful to Gull for his words of warning over a century ago. Whether we would agree with his criteria of good outcome is, however, less certain. One rather amusing aspect of his paper gives insight into the fact that the Victorian ideal of the young woman was somewhat on the plump side. Thus Miss C's general practitioner later wrote to Gull to say 'I trust one day to send you a plump photograph', and then a year afterwards 'you will be delighted to hear that . . . has made a complete recovery, and is getting plump and rosy as of yore'. Perhaps this young woman was merely in an obese phase of the anorexic illness but undoubtedly that would be an uncharitable interpretation.

GULL'S APPROACH IN ITS HISTORICAL SETTING

Whilst Gull was able to recognize the distinct contribution of psychological factors in the cause of anorexia nervosa, his formulation of underlying dynamic mechanisms was rudimentary. In his Oxford address of 1868 his intention was to draw attention to a condition which he called Apepsia Hysterica, but he quickly discarded the term apepsia because 'food, if taken was digested well, except in extreme stages of the disease'. He was also clearly unhappy about using the term 'hysterica', noting that the subjects did not have any of the common symptoms of 'hysteria proper'. Gull envisaged a disorder which originated centrally rather than peripherally, with 'something wrong in the nervous equilibrium . . . something queer in the family history . . . some vagary of the pneumogastric nerve, failure of the gastric branches of the pneumogastric nerves'. He seems to have believed that a central, otherwise ill-defined disorder of mind led to disturbed function of a peripheral autonomic nerve in the abdomen, this in turn causing gastric and intestinal dysfunction. He was unable to lead on to conceptualize that the illness might be entirely psychogenic without specific secondary autonomic nerve dysfunction. In the interval between Gull's Oxford address of 1868 and his paper of October 1873 Laségue quite independently in April 1873 described an identical syndrome which he called anorexia hysterique (Laségue, 1873). Gull had also himself come to the conclusion that 'anorexia' would be a more accurate term than 'apepsia'. Although the term 'hysteria' persisted in an 1873 report in the *British Medical Journal* (1873), he later dropped reference to it and so finally we meet 'anorexia nervosa' at the head of his 1873 paper in which his findings were published in full.

In comparing the papers of Gull and Laségue, remarkable for their appearance at the same time yet each quite independent of the other, certain differences of emphasis was clear. Laségue was more concerned to postulate an active reaction on the part of the patient, leading to early disgust for food, whereas Gull remained preoccupied with morbid forces in peripheral nerves, albeit caused by psychogenic factors. Both highlight the family tensions and dilemmas which quickly follow the onset of anorexia nervosa in one of its members.

Another theme which is clearly discernible in the papers of both Gull and Laségue concerns the medical man's ambivalence in the face of a perplexing, self-induced, life-threatening illness. In spite of invoking illness mechanisms, the pejorative critical approach breaks through time and time again. Early in Gull's paper we find the statement: 'It would be admitted that young women of the ages named are especially obnoxious to mental perversity'. Even though we need to note that 'obnoxious' in Gull's day meant 'susceptible', the criticism resonates still. The young woman's apparent lack of concern was clearly difficult to accommodate. Laségue's attitude is captured in his comment 'The state of quietude—I might almost say a condition of contentment truly pathological. Not only does she sigh for recovery, but she is not ill-pleased with her condition, notwithstanding all the unpleasantires it is attended with. In comparing this satisfied assurance to the obstinacy of the insane, I do not think I am going too far'. The implication was clearly that such patients obtained some perverse gratification by seeking attention through deliberate self-induced starvation.

The background to Gull's paper was undoubtedly dominated by the tragedy of Sarah Jacob, the Welsh fasting girl who died in 1869, a year after he delivered his Oxford address, but prior to his definitive paper of 1873. As early as 1867 Gull may well have been aware of the increasing controversy over Sarah Jacob's alleged miraculous fasting and he must surely have been very disturbed indeed at the events which led to her death. Well-meaning people, including doctors and nurses, had set up a watch committee to decide finally whether this young woman could survive without food or drink, only to precipitate a series of events leading to her death, probably through unintentionally denying her access to nutrients and liquids which she had probably been acquiring in secret. It would be uncharitable in the extreme to look back and criticize this intervention merely as crude and inept, without noting that even as late as the mid-19th century the fasting girl was so poorly understood that some kind of miraculous cause could still be conceived as one possible explanation. The controversy over Sarah Jacob preoccupied the major medical journals of the time and it must have caused Gull, as an eminent contemporary, a great deal of concern that such a situation should have arisen at all. In its annotation which reported the November 1873 meeting of the Clinical Society of London, at which Gull delivered his paper, the *British Medical Journal* (*BMJ*, 1873) quoted Gull as saying 'The Welsh Fasting Girl died not of starvation but of urinaemia, after being deprived of drink for six days'.

THE SIGNIFICANCE OF GULL'S CONTRIBUTIONS

Today we recognize the complex mix of both somatic and psychological factors in the causation of anorexia nervosa. Although our understanding is still very limited, we are nevertheless beset by complex theoretical systems of many kinds, all of which clamour for the prize of ultimate explanation or at least priority over all others. Overweaning enthusiasm for one therapeutic approach clouds our judgement and leads to angry rejection of the patient should she fail to respond favourably to our overtures. Gull's paper helps us to retain a modest· objectivity here. Even though his psychological understanding was not a sophisticated one, his clinical assessment was crystal clear; he emphasized that powerful psychological forces were involved, and he did not indulge in explanations based on undisciplined theoretical fancy.

In Gull's paper we can discern the struggle towards psychological explanation; even Gull, with no formal training in psychological medicine, acknowledged the importance of a morbid mental state. His paper provides us with insight into the early concept of hysteria, and Gull's reluctance to resort to an entirely psychological explanation, holding on as he did to the idea of abnormal forces in the pneumogastric nerve, albeit caused by 'central mechanisms'. Is not all this identical with current dilemmas in psychosomatic medicine?

Gull's paper also remainds us that even today we need to be vigilant concerning our attitudes to persons who starve themselves deliberately. Subsequent writers have continued to show Gull's critical reserve about the motives which may lead to such behaviour. Thus in 1911 Samuel Gee referred to the woodcut of Miss A in Gull's paper as 'the very picture of pathetic resignation worthy of a medieval saint'. In their 1911 *Textbook of Medicine*, Albutt and Rolleston described anorexia nervosa under the heading of hysteria thus: 'Out of such material when the friends and surroundings supply the elements of fraud and credulity, are made the fasting girls who from time to time become notorious and whose exploits have been known to terminate in death'. When even the recent literature can associate anorexia nervosa with deception, ploy, fraud and malingering, are attitudes of today any more objective? According to Naish (1979) 'What the girl is trying to say is "The system doesn't allow me to be as important as I would like to be so let me take the centre of the stage by proving with my body that I am important . . . watch me, Mum, I can dice with death and there isn't a thing you can do about it".' Gull's paper challenges the contemporary practitioner to remove the mote from his own eye. Judging from the way in which the fasting girl of today becomes embroiled in battles between our many complex theoretical approaches, might we indeed at times be less objective than Gull and his contemporaries?

One final and fundamental aspect of Gull's paper needs consideration here. It is widely agreed that identification of a clinical syndrome can produce many useful leads with regard to treatment and further research, and undoubtedly this has been true in the case of anorexia nervosa. Nevertheless such re-ification may also lead to problems. At a time when we concern ourselves with total morbidity throughout the community as well as with hospital declared illness, we must be careful not to exclude minor forms of anorexia nervosa, or atypical variants, merely because they do not conform to a rigid set of diagnostic criteria. Full understanding will only be achieved by consideration of the total clinical spectrum which this puzzling illness still presents to us, and paradoxically if we define the syndrome too narrowly, we will be at risk of misperceiving the insights contained in William Gull's classic papers.

H. G. Morgan

REFERENCES

Albutt, C. and Rolleston, H. D. (1911). In *A System of Medicine*, vol. 8, London, Macmillan, p. 709.

British Medical Journal (1873). Annotation, **2**, 527–528.

Cule, J. (1967). *Wreath on the Crown: The Story of Sarah Jacob The Welsh Fasting Girl Retold*, Gomerian Press, Llandysyl.

Fowler, R. (1871). *A Complete History of the Case of the Welsh Fasting Girl (Sarah Jacob).* Henry Renshaw, London.

Gee, S. J. (1915). Nervous atrophy (atrophia nervosa: anorexia nervosa), in *Medical Lectures and Clinical Aphorisms*, 4th edn, Hodder and Stoughton, London.

Gull, W. W. (1868). *Lancet*, **2**, 171.

Gull, W. W. (1888). Clinical notes, *Lancet,* **1**, 516–517.

Laségue, E. C. (1873). On hysterical anorexia, *Archives Generales de Medicine,* April 1873, in *Evaluation of Psychosomatic Concepts: Anorexia Nervosa a Paradigm*, International Psychoanalytic Library, M. R. Kaufman and M. Helman, (Eds), Hogarth Press, London, 1965.

Naish, J. M. (1979). Problems of deception in medical practice, *Lancet,* **2**, 139–142.

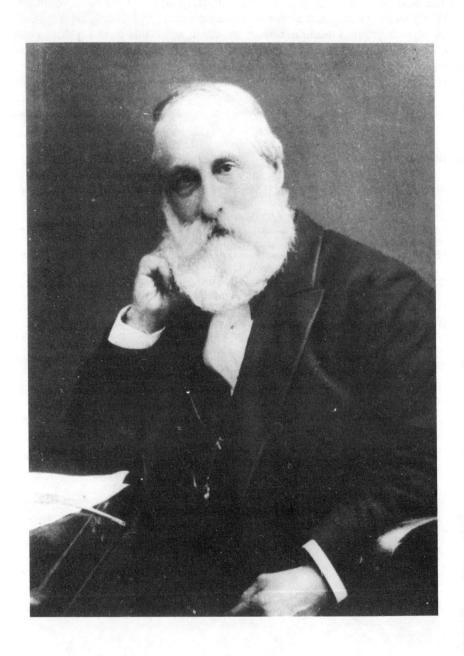

4

Insanity in Ancient and Modern Life with Chapters on its Prevention
D Hack Tuke MD, 1878

FACTS AND FIGURES IN REGARD TO THE INCREASE OF INSANITY

Every year's official return of the numbers of the insane in England and Wales ought to render it more possible to form an opinion in regard to the growth of lunacy and its comparative extent at different periods. At any rate the area grows wider and wider. Taking therefore the last Report of the Lunacy Commissioners, let us review the figures which have accumulated, and endeavour to arrive at some general result.

The question which interests the majority of persons who look at these statistics is whether or not insanity is shown by them to have increased in recent years. Now the first error into which every one falls who is not accustomed to the sources of fallacy which beset such figures is, taking the actual number of lunatics reported to be under care at any given time as representing the liability of a people to insanity, whereas the only certain proof of this liability is to be found in the number who become insane. In other words the existing lunacy at any period is no indication of the occurring lunacy. The same number of persons may have annually become deranged fifty years ago as in 1877, and yet if of the former a larger proportion were neglected and died, the existing number of lunatics would vary greatly in the two periods. This is what has actually happened. The insane succumbed in large numbers from neglect or cruelty half a century ago; now they live on to a fair age, some of them to very advanced life. For instance, an old lady died recently in St. Luke's Hospital in her ninety-eighth year, who would no doubt, under the barbarous system of former days, have died many years earlier. When, attempting to escape from this fallacy, we seek to ascertain the number who became insane half a century ago, and how many become insane now, we are wholly unable to compare the two; because, while our information now is much more nearly exact, we are devoid of trustworthy facts in regard to the former period. A fair comparison is therefore impossible. In proportion as public attention has been drawn to the condition of the insane, have the numbers reported and registered augmented until they amount to the alarming figure of 66,636. Taking the poor insane only, there were no more than 1,765 reported to Parliament in 1807. Twenty years later there were 9,000. Fifteen years afterwards there were 13,868 and in 1860 they were 33,000 in number. After the lapse of another ten years 48,433 were reported; while, lastly, there are at the present time 59,039. This would certainly be a very startling representation of the increase of pauper lunacy in seventy years without the explanation we have given. Returning to the number who *become* insane, we will take the figures since 1859 to show how many patients have been annually admitted into asylums for the insane in England and Wales, for although they cannot safely be taken as indicating exactly the numbers becoming each year insane, they are the nearest approximation available. These show that the number of admissions into asylums has risen from 4.7 to 5.9, or 1.2, in every 10,000 of the population, equal to an increase of 26 per cent; or, to 100,000 persons living, there were 59 persons admitted in 1876 against 47 in 1859, which would be about the same if calculated on the population of twenty years of age and upwards—the period of liability to insanity. Of course if of these admissions a large number prove to be incurable cases, and if through good care, there is a low mortality in the asylums, the accumulation of cases will be very great. If, in short, the recoveries and deaths are less numerous than the admissions, there must be accumulation. On the 1st of January, 1859, there were 23,001 patients under detention in asylums. Between this date and January 1st, 1877, 200,203 were admitted or transferred. There recovered 68,324, and there were discharged not recovered 48,792, while 61,773 died; leaving 44,300 patients remaining in asylums. This is an actual increase on 1859 of 93 per cent; or, taking the increase of the population into account, of 55 per cent. There can be no question, then, that the admissions have far exceeded the discharges, and that an enormous accumulation of lunatics has been the result. For the increase in admissions there are various reasons, apart from the real spread of insanity, into which it would, perhaps, be tedious to the reader to enter very fully; but it may be observed that in several respects the guardians of the poor have not the same inducements they formerly had for keeping pauper patients out of asylums, and therefore they send a large number to them, for whom, twenty years ago, they would have otherwise cared. Briefly summarized, the causes of the increase in and out of lunatic asylums are:- (1) The Act of 1845, obliging counties to build asylums. (2) The Act of 1853, ordering a quarterly return of pauper lunatics not in asylums. (3) The Act of 1862, making pauper lunatics chargeable upon the common fund of the union, instead of the particular parish. (4) The Act of 1874, granting four shillings per head towards the maintenance of paupers in asylums out of the Consolidated Fund. There is also, indeed, some comfort to be derived from the fact that the *rate* of increase of lunatics (wherever cared for) is a declining one. Thus, during the five years ending 1864 the average annual increase (allowing for the increase in the population) was at the rate of nearly 3 (2.97) in a hundred; during the next five years it was less than $2\frac{1}{2}$ (2.31) per cent; in the succeeding quinquennium it was under 2 (1.92) per cent; and since then it has been little more than 1 (1.17) per cent. Or taking two periods—1859–68 and 1868–77—the increase in the total number of lunatics (allowing for population) was in the former period 24.43 per cent, and in the latter period 16.83 per cent, showing a decline in the *increase* of 7.63 per cent, and a decline in the *rate* of increase of as much as 31 per cent. If, for the same two periods, those lunatics only are taken who are certified—that is to say (with slight exceptions) are in asylums and not in work-houses or boarded out—the increase was 30.58 per cent during the first period, and 18.25 during the second, showing a decline in the *increase* of 12.33 per cent, and a decline in the *rate* of increase of no less than 40 per cent.

There undoubtedly is, however, an increase, though it shows a declining rate; and if a man is losing so much money a year, it is not altogether reassuring to be told that the rate of loss is a declining one. As already stated, this increase has taken place mainly among the pauper patients, viz. 49 per cent against 22 per cent among the private ones. Obviously, this is likely to occur as regards lunatics placed in confinement, because insanity among the poor is notorious, while among the rich and educated it is concealed as much as possible; temporary attacks being treated at home, or among friends, or in lodgings, without certificates, and some permanent cases being sent abroad, when not treated in their own houses. On many grounds we must be careful not to be misled into supposing from mere figures that there is only a slight amount of insanity among the opulent and the brain-workers.

It has, indeed, been stated that the proportion of private patients to the population has not increased between 1859 and 1877; and the very natural observation has been based upon it, that the circumstances of modern high life do not produce insanity, and that whatever increase there may have been in the total amount of lunacy in this country, arises from the poorer classes, among whom high pressure, excessive mental strain, and the like, do not exert an influence.

But the number of private patients at the two periods in question, calculated on the population, does show a considerable rise, viz. from 1 in 3,953 to 1 in 3,231; in other words, had the ratio to population remained the same in 1877 as in 1859, there would have been 6,210 of this class, whereas there actually were 7,597, or 1,387 more than there ought to have been, had they increased only *pari passu* with the population. This is no inconsiderable amount, being equivalent to about 22 per cent, and it must not be forgotten that the explanations given of the increase of pauper lunatics possess no force here. Altogether apart from the question of increase, I may here state my belief that there are nearer 12,000 than 7,597 non-pauper lunatics at the present time in this country.

The reader may be interested in knowing how the large number of insane enumerated are distributed. On the 1st of January 1877 by far the majority were in County and Borough Asylums, namely, 35,523; in Registered Hospitals, 2,731; 16,038 were in Workhouses, and 6,312 were outdoor paupers, while 4,722 were placed in Licensed Houses (that is to say, Private Asylums), 358 in Naval and Military Hospitals and the Royal India Asylum, and 494 in the State Criminal Asylum at Broadmoor; 458 were private single patients; making a total of 66,636, exclusive of 252 lunatics found insane by inquisition, and residing in charge of their committees.

In conclusion, it may be said that the increase of recognised insanity in this country during the last half century has been enormous; that the great mass of this is easily explained by the attention of the public and Parliament having been directed to the care and treatment of the insane; by the consequent provision of asylums; by the lower rate of mortality; and by the increased stringency of the Commissioners in regard to certifying patients.

Further, while the striking apparent increase which has taken place in the number of the insane is found to be among the working classes, there are manifest reasons why cases of insanity among them should have become more widely and correctly known than those among the higher classes; and why, therefore, there is actually a greater amount of insanity among the educated and wealthy than appears in the blue books.

Lastly, looking not at the accumulation of lunatics in asylums, but at the admissions, and making every possible allowance for their considerable rise beyond that of the population, it is impossible to deny that there is reason to fear some real increase of occurring insanity.

Hack Tuke was first and foremost a humanitarian concerned with the proper care of the insane. In this he followed his great-grandfather William Tuke, who had founded The Retreat at York in 1792, and his father Samuel, whose *Description of the Retreat* (1813) had been widely acclaimed. But like other philanthropists of the 19th century, he realized that the description of abuses might not of itself be sufficient to gain the attention of a public apt to think that hard cases made bad law. The descriptions should be backed up by evidence of how often and in what circumstances the abuses occurred, that is to say, by statistical evidence. Such statistics strengthened the humanitarian movement and, as Tuke observed[1], helped protect it from the dangers of over-excitement by 'hysterical agitators' and from dilution by philanthropists of the 'fussy intermingling' kind.

In his chapter on Facts and Figures, Tuke gives only a brief account of a complex subject, no doubt appreciating that in a popular book anything more 'would perhaps be too tedious to the reader'. Yet the very general concern that insanity might be increasing required some exposition of the arguments which showed that much, if not all, of the apparent increase could be explained away. Essentially there were three arguments. Insanity was being better recognized, so more cases were being discovered. The insane were now more likely to be admitted to asylums; hence the increase in admission rates. Under the conditions of modern asylum care, those who could not be discharged lived longer than they would have done if they had remained in the community; hence the increase in the asylum population.

Tuke's conclusion here may be compared with those he reached at an earlier, and at a later, date.

In his earlier *Manual of Psychological Medicine*[2], he says the question of increasing insanity cannot be solved because the available statistics do not give the numbers of 'occurring cases' (i.e. new cases). He provides a table of asylum numbers and admission rates and sets out impartially the arguments for and against an increasing rate of insanity. In the Facts and Figures chapter of 1878 he gives only the arguments against an increase, and yet he concludes, 'it is impossible to deny there is reason to fear some real increase of occurring insanity'. In his later article on the statistics of insanity in the *Dictionary of Psychological Medicine* (1892), he discusses in detail the statistical problems involved; and although he does not repeat the arguments, he accepts the authority of a recent article by the statistician Noel Humphries and concludes that 'statistics do not support the opinion that a distinctly larger number of persons in proportion to the population become insane than was formerly the case'. This was to be his last statement on the subject and was perhaps as near to the expression of a decided opinion as his Quaker background would allow. The weight of his authority and the similar conclusion of the Lunacy Commissioners' Special Report of 1897 (two years after his death) seemed finally to settle the matter: the very marked increase in the prevalence of insanity during the 19th century had not been due to any important increase in incidence.

This conclusion seems to have been accepted without question by 20th century sociologists concerned with the evils of capitalism in the industrial revolution, for they never mention (as far as my reading goes) the possibility that the asylum era might have been related to an increase in the incidence of insanity. But this possibility has lately been reconsidered[3]. The case for an increasing incidence has been supported by three types of argument. First, the effects of better recognition, and of increased longevity in asylums, should have flattened out after 20 or 30 years; but the numbers of ascertained insane continued to increase throughout the 19th century. Second, the first admission rate (recorded from 1869) showed a marked and fairly steady increase until after 1900. Third, the asylum death rate did not change greatly, and the recovery rate showed a noticeable fall during the last quarter of the century, suggesting that the increased admission rate was not simply due to a widening of the concept of insanity and the consequent admission of milder cases[4]. Undoubtedly there is more to be said on the subject[5], and it may be that no definite conclusion is possible.

Although statistics serve to stiffen the impact of impression and anecdote, their application is subject to the same weaknesses. Tuke appreciated the value which statistics (in the 19th century sense of numbers of cases) might have for research, but his interpretations show something of the prejudice to be expected of a Victorian moralist. Thus in discussing the greater incidence of insanity in single than in married persons, he observes how difficult it is to distinguish cause from effect in statistical inquiries; but he concludes, without giving any reasons, that 'celibacy is more likely to favour mental disorder than the married condition'. And in noting that the asylum admission rate has recently become higher in females than males, he advises we should wait to see if this difference continues before we draw 'the natural inference' that 'the increased tendency of women to enter into intellectual pursuits and to take part in political life' is the cause of 'injurious results in the direction of mental disorder'[6]. Yet some degree of prejudice is unavoidable; and its opposite form—that of supposing accepted opinion to be commonly mistaken—is likely to have just as much influence on the choice and interpretation of statistical data.

An appreciation of the value of statistics was only a small part of Hack Tuke's contribution to psychiatry. Born at York in 1827, he was a weakly child, and on reaching maturity was not thought strong enough to enter his father's wholesale business in tea and coffee. For two years from the age of 20 he worked as steward at the Retreat, where John Thurnam (author of the *Statistics of Insanity*, 1845) was superintendent. The experience led him to study medicine; and after qualifying from St. Bartholomew's Hospital, he became visiting physician to the Retreat and lecturer in psychology at the York School of Medicine. But his health failed, and a severe haemoptysis forced him to seek a milder climate, that of Falmouth in Cornwall where he remained for 15 years without formal employment. At the time of this move, Charles Bucknill was medical superintendent of the nearby Devon County asylum (a post he took up because he too had been considered phthisical); and together they published in 1858 their famous *Manual of Psychological Medicine*, a book described by Pliny Earle in America as 'by far the best treatise upon insanity in the English language and there is reason to believe it has no superior in any other'[7]. It remained the standard textbook of psychiatry for the rest of the century, going to four editions. At the time of its publication Tuke was 31 years of age and had had no more than three or four years in the practice of psychiatry.

Tuke used his fallow years at Falmouth to collect material for another book which, though soon forgotten, remained a favourite with him. This was *Illustrations of the Influence of the Mind upon the Body* (1872), described by a reviewer as the first scientific attempt to systematize the subject. The illustrations are merely anecdotes, though many of these were drawn from the personal accounts of eminent and trustworthy men. But the concluding chapter describes how the mind might be applied to exert a beneficial influence on the body in ill-health: the chapter is entitled 'Psycho-therapeutics', and this may be the first usage of a term which the Oxford English Dictionary dates only from 1887[8].

By 1875, Tuke's health was sufficiently restored to permit him to take up private practice in London, where he lived for the rest of his life. *Insanity in Ancient and Modern Life* (1878) was written for 'the public at large', and to a modern taste is likely to be the most readable of his books. Its theme is the cause and prevention of insanity. Among uncivilized peoples, the testimony of travellers 'suffices to prove that insanity is rare ... The evidence is so uniform that we cannot but allow it great weight'[9]. Therefore, Tuke says, the principal causes of insanity must lie in the ill-effects of civilization—worry, over-study or idleness among the educated and the rich; intemperance, malnutrition and bad housing among the working poor. The final section of the book deals with 'auto-prophylaxis, or self-preservation from insanity'; and in an age when insanity seemed to be increasing and where general paralysis might strike down a healthy person in the prime of life, the prospect of being able to protect oneself by obedience to 'the laws of mental health' must have been a comfort indeed.

But it is as the historian of lunacy and its humane treatment that Hack Tuke has been best known. In a series of books[10] he describes how the 'shameful abuses' in the care of the insane—abuses which should be 'remembered for ever as the only means of preventing their recurrence'[11]—were exposed and gradually controlled by successive legislation. Tuke is properly proud that reform began at the Retreat in 1792, a year before Pinel's appointment to the Bicêtre. The keynote of the Retreat was humanity: it was a 'Holy Experiment' in the management of insane patients without the moral abuse of chains—and without the medical abuses of bleeding, blistering, purging or vomits[12]. In Tuke's opinion, humane management must come first; medical treatment and scientific study are secondary. He dismisses Haslam's writings with the comment that 'whatever their value and interest, we know but too well the condition of the patients in the asylum of which he was apothecary'[13]; and his warm approbation of Connolly might be contrasted with the dark memoir of Maudsley[14] or the recent bitter, if brilliant, biographical essay of Scull[15].

The *Dictionary of Psychological Medicine* (1892) was Tuke's last and, in the opinion of contemporaries, his greatest achievement. That the project was conceived and completed within two years—to the astonishment of Bucknill—is a testimony both to Tuke's energy and his editorial skills. There were 128 contributors, and Tuke himself wrote 68 original articles for it. Besides its main subject matter, the Dictionary is prefaced by a historical sketch of the insane and an essay on the philosophy of mind, and concludes with a bibliography of English books on insanity from 1584 to 1892. It remains of enduring value to historians and psychiatrists as an index of psychiatric knowledge and opinion at the close of the 19th century.

Tuke brought his erudition and literary skills to the editorship of the *Journal of Mental Science* (from 1880 until his death in 1895). It was said that 'from the benignity of his disposition he accepted too many papers' and that in consequence 'some manuscripts lay a long time unprinted'[16]; but he was in no doubt of the importance of his office. He compared the Medico-Psychological Association and its Journal to a bell and clapper; and it was the editors, he said, who had 'helped to make an otherwise clapperless bell articulate'[17]. Generally regarded as the 'father' of the MPA, Tuke was its president in 1881; and his presidential address, outlining the history and aims of the Association, may very usefully be read today[18]. He contributed many articles to the Journal and two to the new journal *Brain*, on hallucinations of the sane and on folie à deux. He was particularly interested in 'moral insanity'—though admitting he found it difficult to distinguish from moral *depravity*—and discussed its history in a book on Prichard and Symonds (1891)[19].

In addition to his writing and his busy practice, Tuke found time to be a Governor of Bethlem Hospital and is said often to have attended postmortems there, though disappointed that nothing had been found to indicate the material basis of insanity. He was lecturer on insanity at Charing Cross Hospital and examiner in 'mental physiology' for the University of London. He was a founder member of the After-Care Association (1879) and its Chairman from 1886.

When we reflect on the very considerable literary and administrative contributions of Hack Tuke to psychiatry, and when in addition we recall that his younger contemporaries looked up to him as 'the grand old man', and that, at the time of his death, probably no other name was 'so well-known among alienists the world over', we may be surprised that his life and works are not better remembered today. But he belonged to too recent a time for inclusion in the modern biographical accounts of British alienists; and although he was unlike Maudsley in that he had a cheerful and sociable disposition, he was probably like him in disapproving the exposure of a person's private life. Tuke's writings can certainly bear comparison with Maudsley's; but the fact that Maudsley's name is better known today may be due not only to his memorial in the Maudsley Hospital but also to his having had a more original and scientific outlook. In the most detached of Tuke's obituary notices (by an anonymous contributor in the *Lancet*), it is remarked that Tuke did not add much to the purely scientific medical knowledge of his specialty. Moreover Tuke had a *penchant* for those aspects of psychology which have not been comfortably accepted as part of science. As a young man he was attracted by phrenology; his last book was on sleep-walking and hypnotism; and he seems all his life to have maintained a deep interest in mesmerism, auto-suggestion, unconscious cerebration and the power of the mind over the body.

But medicine is by no means all science. The scientific attitude is indeed generally necessary for advances in knowledge and treatment, but it ineluctably entails a degree of detachment from the patient and his sufferings, a detachment which may, in the absence of checks, pass into a disregard. Perhaps this is what happened to Haslam. Tuke's contribution lay in asserting the *moral* side of medical practice. He consistently promoted the view that the patient is more important than the disease and that the humane care of the sick—particularly where the sick have little power to protect themselves—takes precedence over medical treatment and scientific study. These are fundamental truths with which everyone would agree; but the greater the part of science in medicine, the more often they need to be repeated.

E. H. Hare

REFERENCES AND NOTES

1. *Reform in the Treatment of the Insane* (1892), p. 56.
2. Third edition (1874), p. 114.
3. Hare, E. (1983). Was insanity on the increase? *British Journal of Psychiatry*, **142**, 439–455.
4. In *Past and Present Provision for the Insane Poor in Yorkshire* (1889), Tuke provides a table (p. 38) from which it can be seen at a glance how, for that county, the recovery rate fell and the mortality rate showed little change during the century.
5. See: Scull, A. (1984). Was insanity increasing? A response to Edward Hare. *British Journal of Psychiatry*, **146**, 432–436; Turner, T. H. (1985). Was insanity on the increase? *British Journal of Psychiatry*, **146**, 325; Walton, J. K. (1985). Casting out and bringing back in Victorian England: pauper lunatics 1840–1847. In *The Anatomy of Madness: Essays in the History of Medicine*, W. F. Bynum, R. Porter and M. Shepherd (Eds), Tavistock, London, vol. 2, pp. 132–146.
6. *Dictionary of Psychological Medicine* (1892), vol. 2, pp. 1203, 1204.
7. Earle, P. (1877). The curability of insanity. *American Journal of Insanity*, **33**, 483–533.
8. The influence of the mind on the healthy body, says Tuke, may be classed under Psychophysiology; of the mind on the sick body, under Psychopathology; and of the restorative action of the mind on the sick body under Psychotherapeutics (p. 418).
9. Pages 15–16.
10. *Moral Treatment of the Insane* (1854); *History of the Insane in the British Isles* (1882); *The Insane in the United States and Canada* (1885); *Reform in the Treatment of the Insane* (1892).
11. *Reform in the Treatment of the Insane*, p. 27.
12. *Reform in the Treatment of the Insane*, p. 27.
13. *History of the Insane in the British Isles*, p. 142.
14. Maudsley, H. (1866). Memoir of the late John Connolly. *Journal of Mental Science*, **12**, 151–174.
15. Scull, A. (1985). A Victorian alienist: John Connolly, FRCP, DCL, 1794–1866. In *The Anatomy of Madness* (supra), vol. 1, pp. 103–150.
16. Obituary in the *Journal of Mental Science*, 1885, **41**, 377–386, by W. W. Ireland. Other than this obituary, and those in the *Lancet* and *British Journal of Medicine*, I have not found any helpful account of Hack Tuke's life and work.
17. *History of the Insane in the British Isles*, page 500.
18. Presidential address (1881) *Journal of Mental Science*, **31**, 305–341. The address is also printed as Chap. 11, 'Progress of Psychological Medicine during the last 40 years: 1841–1881', in *History of the Insane in the British Isles*.
19. *Prichard and Symonds, with Chapters on Moral Insanity* (1891), page 97.

5

On a Particular Variety of Epilepsy ('Intellectual Aura'): One Case with Symptoms of Organic Brain Disease
Hughlings Jackson, 1888

I have notes of about fifty cases of the variety of epilepsy I am about to speak of. I have seen very many patients with symptoms of local gross organic brain disease (optic neuritis, etc.); in many of the latter, as subsequent necropsies showed, there was intracranial tumour. But one of the cases I am about to relate and remark on is the only one I have seen in my own practice in which this variety of epilepsy was found associated with marked symptoms of local gross organic brain disease. Although necropsy was forbidden, the case is of great clinical importance. The variety of epilepsy alluded to is one in which (1) the so-called "intellectual aura" (I call it "dreamy state") is a striking symptom. This is a very elaborate or "voluminous" mental state. One kind of it is "Reminiscence"; a feeling many people have had when apparently in good health. Along with this voluminous mental state, there is frequently a "crude sensation" ("warning") of (a) smell or (b) taste; (or, when there is no taste, there may be movements, chewing, tasting, spitting, *implying* (?) an epileptic discharge beginning in some part of the gustatory centres), or (c), the "epigastric" or some other "systemic" sensation. The wording of this statement implies, at any rate it is meant to imply, that the "dreamy state" sometimes occurs without any of the crude sensations mentioned, or movements supposed to imply discharges of gustatory elements, and that sometimes those crude sensations and movements occur without the "dreamy state"; this will be exemplified in cases shortly to be given for incidental illustration.

I have been struck by certain non-associations. In my experience vertigo, in the sense of external objects seeming to move to one side, rarely occurs with the "dreamy state." In this paper I have to state exceptions to this. The other variety of vertigo, that is, the feeling of the patient himself turning, does not so rarely occur with the "dreamy state." Again, I have no account of crude sensations of sight (colour projections) associated with the "dreamy state," but I have notes of one case in which the patient, *at other times*, had migrainous paroxysms with visual projections. In cases of epilepsy beginning by colour projections, the much less elaborate mental state "seeing faces" is not uncommon. I have thought that crude sensations of hearing are not associated with the "dreamy state." Until recently I have known of no exception, but I shall have to relate one in a case, the notes of which are supplied to me by Dr. James Anderson. Auditory sensation warnings are not rarely followed by "hearing voices" (really words as if spoken to the patient), a less elaborate state than the "dreamy state." I now return to the variety epilepsy with the "dreamy state."

There is not always *loss*, but there is, I believe, always, at least *defect*, of consciousness co-existing with the over-consciousness ("dreamy state"). *After* some paroxysms in which consciousness has been lost there are exceedingly complex and very purposive-seeming actions during continuing unconsciousness; in a few cases the actions appear to be in accord with the "dreamy state."

It will have been seen that I do not consider the "dreamy state" to be a "warning" ("aura"), that is to say, not a phenomenon of the same order as the crude sensations of smell, etc. Hence my objection to the term "intellectual aura," and adoption of the less question-begging adjective "dreamy," one which is sometimes used by the patients. It is very important in this inquiry to distinguish mental states according to their degree of elaborateness —from crude, such as the crude sensation warnings of smell, etc., to the vastly more elaborate, such as the "dreamy state"—in order that we may infer the physical condition proper to each. The crude sensations are properly called warnings; they occur during *epileptic* (sudden, excessive and rapid) discharges; the elaborate state I call "dreamy state" arises during but slightly raised activities (slightly increased discharges) of healthy nervous arrangements.

* * * *

Just as the most exact knowledge we have of the seats of "discharging lesions" in different epilepti-*form* seizures is from cases of gross organic brain disease, so no doubt our most exact knowledge of the seats of "discharging lesions" in epilep*tic* seizures will be obtained from cases of such kind of disease. Some preliminary remarks on *slight* epileptic fits are necessary. I mean fits commonly called attacks of epilepsy proper.

The slighter paroxysms are, the more deserving are they of minute and precise investigation, both for the patient's sake and for scientific purposes; for the patient's sake since, unless we give more careful attention to the details of them, we shall sometimes altogether overlook epilepsy; for scientific purposes, because the analysis of slight seizures is more easy and fruitful than that of severe ones. It often happens that a patient has sometimes severe seizures of the variety of epilepsy under remark, and at other times severe seizures; and not rarely he has no "warning," in any sense of the term, of the latter. Obviously the clue to the seat of the "discharging lesion" is only given definitely by the "warning" (such as the crude sensations mentioned); so that of the patient's slight seizures we may learn much, of the severe ones without warning very little that is definite.

I urge strongly that the great thing as to the diagnosis of epilepsy is not the "quantity" of the symptoms, nor the severity of the fits, but paroxysmalness. Again, *loss* of consciousness is not essential for the diagnosis of epilepsy; there may be *defect* of consciousness only; and, as we have been saying, there may be "over-conscious-ness" ("dreamy state") co-existing with the defect of consciousness; with defect of consciousness as to present surroundings there may be a rise of consciousness as to some other and often quasi-former surroundings ("dreamy state]); the latter may attract exclusive attention, the co-existing defect of consciousness being ignored. The most seemingly trifling symptoms, when occurring paroxysm-ally, deserve careful analysis in proportion to their paroxysmalness; suddenly "coming over queer" for a moment or two may be a slight epileptic attack and the forerunner of severe attacks. Of course it is a very old story that veritable epileptic fits may be very slight indeed, and, often enough, so slight and transitory that bystanders do not notice them; but there are particular reasons for insisting on this point with regard to cases of the variety of epilepsy the subject of this paper. I particularly wish to remark that, in many of them, the slight seizures are so very slight, that the patient unfortunately disregards or underrates them until a severe fit comes and declares their evil significance. As bearing closely on this neglect I here say that such slight seizures are not always disagreeable, but sometimes positively agreeable. I have heard patients say that they used to "encourage" the feeling, before they knew what it meant. The day I write this, a patient told me that he used to try to bring the feelings on when he first had the attacks; they are now disagreeable. The symptoms often seem to be so fanciful to the patients that they may reckon them for a time as mere oddities. Even when they have found out the bad meaning of their slight attacks, they are often seemingly unwilling to give any details of the "dreamy state." They and their friends do not seem to care for questions as to movements of chewing, smacking the lips, etc., thinking, probably, that such little things have no real bearing on a serious condition. I would go further and say, that some medical men seem to think questionings on the "dreamy state," inquiries about spitting, champing movements, etc., are unpractical. I now stay to illustrate some of the preceding remarks.

One of my patients, a medical man, had seizures of this variety of epilepsy in so slight degree at first, that he took no more notice of them than to make them a subject of joking (to use the words from the report he made of his own case, he "regarded the matter playfully, as of no practical importance"). He now has severe as well as slight fits. I refer also to the case of a medical man who reported it himself under the pseudonym Quærens. The title is, "A Prognostic and Therapeutical Indication in Epilepsy." When he consulted me, February 1880, he had had eighteen severe fits (loss of consciousness, convulsion, tongue-biting), and had had "many hundreds" of slight attacks. The *slight* attacks which he still had when I first saw him were so slight that strangers noticed nothing wrong with him; he is never quite unconscious in them; the severest of these slight fits only "bemaze" him for a minute or two; he can go on talking. Here are epileptic attacks with defect ("bemazement"), but not with loss of consciousness. A medical friend who sees much of Quærens observes a little flushing of the patient's face, that he is "as if considering something," but only to his intimate friends is it known that he has any kind of seizure. The only local symptom I heard of is a peculiar feeling in the right hand. In each slight fit he has that variety of the "dreamy state" which I call Reminiscence; this peculiar feeling occasionally occurs in many people who are supposed to be healthy. Quærens quotes Tennyson, Coleridge, and Dickens about it. I reproduce the quotation from Dickens, and after it the whole of the patient's report of his own case:

"We have all some experience of a feeling which comes over us occasionally, of what we are saying and doing having been said or done before, in a remote time—of our having been surrounded, dim ages ago, by the same faces, objects, and circumstances—of our knowing perfectly what will be said next, as if we suddenly remembered it."—*David Copperfield.*

"Last year I had the misfortune to become, for the first time in my life, subject to occasional epilepsy. I well remember that the sensation above described, with which I had been familiar from boyhood, had, shortly before my first seizures at a time of over-work, become more intense and more frequent than usual. Since my first attack, I have had only few recurrences of the feeling in question. On two occasions, however, it was followed next day by an epileptic seizure, and I have since treated its occurrence as an indication for immediate rest and treatment.

"There seems to me a twofold therapeutic interest in this experience. First that, whatever pretty suggestions Coleridge and Tennyson may make to account for it, and however universal its occurrence may be regarded by Dickens, it probably ought to be regarded as showing disturbance of brain function; and that, perhaps, its recognition and removal might sometimes prevent the development of a more important disorder. Secondly, that inquiry in cases of epilepsy may detect a something of this sort, put aside as not being of sufficient consequence to speak of; and yet in truth being a minimised form of *petit-mal*, warning to precautions against a larger seizure."

The following is also a striking illustration of slight epileptic seizures with the "dreamy state," before severe fits. A man, H., aged 29, who consulted me, March 1882, began to be ill in 1873 or 1874 (he could not be more precise). He had "curious sensations," "a sort of transplantation to another world, lasting a second or so." He otherwise described them by saying that whatever he was doing at the time he (now I use his words) "imagined I have done this before, imagined I was in exactly the same position years ago." He said, too, that it was as if waking from sleep. At first he had these "sensations" at long intervals (he could make statements no more definite), but they became more frequent, two or three a day. He was not quite unconscious in them; he had defect of consciousness only. He thought nothing of them; took no notice of them. Now, suppose he had at this stage consulted a medical man, what would have been said of such seizures? The patient had no crude sensation—warning. I got no more than the facts stated. There might be a natural hesitation to diagnose epilepsy from the "dreamy state" alone, as in this case it was very like, if not quite like, ordinary "reminiscence." I should never, in spite of Quærens' case, diagnose epilepsy from the paroxysmal occurrence of "reminiscence" without other symptoms, although I should suspect epilepsy, if that super-positive mental state began to occur very frequently, and should treat the patient according to these suspicions were I consulted for it. I never have been consulted for "reminiscence" only; there have always been in the cases I have seen, at the time I have seen them, with this and other forms of "dreamy state," ordinary, although often very slight, symptoms in epileptic paroxysms know quite well that its occurrence in healthy people is part of popular knowledge. This case of H. was then, however, most certainly one of epilepsy; the sequel showed it. To go on with the report of this case. One morning (March 1875) he found his tongue bitten; of anything occurring in the night he knew nothing. He did not consult a medical man until he found his tongue bitten another morning. In February 1882 he had a severe fit in the day; twice he fell in a fit in public places. His friends told him of other attacks in the day, of which he knew nothing. In them he became unconscious, and after some of them, whilst continuing unconscious, he acted elaborately and strangely.

Before leaving this part of my subject I remark, by way of recapitulation, that he who neglects the "dreamy state," because it is indefinite and "merely curious," and such symptoms as chewing, etc., movements, and apparent alteration in the size and distance of external objects, because they seem trifling things, may not even surmise that his patient has the serious disease epilepsy in a rudimentary form, until a severe fit comes to tell him so. Even then it may be said that the slight paroxysms "developed into" epilepsy; but I insist that such slight paroxysms are themselves epileptic. Such slight seizures may be erroneously put down as hysterical, or may be fancifully ascribed to indigestion, malaria, etc.

* * * *

In an article, *West Riding Asylum Reports*, vol. v, 1875, pp. 116–17 ("On Temporary Mental Disorders after Epileptic Paroxysms"). I mention the case of an epileptic patient who after some of his slight seizures (he had severe ones, too) would act very elaborately. After one he was found "standing by the table mixing cocoa in a dirty gallipot, half filled with bread and milk intended for the cat, and stirring the mixture with a mustard spoon which I must have gone to the cupboard to obtain." But I omitted to state what I find in my notes of this case, that at the onset of his fits the patient had "a sort of dreamy state coming on suddenly." I fear I then thought this symptom too indefinite to be worth inquiring into and recording, or possibly, to adopt Quærens' words, I put it "aside as not being of sufficient consequence to speak of," though I hope the omission was only a blunder. In this patient's case I have no note of any crude sensation warning.

No better neurological work can be done than the precise investigation of epileptic paroxysms. Whilst epilepti*form* convulsions have been minutely studied, comparatively little attention has been given to the analysis of epilep*tic* fits. Speaking only of epileptic fits and solely of slight seizures of this kind, the endeavour should be not merely to ascertain whether a case is one of "genuine epilepsy" or not, but to describe all that happens in the paroxysm. For although I use the expression "variety of epilepsy" as if there were a clinical entity "epilepsy," with complications, peculiarities, etc., warranting subdivisions of it, there can be no question that there are at least as many epilep*sies* as there are paroxysms beginning with different "warnings." What we call the warning, this being the first event from, or during, the onset of the local, sudden, rapid and excessive (or briefly the "epileptic") discharge, is the clue to the seat of the "discharging lesion." There are at least as many differently seated "discharging lesions" as there are different warnings of the paroxysms. So that I admit that the grouping together of cases of epilepsy which present, in the paroxysms, the "dreamy state" is an entirely arbitrary proceeding, as much so as taking any other striking symptom to mark a group would be; all the more that not only, as I have said and illustrated, does the "dreamy state" sometimes occur without a crude sensation of smell, etc., but that these crude sensations may occur in slight fits without the "dreamy state." And in the group itself, as arbitrarily indicated, there are at least several different epilepsies; certainly a paroxysm beginning with a crude sensation of smell is a subvariety, and one beginning with the "epigastric" sensation is another, although in both cases there may be the "dreamy state."

The "discharging lesion" must be differently seated in the two cases; most likely the former is a "discharging lesion" in some part of Ferrier's centre for smell. But artificial separations, studies of cases as they approach certain tyes, are absolutely necessary for clinical purposes. Hence I shall continue to use the expression "variety of epilepsy" for a group of different epilepsies, each of these agreeing in presenting the "dreamy state;" this will not be harmful if we investigate each case on its own merits. But I hope that this empirical method, one much less empirical than the current method, will aid us towards a scientific classification; that we shall ultimately be able not only to speak of certain symptoms as constituting genuine epilepsy or some variety of it, but of these or those particular symptoms as pointing to a "discharging lesion" of this or that particular part of the cortex. This will be trying to do for epilepsy what has been done to a great extent for epileptiform seizures. We may speak of "varieties of epileptiform seizures," but we speak of each case as showing that there is a "discharging lesion" of this or that part of the cortex in the Rolandic region.

Before we can make good generalisations we must carefully analyse. To group together as "visual warnings" colour projections, apparent alteration in the distance of external objects and "dreamy states" with definite scenes, is generalizing without previous analysis, and is an attempt to organize confusion; they are exceedingly different things. He who is faithfully analysing many different cases of epilepsy is doing far more than studying epilepsy. The highest centres ("organ of mind"), those concerned in such fits, represent all, literally all, parts of the body sensorily and motorily, in most complex ways, in most intricate combinations, etc. A careful study of many varieties of epileptic fits is one way of analysing this kind of representation by the "organ of mind." Again, it is not, I think, an extravagant supposition that there are, after slight epileptic fits of different kinds, many temporary morbid affections resembling those persistent ones produced by destructive lesions of different parts of the cortex. To illustrate for a moment by epileptiform seizures; there is temporary aphasia after some fits beginning in the face or hand (more "elaborate" utterances, I think, when the exact starting-point is in the ulnar fingers); this is the analogue of aplasia from a destructive lesion (suffering, etc.) To return to epilepsy. There is, I am convinced, in, or after, certain paroxysms of epilepsy temporary "word-blindness"; certainly in one patient of mine who had a "warning" by noise. I could not make out that this patient was at the same time "word-deaf," but thought his temporary deafness was ordinary deafness. Still there may have been word-deafness. In another patient, who called his attacks "losses of understanding," there was clearly both "word-deafness" and "word-blindness," with retention of ordinary sight and hearing; this patient's attack used to begin with a warning of noise, but he has recently had his "losses of understanding" without that warning.

I have given brief details of some cases of the variety of epilepsy with the "dreamy state" in the preceding introductory remarks. I now narrate other cases at more length. (Two of Jackson's original five are included.)

CASE 1

—Epileptic attacks with crude sensation warnings, by smells in the nose and by the "epigastric" sensation; "intellectual aura" or "dreamy state"; double optic neuritis. Attacks of left-sided tremor—apoplexy and left hemiplegia. No necropsy.

It is well to say at once, that there was no evidence of disease of the digestive, renal, circulatory, or respiratory systems. There was no history of syphilis. For most of the notes of the case I am indebted to Mr. Wholey.

A. B., a man 37 years of age, was sent from the out-patient room to George Ward, London Hospital, to see me, November 7, 1884. He was subject to attacks of *le petit-mal*. The first attack was in 1882; it only lasted about five minutes. He had no more until May 1884; since which date he had had many, sometimes three or four a week. The attacks began by smells, which he declared to be horrible, but he could give no particular description of them; he wife said that he had likened them to the smell of phosphorus. There was no loss of smell (tested November 17) as there sometimes is in epileptics who have paroxysms beginning with such so-called "subjective" smells. (There was no organic disease of the nose.) The patient had another preluding sensation—one seeming to him to start from the epigastric region. No doubt both these crude sensations were concomitant with the onset of the central discharges causing the fits—of the cells of that part of the cortex risen into that high degree of instability which I call a "discharging lesion." His wife said that for a day or two before an attack he felt drowsy and stupid. In the attacks the patient would become "vacant," and would sometimes lose consciousness altogether for a short time. But besides negative affection of consciousness (that is, when consciousness was only defective), there was at the same time the diametrically opposite, the super-positive, state, "increase of consciousness," that is, there was the so-called "intellectual aura," what I call the "dreamy state." Thinking it very likely, because he had a "warning" of smell, that he had this super-positive state, I urged him to tell us all that he felt in his paroxysms, asking no leading questions. He said that he "began to think of things years gone by," "things intermixed [like all the rest on this matter, these were his own words] with what had occurred recently," "things from boyhood's days." Another account is "peculiar sensations passing through his memory and appearing before his eyes." "He thinks of things he has, might, or will do," "he mentally sees people whom he has not seen for some years." He had also in the paroxysms left-sided movements (he was, it is necessary here to say, right-handed). They were described as "trembling." According to the patient's wife, the movements began after the other paroxysmal symptoms; according to him, with them. He said they began either in the leg or in the arm; according to his wife, they always began in the leg. All that is certain is that they were left-sided, but I have little doubt but that they did, most often at least, start in the leg. On January 12, to anticipate, the following note was made: "Another fit this morning early. Tremor began in the left leg and then 'went up' the side of the body and into the left arm. Trembling was very rapid, and lasted on and off quite an hour. He tried to put bread to his mouth with the left hand, but the trembling prevented him from doing it without using his right hand as well. He tried to walk, and in doing so he says he felt as if he must go to the left, and it was only by dint of a good deal of effort that he could walk at all straight. In some attacks beginning in the left toes there occurred flickering in the left side of the face, and when the arm was gained it was affected after the face." That these attacks should last so long as mentioned in the foregoing note does not invalidate the assertion, that they were owing to central discharges. It is well known that even some severe epileptiform seizures of the common kind last for hours, there being not a mere succession of fits, but one continuous seizure. The "reflexes," superficial and deep, were considered to be normal.

For more than twenty years I have urged the routine examination of the fundus oculi in all cases of nervous disease. But in this case at the first visit I stupidly omitted using the ophthalmoscope. On November 17, Mr. Wholey, my then house physician, discovered double optic neuritis. On that day I for the first time saw double optic neuritis in a case of this variety of epilepsy. As is exceedingly common in physicians' practice, there was no defect of sight to careful testing. A few days later Mr. Couper examined the patient's fundi, and reported as follows:

"*Left eye.*—Considerable capillary redness of disc, with œdematous swelling amounting to $2\frac{1}{2}$ D. The choroidal boundary of the disc is concealed from view. The optic nerve fibre bundles are faintly visible above and below. There are radial streaks; they show no blood-staining. The œdema and greyish opacity extend a short way from the disc into the retina. The veins are large and prominent, and slightly varicose.

Right eye.—There is more œdema of this disk, the swelling amounting to 3 D, also more greyish opacity; the choroidal margin is concealed. The veins are large, very slightly varicose, and this latter change extends far towards the equator throughout several ramifications. There are no visible hæmorrhages or blood-staining of the disc, but there is considerable capillary engorgement, the disc being as red as the adjoining part of the fundus."

Finding double optic neuritis, the conclusion was that all the symptoms were dependent (mostly indirectly) on tumour of the cerebrum, its right half as the left-sided motor symptoms showed. No conclusion was at first come to, as to the nature of the tumour; it was not considered likely to be a syphilitic one.

Under mercurial inunctions the optic neuritis passed off. The fundi were examined again by Mr. Couper, January 5, 1885; the swelling was less. Details of this examination need not be given. On February 19, Mr. Couper examined for the third time, and reported that if he had then examined for the first time he could not have said that there had been neuritis; the discs had become again normal in appearance.

The patient, rid of his optic neuritis, did not seem much better in general. He was slightly bemazed, slightly hesitating, slow rather in speech and suffered from headache. He was, however, up and about, and to an ordinary non-medical observer no decided mental or physical defect would have been at most times observable. But, as often happens in cases of optic neuritis, or, as in this case, in patients who have had it, death occurred rapidly. Mr. Wholey noted, March 25, that the patient had been complaining very much of pain in the head. About 7.30 p.m. the patient went to the lavatory and was no doubt sick there, as some yellowish fluid came from his mouth and nose. He became suddenly pale and fell down unconscious; there was left hemiplegia. He died about six hours after the attack. Necropsy was forbidden.

Commentary on Case 1

—The things to be remarked on are: (1) double optic neuritis and its existence without defect of sight; (2) rapid death in cases of double optic neuritis (from the intracranial disease it signifies); (3) treatment of cases of brain disease with optic neuritis; (4) the left-sided motor paroxysms; (5) crude sensation warnings (smell and the "epigastric sensation"); (6) (a) negative affections of consciousness with (b) super-positive affection of consciousness ("dreamy state").

Of 1, 2, 3, and 4 I intend to say little here. I have written on 1, 2, and 3 many times since 1865; and at very great length in the *Transactions Ophthalmic Society*, vol. i, 1881, pp. 60 *et seq.* The double optic neuritis is clinically the most important thing in the case, certainly a thing of most importance in prognosis as regards life. It is accepted doctrine nowadays that it is (a) the *best* evidence (which means that it is not decisive evidence) of local gross organic disease (tumour, etc.) within the cranium; that (b) it is of no localising value beyond that it points to disease "within the cranium;" that (c) it very often exists with good sight*; that (d) under treatment it may pass off, sight remaining good.

It is certain that double optic neuritis may pass away under treatment when the organic disease within the skull causing it remains, sight continuing good. It is an error to suppose, when a patient is rid of double optic neuritis, of headache, and all other symptoms pointing to intracranial tumour, by antisyphilitic

---

* I very well remember my astonishment on finding for the first time that a patient with double optic neuritis could see well ("Case of Tumour at the Base of the Brain," *Medical Times and Gazette*, June 17, 1865; *Royal London Ophthalmic Hospital Report*, vol. iv, 1865). But nowadays the young medical men I am acquainted with are astonished that anyone doubts that marked optic neuritis often exists with good sight. For all that, although well known, it is not sufficiently known that patients with very striking abnormal changes in the discs may have no visual defect.

treatment, that a syphilitic tumour of the brain has been got rid of. No doubt the organic disease in A. B. (Case 1) remained when the optic neuritis had disappeared, and that this disease afterwards caused his death. I always treat optic neuritis in the same way as I should intracranial syphilis; the cause of it is sometimes a syphilitic tumour of the brain; but could I know that the lesion was not syphilitic. I could give mercurials and iodides. (Of course, cases in which the neuritis occurs in Bright's disease and cases of swelling of the discs in tubercular meningitis are excepted.) I believe that there would be fewer blind people if the ophthalmoscope were used by routine in cases of severe headache; optic neuritis, discovered in its præ-amaurotic stage, presumably the stage most amenable to treatment, would very often yield to treatment. I do not, however, say that optic neuritis will not pass away without drug treatment. For after removal of tumour from the brain (Horsley), optic neuritis has disappeared when no medicines have been given. Ferrier narrates a case of cerebral abscess (*Lancet*, March 10, 1888) in which optic neuritis passed off after operation by Horsley; no drugs were given. Horsley trephined and evacuated a cerebral abscess, the position of which Ferrier had very accurately diagnosed. The patient is now quite well. Yet I should not dare to omit treatment of the kind mentioned in ordinary cases of optic neuritis. If it does nothing for intracranial tumour, it often, I am convinced, prevents blindness. To return to the case of A. B.

It is well known that patients with double optic neuritis often die suddenly or rapidly, as A. B. did. A. B. probably died by hæmorrhage from a vascular tumour of the right cerebral hemisphere (temporo-sphenoidal lobe?). In some cases, as Hilton Fagge has pointed out, patients who have cerebral tumour die by rapid respiratory failure. This may happen when there is no hæmorrhage from the tumour. It is possible that cerebral tumour, besides producing optic neuritis, sometimes produces similar pathological changes in centres in the medulla, the respiratory among others.*

The attacks of one-sided tremor ("diluted convulsion") such as A. B. had, occur, in my opinion, in cases of disease behind the

---

* Some time ago (*Transactions Ophthalmic Society*, vol. i, 1881, p. 98) Dr. Buzzard said: "Was it possible . . . that the vomiting and slowing of the pulse might represent an affection of the pneumogastric brought about by the same cause as that which produced optic neritis, and that the sudden or rapid death Dr. Hughlings Jackson had mentioned as one of the possible contingencies of optic neuritis from intracranial disease, might also be explained by a more severe influence on the same nerve?"

so-called motor regions; if so, there is some little evidence towards showing that the supposed sensory districts are not purely sensory. They were not epileptiform seizures, I mean not like fits I have seen dependent on disease of the so-called motor region. I shall speak of these "diluted convulsions" elsewhere.

Saying again that the topics 1, 2, 3, and 4 are clinically of vast importance, I shall go on to speak of cases of epilepsy with the "dreamy state" more generally. I have only seen three cases (Dr. James Anderson's patient, A. B., and that of a woman) in which with this variety of epilepsy there were strong symptoms of local gross organic disease within the cranium. Before speaking further of the (5) crude sensations and (6) abnormal affection of conscious-ness (*a* and *b*), I will narrate other cases of this variety of epilepsy in which there is no reason to suppose that there exists local *gross* organic disease. I say local *gross* organic disease, meaning such as tumours, abscesses, cysts, etc. That there is some local disease in every epilepsy I have no doubt whatever; there is, beyond question, some *pathological* process productive of high instability, which is a functional change (abnormal physiological change) of a few cells of some part of the cortex. I would here refer to remarks I made on the use and misuse of the term "functional" (*Brain*, vol. x, January 1888, p. 312).

* * * *

CASE 5

—*Slight attacks of epilepsy with the "dreamy state" for some years before severe attacks—mouth movements—automatic actions during unconsciousness (which continued after the slight fits).*

The following is a very important case. It is that of a highly educated medical man, who reports it himself. Names of places are omitted or altered from his original report, the alterations being endorsed by the patient; the alterations make no difference in the medical import of the case. He had first very slight attacks, then severe attacks at long intervals also. I shall comment on the slight attacks only.

What he calls "recollection" is what I have called "reminiscence." I retain his term "aura," putting it between commas, although I do not use it myself for any form of the "dreamy state." The report shows clearly that he has some attacks without *loss* of consciousness (see his remarks on reading poetry and on his glacier expedition). In other attacks he had loss of consciousness, and during unconsciousness continuing after them he acted automatically. The actions related in the closing paragraphs show very complex, special, etc., actions after a fit which was presumably slight. I may refer to remarks on this matter in my part of the discussion on Dr. Mercier's paper on "Inhibition."

He had no crude sensation, but the words I have italicised in his account of his physical state, p. 402, during the slight paroxysms imply, I consider, discharge of cortical elements, serving during taste. (The report was finally sent in July 1888.)

"I first noticed symptoms which I subsequently learnt to describe as *petit-mal* when living at one of our universities, 1871. I was in very good general health, and know of no temporary disturbing causes. I was waiting at the foot of a College staircase, in the open air, for a friend who was coming down to join me. I was carelessly looking round me, watching people passing, etc., when my attention was suddenly absorbed in my own mental state, of which I know no more than that it seemed to me to be a vivid and unexpected 'recollection'—of what, I do not know. My friend found me a minute or two later, leaning my back against the wall, looking rather pale, and feeling puzzled and stupid for the moment. In another minute or two I felt quite normal again, and was as much amused as my friend at finding that I could give no distinct account of what had happened, or what I had 'recollected.'

"During the next two years a few similar but slighter attacks occurred, involving mental states which struck me as like to the first and to each other, but of which I can now recollect no details. I asked medical advice, but gathered no explanation, received no treatment, and regarded the matter playfully as of no practical importance. I have been in the habit of dreaming very little all my life, but during these years noticed a few occasions when I woke in the night with an impression that I had succeeded in recollecting something that I wanted to recollect, but was too sleepy to give any attention to it, and had no definite idea of it in the morning. These feelings were slightly uncomfortable, and usually, I think, accompanied by a slight involuntary escape of saliva found on the pillow in the morning, and once or twice by a soreness of the edge of the tongue, due, I should presume, to its having been slightly bitten. They did not recur after about 1875.

"In 1874 I first had a *haut-mal*, preceded by the mental condition I had felt in *petits-maux*, and after medical advice from a physician in London learnt the nature of the disease, and began to attend a little more carefully to the symptoms, which interested me more, as I had begun to turn my attention to medicine.

"I had a severe attack of pneumonia with pleurisy, and perhaps empyema, beginning in October 1875, and during slow convalescence (December 1875–March 1876) was more frequently affected. The character of the *petits-maux* gradually became more stereotyped, and during the period 1876–1886 varied only within comparatively narrow limits. I will attempt to describe the features which I think were common to all, or nearly all.

Mental Condition

"In a large majority of cases the central feature has been mental and has been a feeling of Recollection, *i.e.* of realising that what is occupying the attention is what has occupied it before, and indeed has been familiar, but has been for a time forgotten, and now is recovered with a slight sense of satisfaction as it had been sought for. My normal memory is bad, and a similar but much fainter feeling of sudden recollection of a forgotten fact is familiar. But in the abnormal states the recollection is much more instantaneous, much more absorbing, more vivid, and for the moment more satisfactory, as filling up a void which I imagine at the time I had previously in vain sought to fill. At the same time, or perhaps I should say more accurately in immediate sequence, I am dimly aware that the recollection is fictitious and my state abnormal. The recollection is always started by another person's voice, or by my own verbalised thought, or by what I am reading and mentally verbalise; and I think that during the abnormal state I generally verbalise some such phrase of simple recognition as, 'Oh yes—I see.' 'Of course—I remember,' etc., but a minute or two later I can recollect neither the words nor the verbalised thought which gave rise to the recognition. I only feel strongly that they resemble what I have felt before under similar abnormal conditions. I re-enter the current of normal life, as a rule, quickly—sometimes, as far as I can judge from my own movements or other people's evidence, within ten or fifteen seconds; there is never, however, as sudden a rush of returning normal consciousness as there has been of incipient abnormal consciousness; it is more gradual, and it is hard to say when it is complete, as it almost always leads up to a passive and non-critical mental attitude in which I feel no originative mental impulse. One point which I almost always feel a tendency to avoid, though I am generally dimly aware of a previous wish to attempt it, is to go over my previous abnormal mental state critically and to give my attention to all its details. But attention seems not to be completely under my control; I sometimes put it off, and delude myself with the impression that remembrance will be just as complete after another five minutes, sometimes let it slip with a feeling of indifference, and sometimes, if I am in company or in any active employment, I have no distinct recollection of any desire for self-criticism or analysis. Accompanying this want of control over reflection I often notice a temporary loss of memory for habitually familiar names or facts, which lasts a minute or two, or sometimes more, after my consciousness seems otherwise normal. This may co-exist, indeed, with so normal a state of consciousness, that I can hardly believe I shall find any difficulty in saying what I want to say, and so I fall now and then into the mistake of beginning without hesitation a sentence which I cannot finish. I have found myself just after a *petit-mal* at a London Railway Booking Office, meaning to go to K—, and asking without hesitation for 'Second return to—to—that school, don't you know—' (or some such words) and being a good deal startled at my forgetfulness.

"A *petit-mal* has two or three times come on when I have been reading poetry aloud—the line I am reading or just going to read seems somehow familiar, or just what I was trying to recollect, though I may never have seen or heard it before. I recognise my morbid condition and stop, though I have generally sense enough to finish the line or even sentence, and remain silent for a minute or so; then go on again where I left off, recovering my sense of rhythm and metre sooner than my capacity of giving attention to or understanding the words. I do not remember to have made any deliberate effort to go on reading aloud, *coûte que coûte*, throughout a *petit-mal*. I have made several rude attempts to go on writing, and have kept four or five specimens of what I have written. They were made in very slight *petits-maux*. The writing was done slowly and in a fairly normal hand. I was in the main occupied with the usual impression of recollection, but was dimly aware that I was morbid, and attempted to criticise what I was writing. My impression at the time that I was writing was that the words and sense were quite reasonable, and that I had kept within very familiar and prudent limits of expression. I had found, I thought, just the words I was seeking for. A minute or two later I could see that some of the words were grotesquely *mal à propos*, though I think the grammatical forms of sentence were always preserved. I could not trace any undercurrent of thought or recollection from which the irrelevant words had come.

Physical conditions

"As to the physical conditions accompanying these mental states I can gather a little from my own consciousness, and I have learnt a little more from friendly observers. At the onset I can rarely notice any physical change in myself, my attention being chiefly occupied with my mental condition; but once or twice when I have been standing near a mirror I have noticed pallor of the face, and I have learnt from others that this is common, and that my eyes have a somewhat staring vacant look as if they were not directed to anything near me, or indeed taking notice of anything particular. In this condition I am told, and in fact occasionally remember, that I often say 'yes,' with an air of complete assent to any remark made to me, whether it is a pertinent answer or not; and further, that I occasionally make a slight half-vocalised sound, whether addressed or not. This latter, I have been told, is *somewhat like a modified and indistinct smacking of the tongue like a tasting movement, and is generally accompanied by a motion of the lower jaw,* and sometimes by some twitching of the muscles round one or both corners of the mouth or of the cheeks, but by no sense of taste in my recollection. I have no clear evidence that one side of the face is affected more than the other, and no clear evidence against it; from what little I can learn, if it is at all unilateral it is rather more on the right side than the left; but the evidence is very scanty. I never notice it myself. I also never notice myself, but learn from others, that sometimes, specially if sitting, I have one or two light stamps on the floor with one foot; and in the only cases where this has been accurately observed it has been with the right foot.

"With the returning normal consciousness I generally feel some superficial flush over the skin, especially over the face, and a slightly quickened and more thumping heart-beat which does not go beyond causing me very slight *malaise*. A very constant symptom is increased urinary secretion, which sometimes makes itself felt in as short a time as five or ten minutes, but usually after a longer interval. The water, if soon passed, is very light in colour, of low specific gravity, once or twice as low as 1005, and contains no albumen.

"The *petits-maux* have not been accompanied or followed by hallucinatory sensations of sight, sound, taste, smell, or feeling. There has been, I think, no loss of balance. I well recollect in 1878 running across a Swiss glacier, and jumping across many small crevasses when the initial stage of 'aura' came on, and a reflection shot through my mind, that if ever I was likely to pay dearly for the imprudence of going on, it would be then. But I had insufficient control to stop myself and felt no fear, but only a slight interest in what would happen. I went through the familiar sensation sof *petit-mal* with such attention as I had to give concentrated on them, and not on the ice, and after a few minutes regained my normal condition without any injury. I looked back with surprise at the long slope of broken ice I had run over unhurt, picking my way, I know not how, over ground that would normally have been difficult to me. In the same way a *petit-mal* when I was playing lawn tennis did not in the opinion of my adversary make my strokes or judgment of pace and position to balls to be struck any worse than normal. I had no recollection of the strokes during a minute or two.

"I had no *haut-mal* before 1874, and since then such attacks have recurred mostly at long intervals, sometimes of as much as eighteen months; during slow convalescence from pneumonia, however, in 1975–6 I had as many as seven or eight in two months. The 'aura' of recollection had preceded all of them, more or less, but is less vivid in my subsequent memory than after a *petit-mal*. My evidence as to the subsequent phenomena of the *haut-mal* is very incomplete. My loss of consciousness has not seemed longer to those who watched me than five or ten minutes as a rule, but my loss of memory has been longer and my return to consciousness more gradual. I have not heard that there has been any epileptic cry; the muscular spasms have been variable but generally slight, and not specially localised (except that once I was told of a constant grasping motion of my right arm and hand). In one or two cases the spasms have not been noticed, and the state has been at first supposed to be one of syncope; but some snoring has almost always been noticed before recovery. My subsequent mental condition has been one of indifference and a sense of fatigue; my bodily sensation is, as a rule, of having been lightly bruised all over.

"During the past year (1887), and more especially during the last four months, there has been some change in the symptoms of the *petits-maux*, which may be shortly summed up by saying that there has been less vivid sense of recollection and there have been longer periods of automatism without memory. I think I had best attempt to explain what I mean by two or three instances.

"(1) In October 1887 I was travelling along the Metropolitan Railway, meaning to get out at the fourth station and walk to a house half a mile off. I remember reaching the second station, and I then recollect indistinctly the onset of an 'aura,' in which the conversation of two strangers in the same carriage seemed to be the repetition of something I had previously known—a recollection, in fact. The next thing of which I have any memory was that I was walking up the steps of the house (about half a mile from the fourth station), feeling in my pocket for a latch-key. I remembered almost at once that I had had a *petit-mal* coming on at the second station, and was surprised to find myself where I was. I recollect that I had meant to reach the house not later than 12.45, and had been rather doubtful in the train whether I should be in time. I looked at my watch and found it within a minute or two of 12-45. I searched my pockets for the ticket, which was to the fourth station, found it gone, and concluded that I must have passed the third station, got out at the fourth, given up my ticket and walked on as I had previously intended, though I had no memory of anything since the second station some ten or twelve minutes previously. I imagine that I had carried out my intention automatically and without memory.

"(2) Again, in November 1887, after dark—about 6 p.m.—I was walking westwards in a London street, when I felt a *petit-mal* coming on of which I can remember no particulars. My intention was to walk westwards for about half a mile; my thoughts were occupied with some books I had been reading in a house which I had just left. With my return of memory (which was incomplete and indistinct) I found myself in a street I did not at first recognise. I was somewhat puzzled, and looked up at the street corners for information as to the name of the street. I read the name 'P— St.' which crossed my path at right angles, and with some difficulty realised that I was walking not westwards, as I had been intending, but eastwards, along the street by which I had come, and had, in fact, retraced my steps some three hundred or four hundred yards. I felt no purpose in doing this, no aim at going anywhere in particular, and to save further difficulty, and because I was puzzled, I got into a hansom which was standing still close by me. I have no recollection of giving the driver any orders, and was in a very unreflective state. My impression is that the cab-driver drove quickly to the right house, and I distinctly remember some slight surprise at finding myself giving him a shilling, when I doubt if I could have explained where he came from. Immediately after entering the house I realised tolerably distinctly what had probably happened, and looking at my watch, I calculated that I had not lost more than five minutes by this, if so much.

"(3) About a fortnight later I was walking by the same route about 10.30 p.m., and again felt a *petit-mal* at a point within a hundred yards or so of the one described above. I cannot be certain that a memory of the previous attack recurred to me, but I think it is very probable. My memory again was a blank until I found myself facing eastwards and looking up at the name 'P— St.' Then the memory of the previous retracing of my steps recurred to me at once. I more quickly than before gathered together full consciousness, felt a cab unnecessary, walked home, and had no difficulty in writing steadily for about three hours without fatigue.

"In the earlier of this pair of cases (2 and 3) I had no thought whatever of going back to the house where I had been reading, or to any point in that direction; but I believe I am correct in saying that I was thinking of what I had just been reading there. As far as I know, this is the first instance of my changing my intended action *ex propio motu* in a mental state of which I have no memory. In the companion case (3) I cannot feel sure how much I was influenced by recollection in the earliest stages of the *petit-mal*.

"(4) A fourth occasion is perhaps worth record. I was attending a young patient whom his mother had brought me with some history of lung symptoms. I wished to examine the chest, and asked him to undress on a couch. I thought he looked ill, but have no recollection of any intention to recommend him to take to his bed at once, or of any diagnosis. Whilst he was undressing I felt the onset of a *petit-mal*. I remember taking out my stethoscope and turning away a little to avoid conversation. The next thing I recollect is that I was sitting at a writing-table in the same room, speaking to another person, and as my consciousness became more complete, recollected my patient, but saw he was not in the room. I was interested to ascertain what had happened, and had an opportunity an hour later of seeing him in bed, with the note of a diagnosis I had made of 'pneumonia of the left base.' I gathered indirectly from conversation that I had made a physical examination, written these words, and advised him to take to bed at once. I re-examined him with some curiosity, and found that my conscious diagnosis was the same as my unconscious—or perhaps I should say, unremembered diagnosis had been. I was a good deal surprised, but not so unpleasantly as I should have thought probable."

If something strange happened to a respectable, late Victorian, citizen it is fairly certain he or she would have visited one of the newly fashionable 'nerve' specialists. Virginia Woolf's first doctors were of that ilk before a true 'alienist' was reluctantly sought. Yet it is often forgotten that neurology is very much one of the offspring of psychiatry. While 'mad doctors' and 'asylum keepers' had been part of the medical landscape for several generations, it was only in the latter half of the 19th century that neuropathology (the world of Meynert, Nissl, Alzheimer et al.) and neurophysiology (pathways, reflexes, epileptiform seizures) had sufficiently advanced to form the basis of a clinical speciality.

In Britain, the leading clinicians in this field were William Gowers (1845–1915) and Hughlings Jackson (1835–1911). But it seems appropriate that Jackson's career should parallel that of the psychiatrist Henry Maudsley in being born in 1835, in Yorkshire, in coming to London to seek his fortune, in being appointed to a senior hospital post in his twenties, and in editing the Journal of his chosen subject. In fact Jackson went one better in being a *founder* editor of *Brain*, in 1878, the same year as Maudsley was resigning from 15 years of coeditorship of the *Journal of Mental Science*. Yet even prior to this, as psychiatry fossilized into the deadening world of overcrowded asylums, Jackson was reporting a rich range of neurological cases and, incidentally, providing a philosophical framework for the Freudian developments which were to seal the separation of psychiatry from neurology. But their eventual reintegration, if it comes, will be via a greater understanding of conditions such as Temporal Lobe Epilepsy (TLE), the 'particular variety' that remains the cornerstone—if not the eponymous one—of the Jacksonian heritage.

Jackson's strength is that, unlike Maudsley, he is still quoted in the medical literature: not because his descriptions of the 'dreamy state', ('intellectual aura'), were particularly well written, as the 1888 paper appended here will show, nor because his notions of dissolution, of positive and negative symptoms, were particularly clear or predominant in the history of psychiatric understanding. (He theorized that psychiatric disorders were usually due to a negative effect, namely the removal of the control of 'higher centres', rather than to a direct disease process causing 'positive' symptoms. In this sense he foreshadows Freud's notion of mental illness as a regression to a more primitive, childhood state, and Freud openly acknowledges the debt). Rather, it is that Jackson wrote about mental states having a parallel in organic pathology.

Although a member of the Medico-Psychological Association (MPA) since 1866 he was temperamentally unable to cope with psychiatric patients. As George Savage (Virginia Woolf's psychiatrist) recalled, 'his mind was one which needed order and precision, and the disorders of mind only perplexed him. . .at times he seems to have had a real physical dread of the patients. . . . He looked upon many of the insane as rather useless cumberers of the ground' (Savage, 1917). Nevertheless, he had the insight to recognize a neural basis for changed behaviour and to accept the essential ordinariness of so many psychiatric symptoms. If 'déjà vu'—which seems to be what was meant by 'intellectual aura'—is an almost universal experience and only pathological when too *frequent*, perhaps the same may be said of auditory hallucinations? Both of these symptoms are now accepted as typical phenomena of temporal lobe seizures (Feindel, 1974), yet the medical response to them is dominated by the specialization gap. However, while providing a broad enough understanding for the integration of neurology and psychiatry, Jackson's own personality exemplifies the characteristics that keep the specialties apart.

Jackson's influence can perhaps be better understood by his chosen method of communication. He wrote papers; papers based on clinical cases. He never wrote a book, and his *Neurological Fragments* (1925) and the *Collected Papers* (1931) are simply collections of the briefer works. Their range is as good as a textbook. For example, by 1888, the year of 'A particular variety. . .' he had published over 60 papers on epilepsy alone, including a description of seizures preceded by a 'disagreeable smell' as early as 1864. Beginning as a virtual medical journalist, reporting cases for the *Medical Times* and *Gazette*, he went on to write more than 10 papers/cases a year throughout the 1860s, 1870s and 1880s. Topics included aphasia, jokes, syphilis (his contributions to the psychiatric *Journal of Mental Science* were almost wholly related to syphilis, even though the treponemal basis for General Paralysis of the Insane (GPI) was not established until 1913), chorea, vertigo, optic neuritis (he was a keen and early exponent of the ophthalmoscope in clinical assessment) and of course much of the case material that is now embedded into routine neurological practice. While it is clear that the multivariate effects of syphilitic infection made this period a 'golden age of neurology', it is no less clear that Jackson, Gowers, Ferrier and their contemporaries mined this seam for every possible insight into the pathology of cerebral and neurological function. The notion of Cerebral Localization had recently been introduced by Pierre Broca (his demonstration of the brain of an aphasic patient had occurred in 1861), and Jackson's combination of these ideas with the evolutionist philosophy of Herbert Spencer formed the basis for the development of his unique neurological perspective. When one considers that this was also the golden age of hysteria, with Charcot putting on his 'demonstrations' and Freud preparing his cases with Breuer (*Studies in Hysteria* was published in 1895) it is to Jackson's credit that he established sound criteria for the strange, subjective sensations that constantly hovered on the edge of hysterical forms. A detailed synthesis of these events (Thornton, 1976) makes fascinating reading, although the attribution of all hysterical/hypnotic phenomena to the effects of TLE is probably over-egging the pudding.

As regards the 1888 paper, 'On a Particular Variety of Epilepsy. . .' it is at first sight a little odd that it remains the standard Jacksonian reference. It is *not* the first report of such phenomena, and the author laments the 'very little attention' paid to previous communications (e.g. Anderson, 1886). Nor is it the best documented case, since the 'one case with symptoms of organic brain disease', does not actually go to necropsy, while the other four cases reported are entirely symptomatic. (N.B. Only cases one and five have been included in this extract.) It was only in 1898 that Jackson was able to associate the 'dreamy state' with a lesion in the uncinate gyrus (Jackson and Colman, 1898). Perhaps the strength of this communication is the discussion on epilepsy, Jackson's insistence on the importance of 'paroxysmalness', and his statement that 'the analysis of slight seizures is more easy and fruitful than that of severe ones'. Unlike the various case reports, this paper discusses the problems of establishing 'the dreamy state' and the need to 'describe all that happens in the paroxysm'. It is essentially a clinical paper, synthesizing the fruits of clinical acumen. 'No better neurological work can be done than the precise investigation of epileptic paroxysms', states the author: a sentiment that remains true today, especially in the psychiatric context.

The immediate impact of the paper is difficult to assess. The readers of *Brain* had no correspondence column to which to address their thoughts, but both Gowers and Ferrier referred to Jackson's work frequently in their lectures and one suspects that word of mouth was the primary means of its dissemination. As to the longer term, there are two major strands of inheritance. On the psychiatric side his colleague George Savage, expounding on the theory of dissolution in 1817 (6 years after Jackson's death) felt his teaching had 'not been sufficiently considered from the psychiatric side', but did admit that 'his close logical mind was not associated with fluency of expression' (Savage, 1917). Jackson's impact on Bleuler and Freud ('the insane is in a dream from which awakening is sometimes impossible') is stressed by Stengel (1963), while Henri Ey (1962), in a paper of forceful Gallic idiosyncrasy shows the influence he had on Adolf Meyer, Sherrington and the 'organo-dynamic concept'.

More obvious though, have been the neurological offshoots. With the development of the EEG in the 1930s and 1940s it became possible to assess dreamy states neurophysiologically, and their ictal basis was established. In a sense this was the first special investigation positively to correlate with functional symptoms. The brilliant work of Wilder Penfield in the temporal localization and operative treatment of psychomotor states (e.g. Feindel and Penfield, 1954) was succeeded by an improved understanding of such states in relation to schizophrenia (Beard and Slater, 1962; Herrington, 1969) and sophisticated assessments of the relationship between behaviour and personality (e.g. Bear and Fedio, 1977). The trend towards neuropsychiatry as a unifying discipline is a broader reflection of this pattern. It is perhaps an odd paradox that Jackson, the evolutionist, philosopher and psychiatrist manque, should not only have helped separate neurology from psychiatry, but should have provided the clinical basis for their subsequent, possible, fusion.

Two books are now available for those wishing to pursue a more detailed study. *Hughlings Jackson on Psychiatry* (Dewhurst, 1982) is an invaluable collection of material summarizing many of Jackson's ideas and with a useful bibliography and outline of his career. *Epilepsy and Psychiatry* (Reynolds and Trimble, 1981) has a good historical introduction by Denis Hill and provides a modern synthesis of our present knowledge. A complete list of Jackson's papers may be found in volume one of the *Selected Writings*.

T. H. Turner

REFERENCES

*Anderson, J. (1886). On sensory epilepsy. A case of basal cerebral tumour, affecting the left temporo-sphenoidal lobe, and giving rise to a paroxysmal taste-sensation and dreamy state. *Brain*, 9, 385–395.
Bear, D. M. and Fedio, P. (1977). Quantitative analysis of inter-ictal behavior in temporal lobe epilepsy, *Archives of Neurology*, **34**, 454–457.
Beard, A. W. and Slater, E. (1962). The schizophrenia-like psychoses of epilepsy, *Proceedings of the Royal Society of Medicine*, **55**, 311–316.

---

* Volumes of *Brain* did not correspond to years: vol. 9 is partly 1886, partly 1887, and usually bound by libraries as 1887.

Dewhurst, K. (1982). *Hughlings Jackson on Psychiatry*, Sandford Publications, Oxford.

Ey, H. (1962). Hughlings Jackson's Principles and the Organo-Dynamic Concept of Psychiatry, *American Journal of Psychiatry,* **118**, 673–682.

Feindel, W. (1974). Temporal lobe seizures, in *Handbook of Clinical Neurology*, P. J. Vinker and G. W. Bruyn (Eds), Elsevier/North Holland, Amsterdam.

Feindel, W. and Penfield, W. (1954). Localization of discharge in temporal lobe automatism, *A. M. A. Archives of Neurology and Psychiatry,* **72**, 605–630.

Herrington, R. N. (Ed.) (1969). *Current Problems in Neuropsychiatry*, B. J. Psych. Special Publication No. 4, Headley Bros., Ashford.

Jackson, J. H. and Colman, W. S. (1898). Case of epilepsy with tasting movements and 'dreamy' state: very small patch of softening in the left uncinate gyrus, *Brain,* **21**, 580–590.

Jackson, J. H. (1925). *Neurological Fragments*, with a Biographical Memoir, J. Taylor (Ed.), Oxford Medical Publications, Oxford.

Jackson, J. H. (1931/2). *Selected Writings*, vols 1 and 2, J. Taylor (Ed.), Hodder and Stoughton, London.

Reynolds, E. H. and Trimble, M. R. (eds) (1981). *Epilepsy and Psychiatry*, Churchill Livingstone, Edinburgh.

Savage, G. (1917). Dr. Hughlings Jackson on mental disorders, *Journal of Mental Science,* **63**, 315–328.

Stengel, E. (1963). Hughlings Jackson's influence on psychiatry, *British Journal of Psychiatry,* **109**, 348–355.

Thornton, E. M. (1976). *Hysteria, Hypnotism and Epilepsy: An Historical Synthesis*, Heinemann, London.

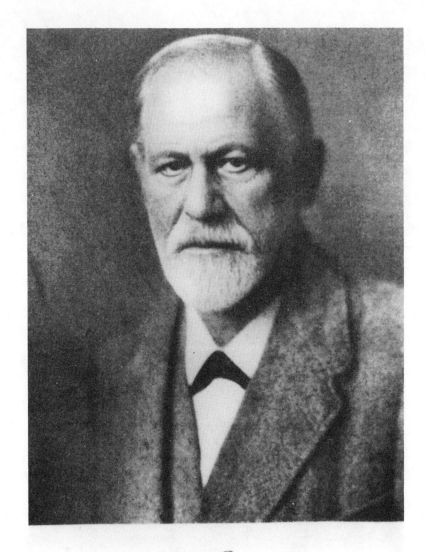

6

On the Psychical Mechanism of Hysterical Phenomena: Preliminary Communication

J. Breuer and S. Freud, 1893

A chance observation has led us, over a number of years, to investigate a great variety of different forms and symptoms of hysteria, with a view to discovering their precipitating cause—the event which provoked the first occurrence, often many years earlier, of the phenomenon in question. In the great majority of cases it is not possible to establish the point of origin by a simple interrogation of the patient, however thoroughly it may be carried out. This is in part because what is in question is often some experience which the patient dislikes discussing; but principally because he is genuinely unable to recollect it and often has no suspicion of the causal connection between the precipitating event and the pathological phenomenon. As a rule it necessary to hypnotize the patient and to arouse his memories under hypnosis of the time at which the symptom made its first appearance; when this has been done, it becomes possible to demonstrate the connection in the clearest and most convincing fashion.

This method of examination has in a large number of cases produced results which seem to be of value alike from a theoretical and a practical point of view.

They are valuable theoretically because they have taught us that external events determine the pathology of hysteria to an extent far greater than is known and recognized. It is of course obvious that in cases of 'traumatic' hysteria what provokes the symptoms is the accident. The causal connection is equally evident in hysterical attacks when it is possible to gather from the patient's utterances that in each attack he is hallucinating the same event which provoked the first one. The situation is more obscure in the case of other phenomena.

Our experiences have shown us, however, that the most various symptoms, which are ostensibly spontaneous and, as one might say, idiopathic products of hysteria, are just as strictly related to the precipitating trauma as the phenomena to which we have just alluded and which exhibit the connection quite clearly. The symptoms which we have been able to trace back to precipitating factors of this sort include neuralgias and anaesthesias of very various kinds, many of which had persisted for years, contractures and paralyses, hysterical attacks and epileptoid convulsions, which every observer regarded as true epilepsy, *petit mal* and disorders in the nature of *tic*, chronic vomiting and anorexia, carried to the pitch of rejection of all nourishment, various forms of disturbance of vision, constantly recurrent visual hallucinations, etc. The disproportion between the many years' duration of the hysterical symptom and the single occurrence which provoked it is what we are accustomed invariably to find in traumatic neuroses. Quite frequently it is some event in childhood that sets up a more or less severe symptom which persists during the years that follow.

The connection is often so clear that it is quite evident how it was that the precipitating event produced this particular phenomenon rather than any other. In that case the symptom has quite obviously been determined by the precipitating cause. We may take as a very commonplace instance a painful emotion arising during a meal but suppressed at the time, and then producing nausea and vomiting which persists for months in the form of hysterical vomiting. A girl, watching beside a sick-bed in a torment of anxiety, fell into a twilight state and had a terrifying hallucination, while her right arm, which was hanging over the back of her chair, went to sleep; from this there developed a paresis of the same arm accompanied by contracture and anaesthesia. She tried to pray but could find no words; at length she succeeded in repeating a children's prayer in English. When subsequently a severe and highly complicated hysteria developed, she could only speak, write and understand English, while her native language remained unintelligible to her for eighteen months.—The mother of a very sick child, which had at last fallen asleep, concentrated her whole will-power on keeping still so as not to waken it. Precisely on account of her intention she made a 'clacking' noise with her tongue. (An instance of 'hysterical counterwill'.) This noise was repeated on a subsequent occasion on which she wished to keep perfectly still; and from it there deveoped a *tic* which, in the form of a clacking with the tongue, occurred over a period of many years whenever she felt excited.—A highly intelligent man was present while his brother had an ankylosed hip-joint extended under an anaesthetic. At the instant at which the joint gave way with a crack, he felt a violent pain in his own hip-joint, which persisted for nearly a year.—Further instances could be quoted.

In other cases the connection is not so simple. It consists only in what might be called a 'symbolic' relation between the precipitating cause and the pathological phenomenon—a relation such as healthy people form in dreams. For instance, a neuralgia may follow upon mental pain or vomiting upon a feeling of moral disgust. We have studied patients who used to make the most copious use of this sort of symbolization. In still other cases it is not possible to understand at first sight how they can be determined in the manner we have suggested. It is precisely the typical hysterical symptoms which fall into this class, such as hemi-anaesthesia, contraction of the field of vision, epileptiform convulsions, and so on. An explanation of our views on this group must be reserved for a fuller discussion of the subject.

Observations such as these seem to us to establish an analogy between the pathogenesis of common hysteria and that of traumatic neuroses, and to justify an extension of the concept of traumatic hysteria. In traumatic neuroses the operative cause of the illness is not the trifling physical injury but the affect of fright—the psychical trauma. In an analogous manner, our investigations reveal, for many, if not for most, hysterical symptoms, precipitating causes which can only be described as psychical traumas. Any experience which calls up distressing affects—such as those of fright, anxiety, shame or physical pain—may operate as a trauma of this kind; and whether it in fact does so depends naturally enough on the susceptibility of the person affected (as well as on another condition which will be mentioned later). In the case of common hysteria it not infrequently happens that, instead of a single, major trauma, we find a number of partial traumas forming a *group* of provoking causes. These have only been able to exercise a traumatic effect by summation and they belong together in so far as they are in part components of a single story of suffering. There are other cases in which an apparently trivial circumstance combines with the actually operative event or occurs at a time of peculiar susceptibility to stimulation and in this way attains the dignity of a trauma which it would not otherwise have possessed but which thenceforward persists.

But the causal relation between the determining psychical trauma and the hysterical phenomenon is not of a kind implying that the trauma merely acts like an *agent provocateur* in releasing the symptom, which thereafter leads an independent existence. We must presume rather that the psychical trauma—or more precisely the memory of the trauma—acts like a foreign body which long after its entry must continue to be regarded as an agent that is still at work; and we find the evidence for this in a highly remarkable phenomenon which at the same time lends an important *practical* interest to our findings.

For we found, to our great surprise at first, that *each individual hysterical symptom immediately and permanently disappeared when we had succeeded in bringing clearly to light the memory of the event by which it was provoked and in arousing its accompanying affect, and when the patient had described that event in the greatest possible detail and had put the affect into words.* Recollection without affect almost invariably produces no result. The psychical process which originally took place must be repeated as vividly as possible; it must be brought back to its *status nascendi* and then given verbal utterance. Where what we are dealing with are phenomena involving stimuli (spasms, neuralgias and hallucinations) these reappear once again with the fullest intensity and then vanish for ever. Failures of function, such as paralyses and anaesthesias, vanish in the same way, though, of course, without the temporary intensification being discernible.

It is plausible to suppose that it is a question here of unconscious suggestion: the patient expects to be relieved of his sufferings by this procedure, and it is this expectation, and not the verbal utterance, which is the operative factor. This, however, is not so. The first case of this kind that came under observation dates back to the year 1881, that is to say to the 'pre-suggestion' era. A highly complicated case of hysteria was analysed in this way, and the symptoms, which sprang from separate causes, were separately removed. This observation was made possible by spontaneous auto-hypnoses on the part of the patient, and came as a great surprise to the observer.

We may reverse the dictum *'cessante causa cessat effectus'* ['when the cause ceases the effect ceases'] and conclude from these observations that the determining process continues to operate in some way or other for years—not indirectly, through a chain of intermediate causal links, but as a *directly* releasing cause—just as a psychical pain that is remembered in waking consciousness still provokes a lachrymal secretion long after the event. *Hysterics suffer mainly from reminiscences.*

2

At first sight it seems extraordinary that events experienced so long ago should continue to operate so intensely—that their recollection should not be liable to the wearing away process to which, after all, we see all our memories succumb. The following considerations may perhaps make this a little more intelligible.

The fading of a memory or the losing of its affect depends on various factors. The most important of these is *whether there has been an energetic reaction to the event that provokes an affect.* By 'reaction' we here understand the whole class of voluntary and involuntary reflexes—from tears to acts of revenge—in which, as experience shows us, the affects are discharged. If this reaction takes place to a sufficient amount a large part of the affect disappears as a result. Linguistic usage bears witness to this fact of daily observation by such phrases as 'to cry oneself out,' and to 'blow off steam'. If the reaction is suppressed, the affect remains attached to the memory. An injury that has been repaid, even if only in words, is recollected quite differently from one that has had to be accepted. Language recognizes this distinction, too, in its mental and physical consequences; it very characteristically describes an injury that has been suffered in silence as 'a mortification' ['*Kränkung*', lit. 'making ill'].—The injured person's reaction to the trauma only exercises a completely 'cathartic' effect if it is an *adequate* reaction—as, for instance, revenge. But language serves as a substitute for action; by its help, an affect can be 'abreacted' almost as effectively. In other cases speaking is itself the adequate reflex, when, for instance, it is a lamentation or giving utterance to a tormenting secret, e.g. a confession. If there is no such reaction, whether in deeds or words, or in the mildest cases in tears, any recollection of the event retains its affective tone to begin with.

'Abreaction', however, is not the only method of dealing with the situation that is open to a normal person who has experienced a psychical trauma. A memory of such a trauma, even if it has not been abreacted, enters the great complex of associations, it comes alongside other experiences, which may contradict it, and is subjected to rectification by other ideas. After an accident, for instance, the memory of the danger and the (mitigated) repetition of the fright becomes associated with the memory of what happened afterwards—rescue and the consciousness of present safety. Again, a person's memory of a humiliation is corrected by his putting the facts right, by considering his own worth, etc. In this way a normal person is able to bring about the disappearance of the accompanying affect through the process of association.

To this we must add the general effacement of impressions, the fading of memories which we name 'forgetting' and which wears away those ideas in particular that are no longer affectively operative.

Our observations have shown, on the other hand, that the memories which have become the determinants of hysterical phenomena persist for a long time with astonishing freshness and with the whole of their affective colouring. We must, however, mention another remarkable fact, which we shall later be able to turn to account, namely, that these memories, unlike other memories of their past lives, are not at the patients' disposal. On the contrary, *these experiences are completely absent from the patients' memory when they are in a normal psychical state, or are only present in a highly summary form.* Not until they have been questioned under hypnosis do these memories emerge with the undiminished vividness of a recent event.

Thus, for six whole months, one of our patients reproduced under hypnosis with hallucinatory vividness everything that had excited her on the same day of the previous year (during an attack of acute hysteria). A diary kept by her mother without her knowledge proved the completeness of the reproduction. Another patient, partly under hypnosis and partly during spontaneous attacks, re-lived with hallucinatory clarity all the events of a hysterical psychosis which she had passed through ten years earlier and which she had for the most part forgotten till the moment at which it re-emerged. Moreover, certain memories of aetiological importance which dated back from fifteen to twenty-five years were found to be astonishingly intact and to possess remarkable sensory force, and when they returned they acted with all the affective strength of new experiences.

This can only be explained on the view that these memories constitute an exception in their relation to all the wearing-away processes which we have discussed above. *It appears, that is to say, that these memories correspond to traumas that have not been sufficiently abreacted;* and if we enter more closely into the reasons which have prevented this, we find at least two sets of conditions under which the reaction to the trauma fails to occur.

In the first group are those cases in which the patients have not reacted to a psychical trauma because the nature of the trauma excluded a reaction, as in the case of the apparently irreparable loss of a loved person or because social circumstances made a reaction impossible or because it was a question of things which the patient wished to forget, and therefore intentionally expressed from his conscious thought and inhibited and suppresed. It is precisely distressing things of this kind that, under hypnosis, we find are the basis of hysterical phenomena (e.g. hysterical deliria in saints and nuns, continent women and well-brought-up children).

The second group of conditions are determined, not by the content of the memories but but by the psychical states in which the patient received the experiences in question. For we find, under hypnosis, among the causes of hysterical symptoms ideas which are not in themselves significant, but whose persistence is due to the fact that they originated during the prevalence of severely paralysing affects, such as fright, or during positively abnormal psychical states, such as the semi-hypnotic twilight state of day-dreaming, auto-hypnoses, and so on. In such cases it is the nature of the states which makes a reaction to the event impossible.

Both kinds of condition may, of course, be simultaneously present, and this, in fact, often occurs. It is so when a trauma which is operative in itself takes place while a severely paralysing affect prevails or during a modified state of consciousness. But it also seems to be true that in many people a psychical trauma *produces* one of these abnormal states, which, in turn, makes reaction impossible.

Both of these groups of conditions, however, have in common the fact that the psychical traumas which have not been disposed of by reaction cannot be disposed of either by being worked over by means of association. In the first group the patient is determined to forget the distressing experiences and accordingly excludes them so far as possible from association; while in the second group the associative working-over fails to occur because there is no extensive associative connection between the normal state of consciousness and the pathological ones in which the ideas made their appearance. We shall have occasion immediately to enter further into this matter.

It may therefore be said that the ideas which have become pathological have persisted with such freshness and affective strength because they have been denied the normal wearing-away processes by means of abreaction and reproduction in states of uninhibited association.

3

We have stated the conditions which, as our experience shows, are responsible for the development of hysterical phenomena from psychical traumas. In so doing, we have already been obliged to speak of abnormal states of consciousness in which these pathogenic ideas arise, and to emphasize the fact that the recollection of the operative psychical trauma is not to be found in the patient's normal memory but in his memory when he is hypnotized. The longer we have been occupied with these phenomena the more we have become convinced that *the splitting of consciousness which is so striking in the well-known classical cases under the form of 'double conscience' is present to a rudimentary degree in every hysteria, and that a tendency to such a dissociation, and with it the emergence of abnormal states of consciousness (which we shall bring together under the term 'hypnoid'), is the basic phenomenon of this neurosis.* In these views we concur with Binet and the two Janets, though we have had no experience of the remarkable findings they have made on anaesthetic patients.

We should like to balance the familiar thesis that hypnosis is an artificial hysteria by another—the basis and *sine qua non* of hysteria is the existence of hypnoid states. These hypnoid states share with one another and with hypnosis, however much they may differ in other respects, one common feature: the ideas which emerge in them are very intense but are cut off from associative communication with the rest of the content of consciousness. Associations may take place between these hypnoid states, and their ideational content can in this way reach a more or less high degree of psychical organization. Moreover, the nature of these states and the extent to which they are cut off from the remaining conscious processes must be supposed to vary just as happens in hypnosis, which ranges from a light drowsiness to somnambulism, from complete recollection to total amnesia.

If hypnoid states of this kind are already present before the onset of the manifest illness, they provide the soil in which the affect plants the pathogenic memory with its consequent somatic phenomena. This corresponds to *dispositional* hysteria. We have found, however, that a severe trauma (such as occurs in a traumatic neurosis) or a laborious suppression (as of a sexual affect, for instance) can bring about a splitting-off of groups of ideas even in people who are in other respects unaffected; and this would be the mechanism of *psychically acquired* hysteria. Between the extremes of these two forms we must assume the existence of a series of cases within which the liability to dissociation in the subject and the affective magnitude of the trauma vary inversely.

We have nothing new to say on the question of the origin of these dispositional hypnoid states. They often, it would seem, grow out of the day-dreams which are so common even in healthy people and to which needlework and similar occupations render women especially prone. Why it is that the 'pathological associations' brought about in these states are so stable and why they have so much more influence on somatic processes than ideas are usually found to do—these questions coincide with the general problem of the effectiveness of hypnotic suggestions. Our observations contribute nothing fresh on this subject. But they throw a light on the contradiction between the dictum 'hysteria is a psychosis' and the fact that among hysterics may be found people of the clearest intellect, strongest will, greatest character and highest critical power. This characterization holds good of their waking thoughts; but in their hypnoid states they are insane, as we all are in dreams. Whereas, however, our dream-psychoses have no effect upon our waking state, the products of hypnoid states intrude into waking life in the form of hysterical symptoms.

4

What we have asserted of chronic hysterical symptoms can be applied almost completely to hysterical *attacks*. Charcot, as is well known, has given us a schematic description of the 'major' hysterical attack, according to which four phases can be distinguished in a complete attack: (1) the epileptoid phase, (2) the phase of large movements, (3) the phase of 'attitudes passionnelles' (the hallucinatory phase), and (4) the phase of terminal delirium. Charcot derives all those forms of hysterical attack which are in practice met with more often than the complete 'grande attaque', from the abbreviation or prolongation, absence or isolation of these four distinct phases.

Our attempted explanation takes its start from the third of these phases, that of the 'attitudes passionnelles'. Where this is present in a well-marked form, it exhibits the hallucinatory reproduction of a memory which was of importance in bringing about the onset of the hysteria—the memory either of a single major trauma (which we find *par excellence* in what is called traumatic hysteria) or of a series of interconnected part-traumas (such as underlie common hysteria). Or, lastly, the attack may revive the events which have become emphasized owing to their *coinciding* with a moment of special disposition to trauma.

There are also attacks, however, which appear to consist exclusively of motor phenomena and in which the phase of *attitudes passionnelles* is absent. If one can succeed in getting into *rapport* with the patient during an attack such as this of generalized clonic spasms or cataleptic rigidity, or during an *attaque de sommeil* [attack of sleep]—or if, better still, one can succeed in provoking the attack under hypnosis—one finds that here, too, there is an underlying memory of the psychical trauma or series of traumas, which usually comes to our notice in a hallucinatory phase.

Thus, a little girl suffered for years from attacks of general convulsions which could well be, and indeed were, regarded as epileptic. She was hypnotized with a view to a differential diagnosis, and promptly had one of her attacks. She was asked what she was seeing and replied 'The dog! the dog's coming!'; and in fact it turned out that she had had the first of her attacks after being chased by a savage dog. The success of the treatment confirmed the choice of diagnosis.

Again, an employee who had become a hysteric as a result of being ill-treated by his superior suffered from attacks in which he collapsed and fell into a frenzy of rage, but without uttering a word or giving any sign of a hallucination. It was possible to provoke an attack under hypnosis, and the patient then revealed that he was living through the scene in which his employer had abused him in the street and hit him with a stick. A few days later the patient came back and complained of having had another attack of the same kind. On this occasion it turned out under hypnosis that he had been re-living the scene to which the actual onset of the illness was related: the scene in the law-court when he failed to obtain satisfaction for his maltreatment.

In all other respects, too, the memories which emerge, or can be aroused, in hysterical attacks correspond to the precipitating causes which we have found at the root of *chronic* hysterical symptoms. Like these latter causes, the memories underlying hysterical attacks relate to psychical traumas which have not been disposed of by abreaction or by associative thought-activity. Like them, they are whether completely or in essential elements, out of reach of the memory of normal consciousness and are found to belong to the ideational content of hypnoid states of consciousness with restricted association. Finally, too, the therapeutic test can be applied to them. Our observations have often taught us that a memory of this kind which had hitherto provoked attacks, ceases to be able to do so after the process of reaction and associative correction have been applied to it under hypnosis.

The motor phenomena of hysterical attacks can be interpreted partly as universal forms of reaction appropriate to the affect accompanying the memory (such as kicking about and waving the arms and legs, which even young babies do), partly as a direct expression of these memories; but in part, like the hysterical stigmata found among the chronic symptoms, they cannot be explained in this way.

Hysterical attacks, furthermore, appear in a specially interesting light if we bear in mind a theory that we have mentioned above, namely, that in hysteria groups of ideas originating in hypnoid states are present and that these are cut off from associative connection with the other ideas, but can be associated among themselves, and thus form the more or less highly organized rudiment of a second consciousness, a *condition seconde*. If this is so, a chronic hysterical symptom will correspond to the intrusion of this second state into the somatic innervation which is as a rule under the control of normal consciousness. A hysterical attack, on the other hand, is evidence of a higher organization of this second state. When the attack makes its first appearance, it indicates a moment at which this hypnoid consciousness has obtained control of the subject's whole existence—it points, that is, to an acute hysteria; when it occurs on subsequent occasions and contains a memory, it points to a return of that moment. Charcot has already suggested that hysterical attacks are a rudimentary form of a *condition seconde*. During the attack, control over the whole of the somatic innervation passes over to the hypnoid consciousness. Normal consciousness, as well-known observations show, is not always entirely repressed. It may even be aware of the motor phenomena of the attack, while the accompanying psychical events are outside its knowledge.

The typical course of a severe case of hysteria is, as we know, as follows. To begin with, an ideational content is formed during hypnoid states; when this has increased to a sufficient extent, it gains control, during a period of 'acute hysteria', of the somatic innervation and of the patient's whole existence, and creates chronic symptoms and attacks; after this it clears up, apart from certain residues. If the normal personality can regain control, what is left over from the hypnoid ideational content recurs in hysterical attacks and puts the subject back from time to time into similar states, which are themselves once more open to influence and susceptible to traumas. A state of equilibrium, as it were, may then be established between the two psychical groups which are combined in the same person: hysterical attacks and normal life proceed side by side without interfering with each other. An attack will occur spontaneously, just as memories do in normal people; it is, however, possible to provoke one, just as any memory can be aroused in accordance with the laws of association. It can be provoked either by stimulation of a hysterogenic zone or by a new experience which sets it going owing to a similarity with the pathogenic experience. We hope to be able to show that these two kinds of determinant, though they appear to be so unlike, do not differ in essentials, but that in both a hyperaesthetic memory is touched on.

In other cases this equilibrium is very unstable. The attack makes its appearance as a manifestation of the residue of the hypnoid consciousness whenever the normal personality is exhausted and incapacitated. The possibility cannot be dismissed that here the attack may have been divested of its original meaning and may be recurring as a motor reaction without any content.

It must be left to further investigation to discover what it is that determines whether a hysterical personality manifests itself in attacks, in chronic symptoms or in a mixture of the two.

It will now be understood how it is that the psychotherapeutic procedure which we have described in these pages has a curative effect. *It brings to an end the operative force of the idea which was not abreacted in the first instance, by allowing its strangulated affect to find a way out through speech; and it subjects it to associative correction by introducing it into normal consciousness (under light hypnosis) or by removing it through the physician's suggestions, as is done in somnambulism accompanied by amnesia.*

In our opinion the therapeutic advantages of this procedure are considerable. It is of course true that we do not cure hysteria in so far as it is a matter of disposition. We can do nothing against the recurrence of hypnoid states. Moreover, during the productive stage of an acute hysteria our procedure cannot prevent the phenomena which have been so laboriously removed from being at once replaced by fresh ones. But once this acute stage is past, any residues which may be left in the form of chronic symptoms or attacks are often removed, and permanently so, by our method, because it is a radical one; in this respect it seems to us far superior in its efficacy to removal through direct suggestion, as it is practised today by psychotherapists.

If by uncovering the psychical mechanism of hysterical phenomena we have taken a step forward along the path first traced so successfully by Charcot with is explanation and artificial imitation of hystero-traumatic paralyses, we cannot conceal from ourselves that this has brought us nearer to an understanding only of the *mechanism* of hysterical symptoms and not of the internal causes of hysteria. We have done no more than touch upon the aetiology of hysteria and in fact have been able to throw light only on its acquired forms—on the bearing of accidental factors on the neurosis.

Vienna, *December* 1892

A paper is considered a classic when it outlives both its author and the ideas of its time. When Breuer and Freud wrote their preliminary communication 'On the psychical mechanism of hysterical phenomena', they essentially wanted to show that the phenomenon of hysteria could scarcely be understood without postulating the existence of the unconscious. They came to this conclusion through hypnosis which they valued both as a research tool and as a therapeutic procedure.

Now, whilst the unconscious is more or less recognized the same could not be said for hypnosis until quite recently. Here the blame lies in great part with Breuer and Freud. The outcome of Breuer's treatment of his hysterical patient Anna O had a lot to do with his personal rejection of hypnosis as a therapeutic tool. Once he had successfully terminated her treatment she developed a phantom pregnancy which drove him to abandon her and take his own wife on a second honeymoon. It also made him resistant to the publication of his findings. Freud, however, saw his friend's apparent disaster as the proof of unconscious feelings which patients project onto those they become involved with; to him this was a manifestation of the phenomenon he later called Transference. Unlike his older colleague, he was spurred on to a further exploration of the human psyche. For personal and theoretical reasons he also abandoned hypnosis as a therapeutic tool and developed his technique of free association: 'Psychoanalysis began with my rejection of the hypnotic technique'. Hypnotherapy is however of growing interest now to psychotherapists and family therapists both in practice and in theory; attempts are being made to define the variations in the state of consciousness and to research into their possible causes.

The two authors make a strong case for linking up the hysterical symptoms, as manifested by hysterical patients, with those hitherto described in traumatic hysteria. In 'traumatic' hysteria 'what provokes the symptoms is the accident'. They then modify this to say: 'in the traumatic neuroses the operative cause of the illness is not the trifling physical injury but the effect of fright, the psychical trauma'. As in traumatic hysteria, with hysterical symptoms, the precipitating causes are psychical traumas such as fright, anxiety, shame or pain. These can be a single experience or many partial ones forming a group of provoking causes. However, 'the causal relation between the determining psychical trauma and the hysterical phenomenon is not of a kind implying that the trauma merely acts like an *agent provocateur* in releasing the symptom, which thereafter leads an independent existence. It is the 'memory of the trauma' which acts like a foreign body which is permanently at work. This is their conclusion after showing that each hysterical symptom (spasms, neuralgias, hallucinations and paralyses), 'immediately and permanently disappeared when we had succeeded in bringing permanently to light the memory of the event by which it was provoked and in arousing its accompanying affect and when the patient had described that event in the greatest possible detail and had put the affect into words.' The discount the possibility of unconscious suggestion since their first case, Anna O, achieved this, to the surprise of Dr Breuer, in states of auto-hypnosis.

The authors proceed to analyse what are the possible contributing factors which make this conversion from a traumatic memory to a hysterical symptom possible. They suggest three potential factors. The first is a disposition or a susceptibility in the patient to hypnoid states such as is shown in the case of Anna O. The second is the nature and the context of the traumatic experience which makes an immediate reaction impossible and which has to be forgotten or, as the authors put it, 'repressed' from the conscious activity of the patient's mind. The third factor is the psychical state of the patient when the trauma occurs; if the patient is in an altered state of consciousness, such as in a twilight state or an auto-hypnotic state, the experience cannot be processed in the normal way, that is to say through the pathways available to the conscious system.

This last statement makes it necessary for the authors to write about their understanding of memory processes, which in some respects are singularly in keeping with present day research findings. They write that the memories which activate the hysterical symptoms 'are not at the patient's disposal'. They note that these memories when acceded to (by hypnosis in their case), appear 'with astonishing freshness and with the whole of their affective colouring'. The psychologists, Weingartner et al. (1977), write that 'the retrieval of information is, in part, dependent on reinstituting the brain context that was present when the to-be-remembered events were encoded and stored in the memory. Information that appears lost in disparate state recall is, in fact, available but temporarily inaccessible.'

Gazzaniga and Le Doux (1978) postulate the existence of a variety of 'memory banks' in the brain. 'The brain has a variety of ways to encode and store information and that given information storage system in the brain is not necessarily accessible to every other network of stored information . . .. As the motivational state changes access to innate or learned behaviour patterns is allowed expression'. This possibility, that memories and their associated affective components can co-exist in the mind, the one being unavailable or 'unconscious' to the other, is the focus of intense research in neuropsychology today.

A phenomenon which struck Freud in particular is what he describes in hysterics as the 'splitting of consciousness'. 'We have become convinced that the splitting of consciousness which is so striking in the well-known classical cases under the form of "double conscience" is present to a rudimentary degree in every hysteria, and that a tendency to such a dissociation, and with it the emergence of abnormal states of consciousness . . . is the basic phenomenon of this neurosis.' Here he concurs with the views of Binet and the two Janets.

Freud and Breuer describe the condition of 'dispositional hysteria' where hypnoid states occur spontaneously and during which ideas and feelings arise which are cut off from the rest of consciousness to varying degrees. They also describe how 'a severe trauma (such as occurs in traumatic neurosis) or a laborious suppression (as of a sexual affect, for instance) can bring about a splitting-off of groups ideas even in people who are in other respects unaffected; and this would be the mechanism of psychically acquired hysteria.'

Right from the beginning of their psychological studies, Freud and Breuer were aware of our capacity to split off from consciousness certain groups of ideas. They also intuitively linked this capacity to split our consciousness with the existence of focalized areas of 'insanity' in our psychic activity, normally confined to our dreams or 'dream psychoses' but which the hysteric cannot ward off except by a conversion of his unconscious manifestations into hysterical symptoms. This fascinating leap from psyche to soma remains one of the most promising areas of research in psychosomatic medicine.

This capacity of the human mind to split within itself was later taken up by Freud in his paper on 'Mourning and Melancholia' (Freud, 1917). Here he described the ego as split to form a 'critical agency' or 'conscience' later defined as the 'super-ego'. He also refers in the same paper to the ego's capacity to identify with the lost object so that in melancholics, 'the object loss is transformed into ego loss and the conflict between the ego and the loved person into a cleavage between the critical activity of the ego and the ego altered by identification'. He thus opens the way for Melanie Klein's work on the internalization of object relationships which in its turn leads on to the appearance of the British object relations theorists such as Balint, Winnicott, Guntrip and Fairbairn. It is the latter who was to finally reject Freud's Instinctual Theory.

This leads us to a second basic assumption in Freud's thinking which is in evidence throughout his writings, including this joint paper he wrote with Breuer. Earlier on we pointed out the reference to the 'laborious suppression (as of sexual affect, for instance,) in hysterical patients'. This is a direct reference to what was to become the basic hypothesis in Freud's theory, the so-called 'principle of constancy' referred to clearly in his later paper: 'Beyond the Pleasure Principle' (Freud, 1920). Both Freud and Breuer were followers of Helmholtz, believing that all rational phenomena are explicable in terms of physical and chemical forces. Freud transposed this hydraulic-like model to his findings in the field of psychology. Thus, in 'Beyond the Pleasure Principle', he writes: 'the moral apparatus endeavours to keep the quantity of excitation present as low as possible or at least to keep it constant.' When Freud began to attribute greater importance to the instincts rather than experience, as the prime activators of human psychic activity, he formulated repression in terms of a need to keep out unpleasurable increases in excitation rather than an attempt to split of the memory of traumatic experiences as he and Breuer first suggested. It was essentially this change of emphasis in Freud towards the importance of the sexual instinct that led to the split between these two co-authors.

In this paper we can see the early manifestations of what were to become two separate conceptual currents present throughout Freud's work and whose contradictory aspects were analysed by Fairbairn in his paper 'Endopsychic structure considered in terms of object-relationships' (Fairbairn, 1954). According to one of Freud's postulates, the unconscious is an undifferentiated mass of undischarged instincts; in the other there is the beginning of a structuralized splitting at the level of the unconscious. It remains a mystery why Freud himself seemed unaware of the potential contradictions between his two conceptual models. The fact is that, to abandon his Instinctual Theory, Freud would have had to put far more weight on the importance of human experiences in terms of human relationships as he did in 'Mourning and Melancholia'. Such an emphasis would have made it more difficult for him to ascribe the incestuous memories of his hysterical female patients to their frustrated sexual instincts. If he had stuck to his original view that these memories were possibly true he could well have been completely ostracized by his Viennese colleagues. Similarly, abandoning the 'Principle of Constancy' would have meant breaking completely with the scientific beliefs of his time.

For those who still doubt the importance of Breuer and Freud's observations, there remains another aspect of their paper which has not yet been commented upon but which has important implications in both the psychoanalytic field and in the field of neuropsychology. When referring to the onset of Anna O's hysterical illness, they clearly describe how she lost the use of her mother-tongue for the 18 months that followed (during which she spoke mainly in English), and how she regained her German after recalling the original experience associated with its loss. Recent findings in neuropsychology and psychoanalytic case studies show how the differential use of languages in neurotic and psychotic patients can be seen as a way of splitting off from traumatic experiences encoded within the language and that such a linguistic shift may be accompanied by changes in hemispheric activity (Zulueta, 1984).

These linguistic dimensions also highlight another aspect of psychoanalysis which had become rather neglected, the importance of language. Its importance is highly stressed by Breuer and Freud who saw it as a valuable substitute for action in their treatment of hysterics. Its importance has re-emerged with the treatment of bilingual patients. Balint (1968) wrote that emotionally charged communications cannot be experienced equally in different languages. He describes each word as 'surrounded by a cluster of associations' which differs with every language and with differing relationships within the same language. It has however been left to the French psychoanalyst, Lacan, to bring language and linguistics back to the centre of the psychoanalytic arena. Not only does he remind us that language is the sole medium of psychoanalysis but also that the human animal is born into language and that it is within the terms of language that the human subject is constructed.

Breuer and Freud's paper can well be seen as a seminal one. Right from the beginning, Freud begins to define the two different conceptual models which run through his later writings. It now behoves his followers to review his work in the light of recent developments in the study of human psychic activity. Whilst Breuer's contribution remains of fundamental importance for Freud we are left guessing as to what his conceptual developments could have been. However his own painful and exciting experience while treating Anna O is a salutary reminder to all clinicians of how difficult it can be to treat hysterical patients.

F. de Zulueta

REFERENCES

Balint, M. (1968). *The Basic Fault,* Tavistock Publications, London.
Fairbairn, W. R. D. (1954). *An Object-Relations Theory of the Personality,* Basic Books, New York.
Freud, S. (1917). Mourning and Melancholia. *Standard Edition.* **14**, p. 239.
Freud, S. (1920). *Beyond the Pleasure Principle,* Standard Edition, **18**, p. 7.
Gazzaniga, M. and Le Doux, (1978). *The Split Brain and the Integrated Mind,* Plenum Press, New York.
Weingartner, H., Miller, H. and Murphy, D. L. (1977). Mood state dependent retrieval of verbal associations. *Journal of Abnormal Psychology,* **86**, 276–284.
Zulueta, F. (1984). The implications of bilingualism in the study and treatment of psychiatric disorders: a review, *Psychological Medicine,* **14**, 541–557.

7
Suicide
E. Durkheim, 1897

SUICIDE AND PSYCHOPATHIC STATES

There are two sorts of extra-social causes to which one may, *a priori*, attribute an influence on the suicide-rate; they are organic-psychic dispositions and the nature of the physical environment. In the individual constitution, or at least in that of a significant class of individuals, it is possible that there might exist an inclination, varying in intensity from country to country, which directly leads man to suicide; on the other hand, the action of climate, temperature, etc., on the organism, might indirectly have the same effects. Under no circumstances can the hypothesis be dismissed unconsidered.

I

The annual rate of certain diseases is relatively stable for a given society though varying perceptibly from one people to another. Among these is insanity. Accordingly, if a manifestation of insanity were reasonably to be supposed in every voluntary death, our problem would be solved; suicide would be a purely individual affliction.

This thesis is supported by a considerable number of alienists. According to Esquirol: "Suicide shows all the characteristics of mental alienation." —"A man attempts self-destruction only in delirium and suicides are mentally alienated." From this principle he concluded that suicide, being involuntary, should not be punished by law. Falret and Moreau de Tours use almost the same terms. The latter, to be sure, in the same passage where he states his doctrine, makes a remark which should subject it to suspicion: "Should suicide be regarded in all cases as the result of mental alienation? Without wishing to dispose here of this difficult question, let us say generally that one is instinctively the more inclined to the affirmative the deeper the study of insanity which he has made, the greater his experience and the greater the number of insane persons whom he has examined."

This theory may be and has been defended in two different ways. Suicide itself is either called a disease in itself, *sui generis*, a special form of insanity; or it is regarded, not as a distinct species, but simply an event involved in one or several varieties of insanity, and not to be found in sane persons. "From what has preceded," Esquirol writes, "suicide may be seen to be for us only a phenomenon resulting from many different causes and appearing under many different forms; and it is clear that this phenomenon is not characteristic of a disease. From considering suicide as a disease *sui generis*, general propositions have been set up which are belied by experience."

The second of these two methods of proving suicide to be a manifestation of insanity is the less rigorous and conclusive, since because of it negative experiences are impossible. A complete inventory of all cases of suicide cannot indeed be made, nor the influence of mental alienation shown in each. Only single examples can be cited which, however numerous, cannot support a scientific generalization; even though contrary examples were not affirmed, there would always be possibility of their existence. The other proof, however, if obtainable, would be conclusive. If suicide can be shown to be a mental disease with its own characteristics and distinct evolution, the question is settled; every suicide is a madman.

But does suicidal insanity exist?

II

Since the suicidal tendency is naturally special and definite if it constitutes a sort of insanity, this can be only a form of partial insanity, limited to a single act. To be considered a delirium it must bear solely on this one object; for, if there were several, the delirium could no more be defined by one of them than by the others. In traditional terminology of mental pathology these restricted deliria are called monomanias. A monomaniac is a sick person whose mentality is perfectly healthy in all respects but one;

he has a single flaw; clearly localized. At times, for example, he has an unreasonable and absurd desire to drink or steal or use abusive language; but all his other acts and all his other thoughts are strictly correct. Therefore, if there is a suicidal mania it can only be a monomania, and has indeed been usually so called.

On the other hand, if this special variety of disease called monomanias is admitted, it is clear why one readily includes suicide among them. The character of these kinds of afflictions, according to the definition just given, is that they imply no essential disturbance of intellectual functions. The basis of mental life is the same in the monomaniac and the sane person; only, in the former, a specific psychic state is prominently detached from this common basis. In short, monomania is merely one extreme emotion in the order of impulses, one false idea in the order of representations, but of such intensity as to obsess the mind and completely enslave it. Thus, ambition, from being normal, becomes morbid and a monomania of grandeur when it assumes such proportions that all other cerebral functions seem paralyzed by it. A somewhat violent emotional access disturbing mental equilibrium is therefore enough to cause the monomania to appear. Now suicides generally seem influenced by some abnormal passion, whether its energy is abruptly expended or gradually developed; it may thus even appear reasonable that some such force is always necessary to offset the fundamental instinct of self-preservation. Moreover, many suicides are completely indistinguishable from other men except by the particular act of self-destruction; and there is therefore no reason to impute a general delirium to them. This is the reasoning by which suicide, under the appellation of monomania, has been considered a manifestation of insanity.

But, do monomanias exist? For a long time this was not questioned; alienists one and all concurred without discussion in the theory of partial deliria. It was not only thought confirmed by clinical observation but regarded as corollary to the findings of psychology. The human intelligence was supposed to consist of distinct faculties and separate powers which usually function cooperatively but may act separately; thus it seemed natural that they might be separately affected by disease.

Today however this opinion has been universally discarded. The non-existence of monomanias cannot indeed be proved from direct observation, but not a single incontestable example of their existence can be cited. Clinical experience has never been able to observe a diseased mental impulse in a state of pure isolation; whenever there is lesion of one faculty the others are also attacked, and if these concomitant lesions have not been observed by the believers in monomania, it is because of poorly conducted observations.

Finally, apart from these special manifestations, there always exists in these supposed monomaniacs a general state of the whole mental life which is fundamental to the disease and of which these delirious ideas are merely the outer and momentary expression. Its essential character is an excessive exaltation or deep depression or general perversion. There is, especially, a lack of equilibrium and coordination in both thought and action. The patient reasons, but with lacunas in his ideas; he acts, not absurdly, but without sequence. It is incorrect then to say that insanity constitutes a part, and a restricted part of his mental life; as soon as it penetrates the understanding it totally invades it.

Moreover, the principle underlying the hypothesis of monomania contradicts the actual data of science. The old theory of the faculties has few defenders left. The different sorts of conscious activity are no longer regarded as separate forces, disunited, and combined only in the depths of a metaphysical substance, but as interdependent functions; thus one cannot suffer lesion without the others being affected. This interpenetration is even closer in mental life than in the rest of the organism; for psychic functions have no organs sufficiently distinct from one another for one to be affected without the others. Their distribution among the different regions of the brain is not well defined, as appears from the readiness with which its different parts mutually replace each other, if one of them is prevented from fulfilling its task. They are too completely interconnected for insanity to attack certain of them without injury to the others. With yet greater reason it is totally impossible for insanity to alter a single idea or emotion without psychic life being radically changed. For representations and impulses have no separate existence; they are not so many little substances, spiritual atoms, constituting the mind by their combination. They are merely external manifestations of the general state of the centers of consciousness, from which they derive and which they express. Thus they cannot be morbid without this state itself being vitiated.

But if mental flaws cannot be localized, there are not, there cannot be monomanias properly so-called. The apparently local disturbances given this name always derive from a more extensive perturbation; they are not diseases themselves, but particular and secondary manifestations of more general diseases. If then there are no monomanias, there cannot be a suicidal monomania and, consequently, suicide is not a distinct form of insanity.

III

It remains possible, however, that suicide may occur only in a state of insanity. If it is not by itself a special form of insanity, there are no forms of insanity in connection with which it may not appear. It is only an episodic syndrome of them, but one of frequent occurrence. Perhaps this frequency indicates that suicide never occurs in a state of sanity, and that it indicates mental alienation with certainty?

The conclusion would be hasty. For though certain acts of the insane are peculiar to them and characteristic of insanity, others are common to them and to normal persons, though assuming a special form in the case of the insane. There is no reason, a priori, to place suicide in the first of the two categories. To be sure, alienists state that most of the suicides known to them show all the indications of mental alienation, but this evidence could not settle the question, for the reviews of such cases are much too summary. Besides, no general law could be drawn from so narrowly specialized an experience. From the suicides they have known, who were, of course, insane, no conclusion can be drawn as to those not observed, who, moreover, are much more numerous.

The only methodical procedure consists of classifying according to their essential characteristics the suicides committed by insane persons, thus forming the principal types of insane suicide, and then trying to learn whether all cases of voluntary death can be included under these systematically arranged groups. In other words, to learn whether suicide is an act peculiar to the insane one must fix the forms it assumes in mental alienation and discover whether these are the only ones assumed by it.

In general, specialists have paid little heed to classifying the suicides of the insane. The four following types, however, probably include the most important varieties. The essential elements of the classification are borrowed from Jousset and Moreau de Tours.

1. Maniacal Suicide

—This is due to hallucinations or delirious conceptions. The patient kills himself to escape from an imaginary danger or disgrace, or to obey a mysterious order from on high, etc. But the motives of such suicide and its manner of evolution reflect the general characteristics of the disease from which it derives—namely, mania. The quality characteristic of this condition is its extreme mobility. The most varied and even conflicting ideas and feelings succeed each other with intense rapidity in the maniac's consciousness. It is a constant whirlwind. One state of mind is instantly replaced by another. Such, too, are the motives of maniacal suicide; they appear, disappear, or change with amazing speed. The hallucination or delirium which suggests suicide suddenly occurs; the attempt follows; then instantly the scene changes, and if the attempt fails it is not resumed, at least, for the moment. If it is later repeated it will be for another motive. The most trivial incident may cause these sudden transformations.

2. Melancholy Suicide

—This is connected with a general state of extreme depression and exaggerated sadness, causing the patient no longer to realize sanely the bonds which connect him with people and things about him. Pleasures no longer attract; he sees everything as through a dark cloud. Life seems to him boring or painful. As these feelings are chronic, so are the ideas of suicide; they are very fixed and their broad determining motives are always essentially the same.

Hallucinations and delirious thoughts often associate themselves with this general despair and lead directly to suicide. However, they are not mobile like those just observed among maniacs. On the contrary they are fixed, like the general state they come from. The fears by which the patient is haunted, his self-reproaches, the grief he feels are always the same. If then this sort of suicide is determined like its predecessor by imaginary reasons, it is distinct by its chronic character. And it is very tenacious. Patients of this category prepare their means of self-destruction calmly; in the pursuit of their purpose they even display incredible persistence and, at times, cleverness. Nothing less resembles this consistent state of mind than the maniac's constant instability. In the latter, passing impulses without durable cause; in the former, a persistent condition linked with the patient's general character.

3. Obsessive Suicide

—In this case, suicide is caused by no motive, real or imaginary, but solely by the fixed idea of death which, without clear reason, has taken complete possession of the patient's mind. He is obsessed by the desire to kill himself, though he perfectly knows he has no reasonable motive for doing so. It is an instinctive need beyond the control of reflection and reasoning, like the needs to steal, to kill, to commit arson, supposed to constitute other varieties of monomania. As the patient realizes the absurdity of his wish he tries at first to resist it. But throughout this resistance he is sad, depressed, with a constantly increasing anxiety oppressing the pit of his stomach. Hence, this sort of suicide has sometimes been called *anxiety-suicide*. Here is the confession once made by a patient to Brierre de Boismont, which perfectly describes the condition: "I am employed in a business house. I perform my regular duties satisfactorily but like an automaton, and when spoken to, the words sound to me as though echoing in a void. My greatest torment is the thought of suicide, from which I am never free. I have been the victim of this impulse for a year; at first it was insignificant; then for about the last two months it has pursued me everywhere, *yet I have no reason to kill myself.* . . . My health is good; no one in my family has been similarly afflicted; I have had no financial losses, my income is adequate and permits me the pleasures of people of my age." But as soon as the patient has decided to give up the struggle and to kill himself, anxiety ceases and calm returns. If the attempt fails it is sometimes sufficient, though unsuccessful, to quench temporarily the morbid desire. It is as though the patient had voided this impulse.

4. Impulsive or Automatic Suicide

—It is as unmotivated as the preceding; it has no cause either in reality or the patient's imagination. Only, instead of being produced by a fixed idea obsessing the mind for a shorter or longer period and only gradually affecting the will, it results from an abrupt and immediately irresistible impulse. In the twinkling of an eye it appears in full force and excites the act, or at least its beginning. This abruptness recalls what has been mentioned above in connection with mania; only the maniacal suicide has always some reason, however irrational. It is connected with the patient's delirious conceptions. Here on the contrary the suicidal tendency appears and is effective in truly automatic fashion, not preceded by any intellectual antecedent. The sight of a knife, a walk by the edge of a precipice, etc. engender the suicidal idea instantaneously and its execution follows so swiftly that patients often have no idea of what has taken place.

In short, all suicides of the insane are either devoid of any motive or determined by purely imaginary motives. Now, many voluntary deaths fall into neither category; the majority have motives, and motives not unfounded in reality. Not every suicide can therefore be considered insane, without doing violence to language. *Of all the suicides just characterized, that which may appear hardest to detect of those observed among the sane is melancholy suicide; for very often the normal person who kills himself is also in a state of dejection and depression like the mentally alienated. But an essential difference between them always exists in that the state of the former and its resultant act are not without an objective cause, whereas in the latter they are wholly unrelated to external circumstances. In short, the suicides of the insane differ from others as illusions and hallucinations differ from normal perceptions and automatic impulses from deliberate acts.* It is true that there is a gradual shading from the former to the latter; but if that sufficed to identify them one would also, generally speaking, have to confuse health with sickness, since the latter is but a variety of the former. Even if it were proved that the average man never kills himself and that only those do so who show certain anomalies, this would still not justify considering insanity a necessary condition of suicide; for an insane person is not simply a man who thinks or acts somewhat differently from the average. Thus, suicide has been so closely associated with insanity only by arbitrarily restricting the meaning of the words.

There are therefore suicides, and numerous ones at that, not connected with insanity. They are doubly identifiable as being deliberate and as springing from representations involved in this deliberation which are not purely hallucinatory. This often debated question may therefore be solved without requiring reference to the problem of freedom. To learn whether all suicides are insane, we have not asked whether or not they act freely; we have based ourselves solely on the empirical characteristics observable in the various sorts of voluntary death.

IV

Since the suicides of insane persons do not constitute the entire genus but only a variety of it, the psychopathic states constituting mental alienation can give no clue to the collective tendency to suicide in its generality. But between mental alienation properly so-called and perfect equilibrium of intelligence, an entire series of intermediate stages exist; they are the various anomalies usually combined under the common name of neurasthenia. Let us therefore see whether they, in cases devoid of insanity, do not have an important role in the origin of the phenomenon we are studying.

What share has this highly individual condition in the production of voluntary deaths? Can it alone, if aided by circumstances, produce them, or does it merely make individuals more accessible to forces exterior to them and which alone are the determining causes of the phenomenon?

To settle the question directly, the variations of suicide would have to be compared with those of neurasthenia. Unfortunately, the latter has not been statistically studied. But the difficulty may be indirectly solved. Since insanity is only the enlarged form of nervous degeneration, it may be granted without risk of serious error that the number of nervous degenerates varies in proportion to that of the insane, and consideration of the latter may be used as a substitute in the case of the former. This procedure would also make it possible to establish a general relation of the suicide-rate to the total of mental abnormalities of every kind.

One fact might lead us to attribute to them an undue influence; the fact that suicide, like insanity, is commoner in cities than in the country. It seems to increase and decrease like insanity, a fact which might make it seem dependent on the latter. But this parallelism does not necessarily indicate a relation of cause to effect; it may very well be a mere coincidence. The latter hypothesis is the more plausible in that the social causes of suicide are, as we shall see, themselves closely related to urban civilization and are most intense in these great centers. To estimate the possible effect of psychopathic states on suicide, one must eliminate cases where they vary in proportion to the social conditions of the latter; for when these two factors tend in the same direction the share of each cannot be determined in the final result. They must be considered only where they are in inverse proportion to one another; only when a sort of conflict exists between them can one learn which is decisive. If mental disorders are of the decisive importance sometimes attributed to them, their presence should be shown by characteristic effects, even when social conditions tend to neutralize them; and, inversely, the latter should be unable to appear when individual conditions contradict them. The following facts show that the opposite is the rule:

		No. of Men and Women to 100 Insane	
	Year	Men	Women
Silesia	1858	49	51
Saxony	1861	48	52
Wurtemberg	1853	45	55
Denmark	1847	45	55
Norway	1855	45*	56*
New York	1855	44	56
Massachusetts	1854	46	54
Maryland	1850	46	54
France	1890	47	53
France	1891	48	52

* As in Durkheim's original, though equalling more than 100 together.—Ed.

1. All statistics prove that in insane asylums the female inmates are slightly more numerous than the male. The proportion varies by countries, but as appears in the table on the preceding page, it is in general 54 or 55 for the women to 46 or 45 for the men.

Koch has compared the results of the census taken of the total insane population in eleven different states. Among 166,675 insane of both sexes, he found 78,584 men and 88,091 women, or 1.18 insane per 1,000 male and 1.30 per 1,000 female inhabitants.† Mayr has discovered similar figures.

There is the question, to be sure, whether the excess of women is not simply due to the mortality of the male being higher than that of the female insane. In France, certainly, of every 100 insane who die in asylums, about 55 are men. The larger number of women recorded at a given time would therefore not prove that women have a greater tendency to insanity, but only that, in this condition as in all others, they outlive men. It is none the less true that the actual insane population includes more women than men;

† Koch zur Statistik der Geisteskrankenheiten, Stuttgart 1878, p. 73.

if, then, as seems reasonable, we apply the argument from the insane to the nervous, more neurasthenics must be admitted to exist at a given moment among females than among men. So, if there were a causal relation between the suicide-rate and neurasthenia, women should kill themselves more often than men. They should do so at least as often. For, even considering their lower mortality and correcting the census figures accordingly, our only conclusion would be that they have a predisposition to insanity at least as great as that of men; their lower figure of mortality and their numerical superiority in all censuses of the insane almost exactly cancel each other. But far from their aptitude

Table IV* Share of Each Sex in the Total Number of Suicides

	Absolute Numbers of Suicides		To 100 Suicides Number of	
	Men	Women	Men	Women
Austria (1873–77)	11,429	2,478	82.1	17.9
Prussia (1831–40)	11,435	2,534	81.9	18.1
Prussia (1871–76)	16,425	3,724	81.5	18.5
Italy (1872–77)	4,770	1,195	80	20
Saxony (1851–60)	4,004	1,055	79.1	20.9
Saxony (1871–76)	3,625	870	80.7	19.3
France (1836–40)	9,561	3,307	74.3	25.7
France (1851–55)	13,596	4,601	74.8	25.2
France (1871–76)	25,341	6,839	79.7	21.3
Denmark (1845–56)	3,324	1,106	75.0	25.0
Denmark (1870–76)	2,485	748	76.9	23.1
England (1863–67)	4,905	1,791	73.3	26.7

* According to Morselli.

for voluntary death being either higher or equal to that of men, suicide happens to be an essentially male phenomenon. To every woman there are on the average four male suicides (Table IV). Each sex has accordingly a definite tendency to suicide which is even constant for each social environment. But the intensity of this tendency does not vary at all in proportion to the psychopathic factor, whether the latter is estimated by the number of new cases registered annually or by that of census subjects at a given moment.

2. Table V shows the comparative strength of the tendency to insanity among the different faiths.

Insanity is evidently much more frequent among the Jews than among the other religious faiths; we may therefore assume that

Table V* Tendency to Insanity Among the Different Religious Faiths

	Number of Insane per 1,000 Inhabitants of Each Faith		
	Protestants	Catholics	Jews
Silesia (1858)	0.74	0.79	1.55
Mecklenburg (1862)	1.36	2.00	5.33
Duchy of Baden (1863)	1.34	1.41	2.24
Duchy of Baden (1873)	0.95	1.19	1.44
Bavaria (1871)	0.92	0.96	2.86
Prussia (1871)	0.80	0.87	1.42
Wurtemberg (1832)	0.65	0.68	1.77
Wurtemberg (1853)	1.06	1.06	1.49
Wurtemberg (1875)	2.18	1.86	3.96
Grand Duchy of Hesse (1864)	0.63	0.59	1.42
Oldenburg (1871)	2.12	1.76	3.37
Canton of Bern (1871)	2.64	1.82	. . .

* According to Koch, *op. cit.*, pp. 108–119.

the other affections of the nervous system are likewise in the same proportion among them. Nevertheless, the tendency to suicide among the Jews is very slight. We shall even show later that it is least prominent in this religion. *In this case accordingly suicide varies in inverse proportion to psychopathic states*, rather than being consistent with them. Doubtless this does not prove that nervous and cerebral weaknesses have ever been preservatives against suicide; but they must have very little share in determining it, since it can reach so low a figure at the very point where they reach their fullest development.

If Catholics alone are compared with Protestants, the inverse proportion is less general; yet it is very frequent. The tendency of Catholics to insanity is only one-third lower than that of Protestants and the difference between them is therefore very slight. On the other hand, the former kill themselves much less often than the latter, without exception anywhere.

3. In all countries the suicidal tendency increases regularly from childhood to the most advanced old age. If it occasionally retrogresses after the age of 70 or 80, the decrease is very slight; it still remains at this time of life from two to three times greater than at maturity. On the other hand, insanity appears most frequently at maturity. The danger is greatest at about 30; beyond

that it decreases, and is weakest by far in old age. Such a contrast would be inexplicable if the causes of the variation of suicide and those of mental disorders were not different.

If the suicide-rate at each age is compared, not with the relative frequency of new cases of insanity appearing during this same period, but with the proportional number of the insane population, the lack of any parallelism is just as clear. The insane are most numerous in relation to the total population at about the age of 35. The proportion remains about the same to approximately 60; beyond that it rapidly decreases. It is minimal, therefore, when the suicide-rate is maximal, and prior to that no regular relation can be found between the variations of the two.

4. If different societies are compared from the double point of view of suicide and insanity, no greater relation is found between the variations of these two phenomena. True, statistics of mental alienation are not compiled accurately enough for these international comparisons to be very strictly exact. Yet it is notable that the two following tables, taken from two different authors, offer definitely concurring conclusions.

Thus the countries with the fewest insane have the most suicides; the case of Saxony is especially striking. In his excellent study on suicide in Seine-et-Marne, Dr. Leroy had already observed the same fact. "Usually," he writes, "the places with a large number of mental diseases also have many suicides. However these two maxima may be completely distinct. I should even be inclined to believe that, side by side with some countries fortunate enough to have neither mental diseases nor suicides . . . there are others where mental diseases only are found." The reverse occurs in other localities.

Morselli, to be sure, reaches slightly different conclusions. But this is because, first, he has combined the insane proper and idiots under the common name of alienated. Now, the two afflictions are very different, especially in regard to the influence upon suicide provisionally attributed to them. Far from predisposing to suicide, idiocy seems rather a safeguard against it; for idiots are much more numerous in the country than in the city, while suicides are much rarer in the country. Two such different conditions must therefore be distinguished in seeking to determine the share of different neuropathic disorders in the rate of voluntary deaths. But

---

* Koch, *op. cit.*

Table VI Relations of Suicide and Insanity in Different European Countries

	No. Insane per 100,000 Inhabitants	A No. Suicides per 1,000,000 Inhabitants	Ranking Order of Countries for Insanity	Suicide
Norway	180 (1855)	107 (1851–55)	1	4
Scotland	164 (1855)	34 (1856–60)	2	8
Denmark	125 (1847)	258 (1846–50)	3	1
Hannover	103 (1856)	13 (1856–60)	4	9
France	99 (1856)	100 (1851–55)	5	5
Belgium	92 (1858)	50 (1855–60)	6	7
Wurtemburg	92 (1853)	108 (1846–56)	7	3
Saxony	67 (1861)	245 (1856–60)	8	2
Bavaria	57 (1858)	73 (1846–50)	9	6

	No. Insane per 100,000 Inhabitants	B* No. Suicides per 1,000,000 Inhabitants	Averages of Suicides
Wurtemburg	215 (1875)	180 (1875)	
Scotland	202 (1871)	35	107
Norway	185 (1865)	85 (1866–70)	
Ireland	180 (1871)	14	
Sweden	177 (1870)	85 (1866–70)	
England and Wales	175 (1871)	70 (1870)	63
France	146 (1872)	150 (1871–75)	
Denmark	137 (1870)	277 (1866–70)	
Belgium	134 (1868)	66 (1866–70)	164
Bavaria	98 (1871)	86 (1871)	
Cisalpine Austria	95 (1873)	122 (1873–77)	
Prussia	86 (1871)	133 (1871–75)	
Saxony	84 (1875)	272 (1875)	153

* The first part of the table is borrowed from the article, "*Alienation mentale,*" in the *Dictionnaire* of Dechambre (v. III, p. 34); the second from Oettingen, *Moralstatistik*, Table appendix 97.

even by combining them no regular parallelism is found between the extent of mental alienation and that of suicide. If indeed, accepting Morselli's figures unreservedly, the principal European countries are separated into five groups according to the importance of their alienated population (idiots and insane being combined in the same classification), and if then the average of suicides in each of these groups is sought, the following table is obtained:

	Mentally Alienated per 100,000 Inhabitants	Suicides per 1,000,000 Inhabitants
1st Group (3 countries)	from 340 to 280	157
2nd Group (3 countries)	from 261 to 245	195
3rd Group (3 countries)	from 185 to 164	65
4th Group (3 countries)	from 150 to 116	61
5th Group (3 countries)	from 110 to 100	68

On the whole it appears that there are many suicides where the insane and idiots are numerous, and that the inverse is true. But there is no consistent agreement between the two scales which would show a definite causal connection between the two sets of phenomena. The second group, which should show fewer suicides than the first, has more; the fifth, which from the same point of view should be less than all the others, is on the contrary larger than the fourth and even than the third. Finally, if for Morselli's statistics of mental alienation those of Koch are substituted, which are much more complete and apparently more careful, the lack of parallelism is much more pronounced. The following in fact is the result:

	Insane and Idiots per 100,000 Inhabitants	Average of Suicides per 1,000,000 Inhabitants
1st Group (3 countries)	from 422 to 305	76
2nd Group (3 countries)	from 305 to 291	123
3rd Group (3 countries)	from 268 to 244	130
4th Group (3 countries)	from 223 to 218	227
5th Group (4 countries)	from 216 to 146	77

5. In short, as insanity is agreed to have increased regularly for a century and suicide likewise, one might be tempted to see proof of their interconnection in this fact. But what deprives it of any conclusive value is that in lower societies where insanity is rare, suicide on the contrary is sometimes very frequent.

The social suicide-rate therefore bears no definite relation to the tendency to insanity, nor, inductively considered, to the tendency to the various forms of neurasthenia.

V

But there is a special psychopathic state to which for some time it has been custom to attribute almost all the ills of our civilization. This is alcoholism. Rightly or wrongly, the progress of insanity, pauperism and criminality have already been attributed to it. Can it have any influence on the increase of suicide? *A priori* the hypothesis seems unlikely, for suicide has most victims among ·the most cultivated and wealthy classes and alcoholism does not have its most numerous followers among them. But facts are unanswerable. Let us test them.

If the French map of suicides is compared with that of prosecutions for alcoholism, almost no connection is seen between them. Characteristic of the former is the existence of two great centers of contamination, one of which is in the Ile-de-France, extending from there eastward, while the other lies on the Mediterranean, stretching from Marseilles to Nice. The light and dark areas on the maps of alcoholism have quite a different distribution. Here three chief centers appear, one in Normandy, especially in Seine-Inférieure, another in Finisterre and the Breton departments in general, and the third in the Rhone and the neighbouring region. From the point of view of suicide, on the other hand, the Rhone is not above the average, most of the Norman departments are below it and Brittany is almost immune. So the geography of the two phenomena is too different for us to attribute to one an important share in the production of the other.

The same result is obtained by comparing suicide not with criminal intoxication but with the nervous or mental diseases caused by alcoholism. After grouping the French departments in eight classes according to their rank in suicides, we examined the average number of cases of insanity due to alcoholism in each class, using Dr. Lunier's figures. We got the result shown in the table opposite.

The two columns do not correspond. Whereas suicides increase sixfold and over, the proportion of alcoholic insane barely increases by a few units and the growth is not regular; the second class surpasses the third, the fifth the sixth, the seventh the eighth. Yet if alcoholism affects suicide as a psychopathic condition it can do so only by the mental disturbance it causes.

---

* Koch, *op. cit.*

	Suicides per 100,000 Inhabitants (1872–76)	Alcoholic Insane per 100 Admissions (1867–69 and 1874–76)
1st Group (5 departments)	Below 50	11.45
2nd Group (18 departments)	From 51 to 75	12.07
3rd Group (15 departments)	From 76 to 100	11.92
4th Group (20 departments)	From 101 to 150	13.42
5th Group (10 departments)	From 151 to 200	14.57
6th Group (9 departments)	From 201 to 250	13.26
7th Group (4 departments)	From 251 to 300	16.32
8th Group (5 departments)	Above	13.47

At first sight there seems to be a closer relation between the quantity of alcohol consumed and the tendency to suicide, at least for our country. Indeed most alcohol is drunk in the northern departments and it is also in this same region that suicide shows its greatest ravages. But, first, the two areas have nothing like the same outline on the two maps. The maximum of one appears in Normandy and the North and diminishes as it descends toward Paris; that of alcoholic consumption. The other is most intense in the Seine and neighbouring departments; it is already lighter in Normandy and does not reach the North. The former tends westward, and reaches the Atlantic coast; the other has an opposite direction. It ends abruptly in the West, at Eure and Eure-et-Loir, but has a strong easterly tendency. Moreover, the dark area on the map of suicides formed in the Midi by Var and Bouches-du-Rhone does not appear at all on the map of alcoholism.

In short, even to the extent that there is some coincidence it proves nothing, being random. Leaving France and proceeding farther North, for example, the consumption of alcohol increases almost regularly without the appearance of suicide. Whereas only 2.84 liters of alcohol per inhabitant were consumed on the average in France in 1873, the figure rises in Belgium to 8.56 for 1870, in England to 9.07 (1870–71), in Holland to 4 (1870), in Sweden to 10.34 (1870), in Russia to 10.69 (1866) and even, at Saint Petersburg to 20 (1855). And yet whereas, in the corresponding periods, 150 suicides per million inhabitants occurred in France, Belgium had only 68, Great Britain 70, Sweden 85, Russia very few. Even at Saint Petersburg from 1864 to 1868 the average annual rate was only 68.8. Denmark is the only northern country where there are both many suicides and a large consumption of alcohol (16.51 liters in 1845). If then our northern departments are distinguished both by their tendency to suicide and their addiction to alcohol, it is not because the former arises from the latter and is explained by it. The conjunction is accidental. In general, much alcohol is drunk in the North because a special nourishment calculated to maintain the organism's temperature is more necessary there than elsewhere; and on the other hand the originating causes of suicide are especially concentrated in the same region of our country.

Alcoholism and Suicide in Germany

	Consumption of Alcohol (1884–86) Liters per Capita	Average of Suicides per 1,000,000 Inhabitants	Country
1st Group	13 to £0.8	206.1	Posnania, Silesia, Brandenburg, Pomerania
2nd Group	9.2 to 7.2	208.4	East and West Prussia, Hanover, Province of Saxony, Thuringia, Westphalia
3rd Group	6.4 to 4.5	234.1	Mecklenburg, Kingdom Saxony, Schleswig-Holstein, Alsace, Grand Duchy Hesse
4th Group	4 and less	147.9	Rhine provinces, Baden, Bavaria, Wurtemburg

The comparison of the different states of Germany confirms this conclusion. If they are classified both in regard to suicide and to alcoholic consumption, (see above), it appears that the group showing most suicidal tendency (the third) is one of those where least alcohol is consumed. Genuine contrasts are even found in certain details: the province of Posen is almost the least affected by suicide of the entire Empire (96.4 cases per million inhabitants), yet it is the one where most alcoholism is found (13 liters per capita); in Saxony, where suicide is almost four times as common (348 per million), only half as much alcohol is consumed. It is to be noted, finally, that the fourth group, that of the lowest consumption of alcohol, is composed almost exclusively of southern states. From another standpoint, if suicide occurs there less than in the rest of Germany, this is because its population is either Catholic or contains large Catholic minorities.

Thus no psychopathic state bears a regular and indisputable relation to suicide. A society does not depend for its number of suicides on having more or fewer neuropaths or alcoholics. Although the different forms of degeneration are an eminently suitable psychological field for the action of the causes which may lead a man to suicide, degeneration itself is not one of these causes. Admittedly, under similar circumstances, the degenerate is more apt to commit suicide than the well man; but he does not necessarily do so because of his condition. This potentiality of his becomes effective only through the action of other factors which we must discover.

THE SOCIAL ELEMENT OF SUICIDE

I

The individual conditions on which suicide might, *a priori*, be supposed to depend, are of two sorts.

There is first the external situation of the agent. Sometimes men who kill themselves have had family sorrow or disappointments to their pride, sometimes they have had to suffer poverty or sickness, at others they have had some moral fault with which to reproach themselves, etc. But we have seen that these individual peculiarities could not explain the social suicide-rate; for the latter varies in considerable proportions, whereas the different combinations of circumstances which constitute the immediate antecedents of individual cases of suicide retain approximately the same relative frequency. They are therefore not the determining causes of the act which they precede. Their occasionally important role in the premeditation of suicide is no proof of being a causal one. Human deliberations, in fact, so far as reflective consciousness affects them are often only purely formal, with no object but confirmation of a resolve previously formed for reasons unknown to consciousness.

Besides, the circumstances are almost infinite in number which are supposed to cause suicide because they rather frequently accompany it. One man kills himself in the midst of affluence, another in the lap of poverty; one was unhappy in his home, and another had just ended by divorce a marriage which was making him unhappy. In one case a soldier ends his life after having been punished for an offense he did not commit; in another, a criminal whose crimes has remained unpunished kills himself. The most varied and even the most contradictory events of life may equally serve as pretexts for suicide. This suggests that none of them is the specific cause. Could we perhaps at least ascribe causality to those qualities known to be common to all? But are there any such? At best one might say that they usually consist of disappointments, of sorrows, without any possibility of deciding how intense the grief must be to have such tragic significance. Of no disappointment in life, no matter how insignificant, can we say in advance that it could not possibly make existence intolerable; and, on the other hand, there is none which must necessarily have this effect. We see some men resist horrible misfortune, while others kill themselves after slight troubles. Moreover, we have shown that those who suffer most are not those who kill themselves most. Rather it is too great comfort which turns a man against himself. Life is most readily renounced at the time and among the classes where it is least harsh. At least, if it really sometimes occurs that the victim's personal situation is the effective cause of this resolve, such cases are very rare indeed and accordingly cannot explain the social suicide-rate.

Accordingly, even those who have ascribed most influence to individual conditions have sought these conditions less in such external incidents than in the intrinsic nature of the person, that is, his biological constitution and the physical concomitants on which it depends. Thus, suicide has been represented as the subject of a certain temperament, an episode of neurasthenia, subject to the effects of the same factors as neurasthenia. Yet we have found no immediate and regular relationship between neurasthenia and the social suicide-rate. The two facts even vary at times in inverse proportion to one another, one being at its minimum just when and where the other is at its height. We have not found, either, any definite relation between the variations of suicide and the conditions of physical environment supposed to have most effect on the nervous system, such as race, climate, temperature. Obviously, though the neuropath may show some inclination to suicide under certain conditions, he is not necessarily destined to kill himself; and the influence of cosmic factors is not enough to determine in just this sense the very general tendencies of his nature.

Wholly different are the results we obtained when we forgot the individual and sought the causes of the suicidal aptitude of each society in the nature of the societies themselves. The relations of suicide to certain states of social environment are as direct and constant as its relations to facts of a biological and physical character were seen to be uncertain and ambiguous. Here at last we are face to face with real laws, allowing us to attempt a methodical classification of types of suicide. The sociological causes thus determined by us have even explained these various concurrences often attributed to the influence of material causes, and in which a proof of this influence has been sought. If women kill themselves much less often than men, it is because they are much less involved than men in collective existence; thus they feel its influence—good or evil—less strongly. So it is with old persons and children, though for other reasons. Finally, if suicide increases from January to June but then decreases, it is because social activity shows similar seasonal fluctuations. It is therefore natural that the different effects of social activity should be subject to an identical rhythm, and consequently be more pronounced during the former of these two periods. Suicide is one of them.

The conclusion from all these facts is that the social suicide-rate can be explained only sociologically. At any given moment the moral constitution of society establishes the contingent of voluntary deaths. There is, therefore, for each people a collective force of a definite amount of energy, impelling men to self-destruction. The victim's acts which at first seem to express only his personal temperament are really the supplement and prolongation of a social condition which they express externally.

It is not mere metaphor to say of each human society that it has a greater or lesser aptitude for suicide; the expression is based on the nature of things. Each social group really has a collective inclination for the act, quite its own, and the source of all individual inclination, rather than their result. It is made up of the currents of egoism, altruism or anomy running through the society under consideration with the tendencies to languorous melancholy, active renunciation or exasperated weariness derivative from these currents. These tendencies of the whole social body, by affecting individuals, cause them to commit suicide. The private experiences usually thought to be the proximate causes of suicide have only the influence borrowed from the victim's moral predisposition, itself an echo of the moral state of society. To explain his detachment from life the individual accuses his most immediately surrounding circumstances; life is sad to him because he is sad. Of course his sadness comes to him from without in one sense, however not from one or another incident of his career but rather from the group to which he belongs. This is why there is nothing which cannot serve as an occasion for suicide. It all depends on the intensity with which suicidogenetic causes have affected the individual.

II

Usually when collective tendencies or passions are spoken of, we tend to regard these expressions as mere metaphors and manners of speech with no real signification but a sort of average among a certain number of individual states. They are not considered as things, forces *sui generis* which dominate the consciousness of single individuals. None the less this is their nature, as is brilliantly shown by statistics of suicide. The individuals making up a society change from year to year, yet the number of suicides is the same so long as the society itself does not change. The population of Paris renews itself very rapidly; yet the share of Paris in the total of French suicides remains practically the same. Although only a few years suffice to change completely the personnel of the army, the rate of military suicides varies only very slowly in a given nation. In all countries the evolution of collective life follows a given rhythm throughout the year; it grows from January to about July and then diminishes. Thus, though the members of the several European societies spring from widely different average types, the seasonal and even monthly variations of suicide take place in accordance with the same law. Likewise, regardless of the diversity of individual temperaments, the relation between the aptitude for suicide of married persons and that of widowers and widows is identically the same in widely differing social groups, from the simple fact that the moral condition of widowhood everywhere bears the same relation to the moral constitution characteristic of marriage. The causes which thus fix the contingent of voluntary deaths for a given society or one part of it must then be independent of individuals, since they retain the same intensity no matter what particular persons they operate on. One would think that an unchanging manner of life would produce unchanging effects. This is true; but a way of life is something, and its unchanging character requires explanation. If a way of life is unchanged while changes occur constantly among those who practise it, it cannot derive its entire reality from them.

Collective tendencies have an existence of their own; they are forces as real as cosmic forces, though of another sort; they, likewise, affect the individual from without, though through other channels. The proof that the reality of collective tendencies is no less than that of cosmic forces is that this reality is demonstrated in the same way, by the uniformity of effects. When we find that the number of deaths varies little from year to year, we explain this regularity by saying that mortality depends on the climate, the temperature, the nature of the soil, in brief on a certain number of material forces which remain constant through changing generations because independent of individuals. Since, therefore, moral acts such as suicide are reproduced not merely with an equal but with a greater uniformity, we must likewise admit that they depend on forces external to individuals. Only, since these forces must be of a moral order and since, except for individual men, there is no other moral order of existence in the world but society, they must be social. But whatever they are called, the important thing is to recognize their reality and conceive of them as a totality of forces which cause us to act from without, like the physico-chemical forces to which we react. So truly are they things *sui generis* and not mere verbal entities that they may be measured, their relative sizes compared, as is done with the intensity of electric currents or luminous foci. Thus, the basic proposition that social facts are objective finds a new and especially conclusive proof in moral statistics and above all in the statistics of suicide. Of course, it offends common sense. But science has encountered incredulity whenever it has revealed to men the existence of a force that has been overlooked. Since the system of accepted ideas must be modified to make room for the new order of things and to establish new concepts, men's minds resist through mere inertia. Yet this understanding must be reached. If there is such a science as sociology, it can only be the study of a world hitherto unknown, different from those explored by the other sciences. This world is nothing if not a system of realities.

Observation confirms our hypothesis. The regularity of statistical data, on the one hand, implies the existence of collective tendencies exterior to the individual, and on the other, we can directly establish this exterior character in a considerable number of important cases. Besides, this exteriority is not in the least surprising for anyone who knows the difference between individual and social states of consciousness. By definition, indeed, the latter can reach none of us except from without, since they do not flow from our personal predispositions. Since they consist of elements foreign to us they express something other than ourselves. To be sure in so far as we are solitary with the group and share its life, we are exposed to their influence; but so far as we have a distinct personality of our own we rebel against and try to escape them. Since everyone leads this sort of double existence simultaneously, each of us has a double impulse. We are drawn in a social direction and tend to follow the inclinations of our own natures. So the rest of society weighs upon us as a restraint to our centrifugal tendencies, and we for our part share in this weight upon others for the purpose of neutralizing theirs. We ourselves undergo the pressure we help to exert upon others. Two antagonistic forces confront each other. One, the collective force, tries to take possession of the individual; the other, the individual force, repulses it. To be sure, the former is much stronger than the latter, since it is made of a combination of all the individual forces; but as it also encounters as many resistances as there are separate persons, it is partially exhausted in these multifarious contests and reaches us disfigured and enfeebled. When it is very strong, when the circumstances activating it are of frequent recurrence, it may still leave a deep impression on individuals; it arouses in them mental states of some vivacity which, once formed, function with the spontaneity of instinct; this happens in the case of the most essential moral ideas. But most social currents are either too weak or too intermittently in contact with us to strike deep roots in us; their action is superficial. Consequently, they remain almost completely external. Hence, the proper way to measure any element of a collective type is not to measure its magnitude within individual consciences and to take the averge of them all. Rather, it is their sum that must be taken. Even this method of evaluation would be much below reality, for this would give us only the social sentiment reduced by all its losses through individuation.

Nothing is more reasonable, then, than this proposition that a belief or social practice may exist independently of its individual expressions. We clearly did not imply by this that society can exist without individuals, an obvious absurdity we might have been spared having attributed to us. But we did mean: 1. that the group formed by associated individuals has a reality of a different sort from each individual considered singly; 2. that collective states exist in the group from whose nature they spring, before they affect the individual as such and establish in him in a new form a purely inner existence.

III

Let us apply these ideas to the question of suicide; the solution we gave at the beginning of this chapter will become more precise if we do so.

No moral idea exists which does not combine in proportions varying with the society involved, egoism, altruism and a certain anomy. For social life assumes both that the individual has a certain personality, that he is ready to surrender it if the community requires, and finally, that he is to a certain degree sensitive to ideas of progress. This is why there is no people among whom these three currents of opinion do not co-exist, bending men's inclinations in three different and even opposing directions. Where they offset one another, the moral agent is in a state of equilibrium which shelters him against any thought of suicide. But let one of them exceed a certain strength to the detriment of the others, and as it becomes individualized, it also becomes suicidogenetic, for the reasons assigned.

Of course, the stronger it is, the more agents it contaminates deeply enough to influence them to suicide, and inversely. But this very strength can depend only on the three following sorts of causes: 1. the nature of the individuals composing the society; 2. the manner of their association, that is, the nature of the social organization; 3. the transitory occurrences which disturb the functioning of the collective life without changing its anatomical constitution, such as national crises, economic crises, etc. As for the individual qualities, they can play a role only if they exist in all persons. For strictly personal ones or those of only small minorities are lost in the mass of the others; besides, from their differences from one another they neutralize one another and are mutually eradicated during the elaboration resulting in the collective phenomenon. Only general human characteristics, accordingly, can have any effect. Now these are practically immutable; at least, their change would require more centuries than the life of one nation can occupy. So the social conditions on which the number of suicides depends are the only ones in terms of which it can vary; for they are the only variable conditions. This is why the number of suicides remains stable as long as society does not change. This stability does not exist because the state of mind which generates suicide is found through some chance in a definite number of individuals who transmit it, for no recognizable reason, to an equal number who will imitate the act. It exists because the impersonal causes which gave it birth and which sustain it are the same. It is because nothing has occurred to modify either the grouping of the social units or the nature of their concurrence. The actions and reactions interchanged among them therefore remain the same; and so the ideas and feelings springing from them cannot vary.

To be sure, it is very rare, if not impossible, for one of these currents to succeed in exerting such preponderant influence over all points of the society. It always reaches this degree of energy in the midst of restricted surroundings containing conditions specially favorable to its development. One or another social condition, occupation, or religious faith stimulates it more especially. This explains suicide's twofold character. When considered in its outer manifestations, it seems as though these were just a series of disconnected events; for it occurs at separated places without visible interrelations. Yet the sum of all these individual cases has its own unity and its own individuality, since the social suicide-rate is a distinctive trait of each collective personality. That is, though these particular environments where suicide occurs most frequently are separate from one another, dispersed in thousands of ways over the entire territory, they are nevertheless closely related; for they are parts of a single whole, organs of a single organism, as it were. The condition in which each is found therefore depends on the general condition of society. There is a close solidarity between the virulence achieved by one or another of its tendencies and the intensity of the tendency in the whole social body. Altruism is more or less a force in the army depending on its role among the civilian population, intellectual individualism is more developed and richer in suicides in Protestant environments the more pronounced it is in the rest of the nation, etc. Everything is tied together.

But though there is no individual state except insanity which may be considered a determining factor of suicide, it seems certain that no collective sentiment can affect individuals when they are absolutely indisposed to it. The above explanation might be thought inadequate for this reason, until we have shown how the currents giving rise to suicide find at the very moment and in the very environments in which they develop a sufficient number of persons accessible to their influence.

If we suppose, however, that this conjunction is really always necessary and that a collective tendency cannot impose itself by brute force on individuals with no preliminary predisposition, then this harmony must be automatically achievcd; for the causes determining the social currents affect individuals simultaneously and predispose them to receive the collective influence. Between these two sorts of factors there is a natural affinity, from the very fact that they are dependent on, and expressive of the same cause: this makes them combine and become mutually adapted. The hypercivilization which breeds the anomic tendency and the egoistic tendency also refines nervous systems, making them excessively delicate; through this very fact they are less capable of firm attachment to a definite object, more impatient of any sort of discipline, more accessible both to violent irritation and to exaggerated depression. Inversely, the crude, rough culture implicit in the excessive altruism of primitive man develops a lack of sensitivity which favors renunciation. In short, just as society largely forms the individual, it forms him to the same extent in its own image. Society, therefore, cannot lack the material for its needs, for it has, so to speak, kneaded it with its own hands.

The role of individual factors in the origin of suicide can now be more precisely put. If, in a given moral environment, for example, in the same religious faith or in the same body of troops or in the same occupation, certain individuals are affected and certain others not, this is undoubtedly, in great part, because the formers' mental constitution, as elaborated by nature and events, offers less resistance to the suicidogenetic current. But though these conditions may share in determining the particular persons in whom this current becomes embodied, neither the special qualities nor the intensity of the current depend on these conditions. A given number of suicides is not found annually in a social group just because it contains a given number of neuropathic persons. Neuropathic conditions only cause the suicides to succumb with greater readiness to the current. Whence comes the great difference between the clinicians's point of view and sociologist's. The former confronts exclusively particular cases, isolated from one another. He establishes, very often, that the victim was either nervous or an alcoholic, and explains the act by one or the other of these psychopathic states. In a sense he is right; for if this person rather than his neighbours committed suicide, it is frequently for this reason. But in a general sense this motive does not cause people to kill themselves, *nor, especially, cause a definite number to kill themselves in each society in a definite period of time.* The productive cause of the phenomenon naturally escapes the observer of individuals only; for it lies outside individuals. To discover it, one must raise this point of view above individual suicides and perceive what gives them unity. It will be objected that if enough neurasthenics did not exist, social causes would not produce all their effects. But no society exists in which the various forms of nervous degeneration do not provide suicide with more than the necessary number of candidates. Only certain ones are called, if this manner of speech is permitted. These are the ones who through circumstances have been nearer the pessimistic currents and who consequently have felt their influence more completely.

But a final question remains. Since each year has an equal number of suicides, the current does not strike simultaneously all those within its reach. The persons it will attack next year already exist; already, also, most of them are enmeshed in the collective life and therefore come under its influence. Why are they provisionally spared? It may indeed be understood why a year is needed to produce the current's full action; for since the conditions of social activity are not the same according to season, the current too changes in both intensity and direction at different times of the year. Only after the annual cycle is complete have all the combinations of circumstances occurred, in terms of which it tends to vary. But since, by hypothesis, the next year only repeats the last and causes the same combinations, why was not the first enough? Why, to use the familiar expression, does society pay its bill only in installments?

What we think explains this delay is the way time affects the suicidal tendency. It is an auxiliary but important factor in it. Indeed, we know that the tendency grows incessantly from youth to maturity, and that it is often ten times as great at the close of life as at its beginning. The collective force impelling men to kill themselves therefore only gradually penetrates them. All things being equal, they become more accessible to it as they become older, probably because repeated experiences are needed to reveal the complete emptiness of an egoistic life or the total vanity of limitless ambition. Thus, victims of suicide complete their destiny only in successive layers of generations.

Emile Durkheim was a pioneer of sociology. He published *Suicide—a study in sociology* in France in 1899 (see Durkheim, 1952). The purpose of the work was to develop the sociological method and he chose suicide as a vehicle for this because:

> "few (subjects) are more accurately defined and because it seems to us particularly timely. . ."
> His basic thesis was that
> "suicide. . .is precisely one of the forms through which the collective affliction from which we suffer is transmitted; thus it will aid us to understand this".

In essence he proposed that suicide is an affliction of society manifest in individuals and might therefore be amenable to social, rather than individual, intervention. If he was correct then in a utopian society there would be no suicide. By implication he judged suicide to be undesirable within a society, a view that is common today and owes much to the morality of western society.

In view of Durkheim's basic thesis, it is perhaps surprising that he discussed the relation between suicide and psychopathic states at such great length, for he stated that insanity is a characteristic of the individual rather than one of the society. In fact what he did in this chapter was to attempt to dismiss the hypothesis that on a social level there is a direct relationship between the two phenomena. His conclusion was that "no psychopathic state bears a regular and indisputable relation to suicide" with the caveat that "under similar circumstances the degenerate is more apt to commit suicide than a well man; but he does not necessarily do so because of his condition. This potentiality of his becomes effective only through the action of other factors which we must discover" and is used as supportive evidence for his original proposition. Although the work as a whole represents a milestone in the development of the sociological method this chapter is one the weakest parts as Durkheim tended to be uncritical about much of the data and used proxies that cannot be supported.

The first part of the chapter is concerned with the hypothetical framework within which the available data would be analysed. The statement that 'if a manifestation of insanity were reasonably to be supposed in every voluntary death our problem would be solved; suicide would be a purely individual affliction' is straightforward and reasonable. He argued that it could not be supported either on the grounds that suicide is a manifestation of insanity (a species of insanity) or on the basis that all suicides suffer from a recognisable form of insanity. In effect he proposed that not all individuals who kill themselves are insane.

In this section Durkheim drew the reader's attention to a fundamental problem inherent in the investigation of suicide: he noted that 'alienists' stated that most suicides known to them show all the indications of alienation but pointed out that no general conclusion could be drawn from those not observed. The fact that the only suicides known to the 'alienists' are alienated said less about the aetiology of suicide than it did about the selection of patients by the 'alienists'. Despite the fact that Durkheim stated this with such clarity, it has not stopped research workers of successive generations making the mistake with alarming regularity. The problem with suicide is that the victim is dead; it is impossible to assess the dead using the same methodology as that adopted for the living. This methodological problem cannot be overcome by assuming that had it been possible to conduct an interview before death, the diagnosis would have been the same as in persons who had achieved their own death after a diagnosis had been made.

Durkheim presented a classification of suicides amongst the insane; it added little to his argument but gave some insight into the way in which insanity was regarded in the 19th century. The four main categories he defined were:

1. Maniacal suicide: the patient was characterized by having what would now be described as psychotic hallucinations.
2. Melancholy suicide, the depressed.
3. Obsessive suicide.
4. Impulsive suicide.

The notion of impulsive suicide had been proposed as early as 1863 by William Farr, an English epidemiologist who, for many years wrote the commentary on the country's vital statistics. In one of his letters to the Registrar General he postulated:

In certain states the mind appears to be fascinated by the presence of a fatal instrument, such, for example, as prussic acid, a pistol, a rope or a razor; and the withdrawal of the means of death suffices to save the life.

The wording in Durkheim's monograph is similar:

> The sight of a knife, a walk by the edge of a precipice, etc. engender the suicidal idea instantaneously and its execution follows so swiftly that patients often have no idea of what has taken place.

It is not clear why Durkheim includes this type of suicide within the classification of insane suicides, having already dismissed the notion that suicide itself may be a form of insanity. The next step in the argument is much the most difficult to accept. Durkheim stated that 'insane suicides' exist, but that not all suicides are insane and continued:

> '... if a deep affection of the nervous system is enough to create suicide a lesser affection ought to exercise the same influence to a lesser degree. Neurasthenia is a sort of lesser insanity; it must therefore have the same effects in part.'

It is likely that the term 'insanity' is the equivalent of today's 'psychotic illnesses' and that 'neurasthenia' is the equivalent of neurosis. Durkheim's view of mental illness displays a lack of contact with contemporary developments in psychology. It is true that much of his work was completed before Freud and his school published their major works on psychopathology and before the development of a comprehensible taxonomy of mental illness, but the notion that there was a distinction between the two types of mental illness was being discussed and would have been known to many practising psychologists and medical men of the time. The unsubstantiated belief that insanity and neurasthenia formed part of a continuum led Durkheim to use the incidence and prevalence of insanity as a proxy for the incidence and prevalence of neurasthenia and the argument from here onwards becomes weak.

The index of insanity Durkheim used was the numbers of people certified as resident insane in institutions. It is unlikely that all the individuals in a society who complied with the contemporary definition of insane would be so certified; it is however likely that all people certified as insane would be in licensed institutions. Moreover, it is unlikely that similar proportions of the insane would be so certified throughout the countries and societies that Durkheim studied indirectly. Thus the rates of insanity are not valid measures. The same problem exists today. There is no national index of mental illness and the only way to establish the prevalence rate of mental illness is to conduct population-based surveys; it is even more difficult to quantify the incidence rate of mental illness. Both incidence rates and prevalence rates remain difficult to interpret because of the problems of imposing a standard taxonomy on large numbers of clinicians each with their own views of illness. This highlights the problem of population studies of mental illness. Unlike many physical illnesses, treatment is not inevitable and thus there is no single institution through which all the mentally ill will pass; many people who suffer from mental illness may recover without formal intervention.

It is interesting to consider why Durkheim did not use mental illness as the subject of his study as it is likely that variations in rates may have revealed as much about the societies as did his investigation of suicide.

The second section of this chapter is concerned with the presentation and analysis of the data. It is likely that the variations in the numbers of insane in different communities reflected the differing legislative systems in those countries to a much greater extent than it gave a true reflection of the numbers of insane or psychotic individuals. They are presented uncritically and without full references to their sources.

·Analysis of the data suffers from the inadequacies of the statistical methodology that was available in the 19th century. Durkheim was able to establish that there was an association between suicide rates in populations and certain other characteristics such as religion, climate, race and wealth. However, it was only possible to use very crude correlation techniques.

THE SOCIAL ELEMENT OF SUICIDE

Psychiatrists, and most other people, view suicide as an intensely personal act by an individual. It might be precipitated by a crisis, by the result of mental illness or represent a statement of hopelessness. For Durkheim suicide rates are measures of the 'health' of the social body or community. Throughout his monograph he was concerned to demonstrate that the tendency to suicide in populations was primarily influenced by their economic and social characteristics, their geography, climatic conditions and other factors not directly under the control of the individuals who kill themselves.

The chapter entitled *Suicide and Psychopathic States* is devoted to an analysis of psychopathic states. It attempted, and in the view of this commentator, failed, to demonstrate that suicide is not substantially influenced by what would now be called mental illness. The chapter entitled *Social Elements of Suicide* seeks to prove that the suicide rates are determined by social conditions. Again the data cannot support the contention. A basic flaw in the whole work is that Durkheim appeared to be looking for data to support his predetermined conclusions. This criticism has often been made of the work; see, for example, Pope (1976). However, it should be remembered that '*Suicide*' was written as an example of the methodology of sociology and used suicide as its vehicle rather than as a research project on the subject itself.

Durkheim began the chapter by drawing the reader's attention to the fact that he has been unable to demonstrate a 'regular' relationship between 'neurasthenia' and suicide nor between 'race or climate' and suicide. He followed with the bold statement:

'Wholly different are the results we obtained when we forgot the individual and sought the causes of the suicidal aptitude of each society in the nature of the societies themselves. . . Here we are face to face with real laws'.

His contention that there was no regular relationship between neurasthenia and suicide was based on observations of certification rates rather than on a careful examination of the individuals themselves. His argument that the social conditions are the underlying determinant of the tendency to suicide was supported by a simple analysis of official statistics. He connected the act of the individual to the nature of society in the sentence:

'The private experiences usually thought to be the proximate causes of suicide have only the influence borrowed from the victim's moral predisposition, itself an echo of the moral state of society'.

This hypothesis is not proven in the monograph.

The work is of historical rather than scientific interest. Its importance lies in its pioneering contribution to the development of sociology as a science. Durkheim was limited by inadequate and inconsistent data and by the lack of sophisticated mathematical and statistical methods for the analysis of data.

The limitations of much contemporary data are at least as serious as they were in Durkheim's time. Although it is possible to debate the definition of suicide and even arrive at one that is agreeable to all who research the subject, the data available for population studies are the 'certified suicides' within a population. Whether a death is, or is not, certified as suicide is determined by the definitions imposed upon certifying officers (Coroners, Medical Examiners, the police) and the ways in which these certifying officers interpret these definitions. Even today international comparative studies are fraught with difficulties (see Boor, 1980; Sainsbury et al., 1980; Walsh et al., 1984). It is unlikely that modern data between states are any more consistent or complete than they were in the 19th century. The difference is that the modern researcher is more critical of the data than was Durkheim. The independent variables considered by Durkheim such as religion, economic and political indicators, family structure, certification rates, etc., differ in their consistency and accuracy now as they did in the 19th century. However, we are probably more aware of their limitations and thus more circumspect about the interpretation of apparent correlations or lack of correlation than was Durkheim!

Notwithstanding the criticisms of the data, the greatest problem with Durkheim's work is the simplicity of the analytic method he was able to use. On the whole, he sought correlations between pairs of variables; for example, suicide and season of year; suicide and religious affiliation; suicide and marriage; rather than using a multivariable technique. He did this because multivariable analysis was not available to him. Contemporary work in this field involves examining the associations between suicide and a number of variables at the same time in order to establish whether or not the incidence of suicide is influenced by a combination of factors. If it can be established that a combination of factors are involved, then the researcher will attempt to identify the relative importance of each factor. Sainsbury (1955), Kreitman and Platt (1984), Beck *et al.* (1974), Brown and Sharan (1972), and Brown (1979), among others, have applied multivariate technique to research the causes of suicide. From this type of work, it becomes apparent that suicide rates are determined directly or indirectly by a number of factors and that the relative importance of the factors vary in time and place. These observations lead the researcher to be more circumspect in the interpretation of their results so that contemporary monographs or papers on the social influences on suicide lack the dogmatism of Durkheim's work. On close examination, Durkheim's constructs on suicide are a series of poorly substantiated hypotheses that are of historical and philosophical interest rather than statements of scientific truth.

R. D. T. Farmer

REFERENCES

Barraclough, B. M. (1972). *Are Scottish and English Suicide rates really different?* *Br. J. Psy.,* **120**, 267–274.
Beck, A. T., Schuyler, D. and Heran, I. (1974). *Prediction of Suicide,* A. T. Beck (Ed.), Charles Press, Bowie, Maryland, 45–56.
Boor, M. (1980). *Relationships between unemployment rates and suicide rates in eight countries* 1962–1976, Psychol. Rep., **47**, 1905–1911.
Brown, J. H. (1979). *Suicide in Britain—more attempts, fewer deaths—lessons for public policy, Arch. Gen. Psych.,* **36**, 1119–1124.
Brown, T. and Sheran, T. (1972). Suicide prediction: A review, Suicide Life Threat Behaviour, **2**, 67–98.
Durkheim, E. (1952). *Suicide A Study in Sociology,* Routledge and Kegan Paul, London.
Kreitman, N. and Platt, S. (1984). Suicide, unemployment and domestic gas detoxification in Britain. *J. Epid. Comm. Health,* **38**, 1–6.
Pope, W. (1976). *Durkheim's Suicide. A Classic Analyzed,* University of Chicago Press, Chicago, London.
Sainsbury, P. (1955). *Suicide in London: An Ecological Study,* Chapman Hall, London.
Sainsbury, P., Jenkins, J. and Levey, A. (1980). *The Social Correlates of Suicide in Europe. The Suicide Syndrome,* R. Farmer and O. Hirsch (Eds), Croom Helm, London, 38–53.
Walsh, D., Mosbech, J., Adelstein, A. and Spooner, J. (1984). *Suicide and self-poisoning in three countries—a study from Ireland, England and Wales and Denmark. Int. J. Epid.,* **13**(4), 472–474.

8

The Causation and Prevention of Insanity

Henry Maudsley MD, 1899

ETIOLOGICAL

The causes of mental derangement, as they are usually described in books, are so vague and general, so little serviceable for use, that the knowledge of them yields us very little help when we are brought face to face with a concrete case and endeavour to gain a clear conception of its causation. The impossibility of getting precise information arises in most instances from the insuperable difficulties under which we are of knowing a person's character and history fully, intimately, and exactly. We cannot go through the complex and often tangled web of his whole life, following the manifold changes and chances of it, and, seizing the single threads out of which its texture has been woven, unravel the pattern of it. No man knoweth his own character, which is ever under his inspection: how then can he know that of his neighbour, when he has only brief and passing glimpses into it?

Great mistakes are oftentimes made in fixing upon the supposed causes of the disease in particular cases; some single prominent event, which was perhaps one in a train of events, being selected as fitted by itself to explain the catastrophe. The truth is that in the great majority of cases there has been a concurrence of steadily operating conditions within and without, not a single effective cause. All the conditions, whether they are called passive or active, which conspire to the production of an effect are alike causes, alike agents; all the conditions, therefore, which co-operate in a given case in the production of disease, whether they lie in the individual or in his surroundings, must be regarded as alike causes. When we are told that a man has become mentally deranged from sorrow, need, sickness, or any other adversity, we have not learned much if we are content to stay there: how is it that another man who undergoes an exactly similar adversity does not go mad? The entire causes could not have been the same where the effects were so different. What we want to have laid bare is the conspiracy of conditions, in the individual and outside him, by which a mental pressure, inoperative in the one case, has weighed so disastrously in the other; and that is information which a complete and exact biography of him, such as never yet has been written of any person, not neglecting the consideration of his hereditary antecedents, could alone give us. Were all the circumstances, internal and external, scanned closely and weighed accurately it would be seen that there is no accident in madness; the disease, whatever form it had, and however many the concurrent conditions or successive links of its causation, would be traced as the inevitable consequence of its antecedents, just as the explosion of a train of gunpowder may be traced to its causes, whether the train of events of which it is the issue be long or short. The germs of insanity are most often latent in the foundations of the character, and the final outbreak is the explosion of a long train of antecedent preparations.

As the causation of insanity may thus reach back through a lifetime, and even have its root far back in foregoing generations, it is easy to perceive how little is taught by specifying a single moral cause, such as grief, vanity, ambition, which may after all be, and often is, a prominent early symptom of the desease which, striking the attention of observers, gets credit for having caused it. I am apt to think that we may learn more of its real causation by the study of a tragedy like *Lear* than from all that has yet been written thereupon in the guise of science. A great artist like Shakespeare, penetrating with subtle insight the character of the individual and discerning the relations between him and his circumstances, apprehending the order which there is amidst so much seeming disorder, and disclosing the necessary mode of evolution of the events of life, embodies in the work of his creative art more real information than can be obtained from the vague and general statements which science in its defective state is compelled to put up with.

Life in all its forms, physical and mental, morbid and healthy, is a relation; its phenomena result from the reciprocal action of an individual organism and of external forces: health is the consequence and the evidence of a successful adaptation to the conditions of existence, and imports the preservation, the well-being, and the development of the organism, while disease marks a failure in organic adaptation to external conditions and leads to disorder, decay, and death. It is obvious that the harmonious relation between the organism and its environment which is the condition of health may be disturbed either by a cause in the organism or by a cause in the environment, or by a cause, or rather a concurrence of causes, arising partly from the one and partly from the other. When it is said then that a person's mind has broken down in consequence of adverse conditions of life, social or physical, there is presupposed tacitly some infirmity of nerve element, inherited or acquired, which has co-operated; were the nervous system in a state of perfect soundness, and in possession of that reserve power which it then has to adapt itself within certain limits to varying external conditions, it is not likely that unfavourable circumstances would be sufficient so far to disturb the relation as to initiate mental disease. But when unfavourable action from without conspires with an infirmity of nature within, then the conditions of disorder are established, and the discord, which a madman is, is produced.

It has been the custom to treat of the causes of insanity as physical and moral, but it is not practicable to make the discrimination in many cases. Where the existence of a hereditary taint, for example, is the physical cause of some moral defect or peculiarity of character which issues at last in insanity, one writer, looking to the mental aspect, will describe the cause as moral, while another, looking to the bad inheritance, describes it as physical. Certainly, where there is visible defective development of brain in consequence of a bad inheritance, as in idiocy sometimes, all persons are agreed as to the physical nature of the defect; but when the cerebral defect is not gross and patent, making itself known only by some vice of disposition, most people will consider it to be of a moral nature. The truth is, on the one hand, that in the great majority of cases in which a so-called moral cause operates there is something in the physical constitution which co-operates essentially, and, on the other hand, that every moral cause operates in the last resort through the physical changes which it produces in the nerve-centres.

With these preliminary remarks I go on to consider those general conditions which are thought to predispose in some way or other to insanity. In the outset I may make two general assertions: that a man is what he is at any period of life, first, by virtue of the

141

original qualities which he has received from his ancestors, and, secondly, by virtue of the modifications which have been effected in his original nature by the influence of education and of the conditions of life. But what a complex composition of causes and conditions do these simple statements import! Hereditary predisposition is a general term which connotes, but certainly does not yet denote, various intimate conditions of which we know nothing definite; we are constrained, therefore, to deal in general disquisitions concerning it instead of describing exactly its varieties and setting forth precisely the laws of its action.

Heredity

—Whether it be true or not, as is sometimes said, that no two leaves nor two blades of grass are exactly alike, there can be little doubt that no two persons in the world are now or ever have been exactly alike. However close the resemblance between them, each one has some characteristic marking his individuality which distinguishes him from everybody else, and which affects the course of his destiny. By the circumstances of life the development of this intrinsic quality may be checked in one direction or fostered in another direction, but it can never be got rid of; it is always there, a leaven leavening the whole bump.

Whence comes this individuality of nature? Without doubt it comes from the same source as the individuality of bodily conformation, of gait, of features—that is to say, from ancestors. There is a destiny made for each one by his inheritance; he is the necessary organic consequent of certain organic antecedents; and it is impossible he should escape the tyranny of his organization. The dread, inexorable destiny which plays so grand and terrible a part in Grecian tragedy, and which Grecian heroes are represented as struggling manfully against, knowing all the while that their struggles were foredoomed to be futile, embodied an instinctive perception of the law by which the sins of the father are visited upon the children unto the third and fourth generations. Deep in his inmost heart everybody has an instinctive feeling that he has been predestined from all eternity to be what he is, and could not, antecedent conditions having been what they were, have been different. In village communities, where the people remain station-ary, and where the characters of fathers and grandfathers are remembered or are handed down by tradition, peculiarities of character in an individual are often attributed to some hereditary bias, and so accounted for: he got it from his fore-elders, it is said, and the aberration has allowance made for it.

In modern days we hardly take due account of this great truth which ancient sages recognised, and which the experience of all ages has confirmed, but it is vastly important to us, if we would do well for our race, to acknowledge and confess it: we are determining in our generation much of what shall be predetermined in the constitution of the generation that will come after us, and it depends greatly upon us whether it shall be well or ill with it. Certainly no one has power to change materially the fundamental tendencies of his own nature; the decrees of destiny have gone forth, and he cannot withstand nor reverse them; but if he contends manfully against bad impulses, as the hero of Greek tragedy who, in the grasp of fatality and foredoomed to failure, abated no effort to win an impossible victory, he will by degrees modify his character in part, and at any rate he will do that which, being embodied as an aptitude in the constitution of his posterity, may happily be a stay and present help to them in time of trouble and temptation. His efforts to overcome what he cannot overcome successfully may haply endow their natures with strength to be victorious in a similar struggle, his pains being their gain, his sowing their harvest.

I might say, perhaps, that every human being has four natures—his animal nature, his human nature, his family nature, and his individual nature. Beneath the individual characteristics lies the family nature, so that it will happen that in two brothers whose every feature differs we perceive intuitively the family identity—a fundamental identity in diversity, and, on the other hand, in two strangers who are very like in features we perceive intuitively a fundamental difference, albeit we cannot describe it in words. Beneath the family nature is the more general human nature, and beneath that again the still deeper lying and more general animal nature, which, long way as man is from his nearest of animal kin, has by no means been worked out of him. Here we have to do only, but enough to do, with the inheritance of the family.

Many familiar examples go to prove that a person inherits not only the general characters of the family, but peculiarities of manner and of disposition: tricks of thought, like tricks of manner, moods of feeling like humours of body, are inborn and come out

143

usually at one period of another of this life. Not only are the ways and looks of immediate ancestors thus reproduced sometimes, but those of ancestors who are remote and not perhaps in the direct line of descent; it would seem in fact that every parent has latent in him the abstract potentialities of his ancestors, for I know not how many generations back along the line of descent, and that these may undergo development again in his posterity if they chance to meet with suitable stimuli. To understand what these latent potentialities are, he would do well to study their developments in father, brothers, sisters, uncles, children—in all branches of the family tree: explicit in them he shall read what is implicit in himself. And here I may fitly take notice that inherited qualities shall appear only at certain epochs of life, the ancestral nervous substrata being then stirred to function for the first time. At puberty, for example, a bodily and mental revolution takes place, new mental substrata are aroused to function, and ancestral characters show themselves which were not noticed before, and probably never would have been noticed had the person been made a eunuch; during pregnancy there may be distinct manifestations of her mother's character in a daughter which no one had observed before; and at the change of life, when a woman's special functions are over, and she tends towards a masculine character of body and mind, there may be evinced peculiarities which call to mind a male ancestor. It is easy to understand that particular experiences in life may, like these changes in the bodily evolution, be fitted to awaken to function latent or quiescent ancestral nervous substrata, and that in this way the accident of an accident in life may chance to bring out an ancestral character which otherwise, like a seed not brought to bear, would have remained dormant.

Very little observation, however, is needed to show that the reproductions of the qualities of ancestors is but one side of the action of heredity—that it does not copy merely, but also invents; so that an individual often exhibits marked differences from any known ancestor. Its operation includes a law of variation as well as the reproduction of the like. It is true it might be said that the variations which an individual presents are not what they seem, but repetitions of qualities of remote ancestors who have been forgotten, but it is an assertion which is opposed to what we know of the correlations between variety of character and increasing complexity of social conditions, and to the evident fact that men in the long run advance by evolutionary variations upon what they have inherited from their forefathers, or go back upon it by retrograde morbid varieties. The existence of different moral dispositions and the intellectual capacities in twins and in double monsters is sufficient proof that hereditary action is not of the nature of a mere mechanical copy; it is rather of the nature of a complex chemical combination, whereby compounds not resembling in properties their constituents are oftentimes produced. There is not an organ of the parent's body, we have reason to think, not a tissue of which an organ is formed, not an element probably of a tissue, which has not its idiosyncrasy represented in the minute germ in some latent and mysterious way, and which may not therefore come out in its full traits of character in the developed offspring. Moreover, if it is neither developed after its own kind nor utilised in combinations, it may lie completely dormant in that generation and come out in the offspring's offspring, or even in a later generation; for we know not in the least how long it may remain latent before it is extinct.

This skipping of one generation and reappearance in a succeeding one has been called Atavism, and has excited surprise when it has been observed in morbid heredity: it is so striking sometimes in insanity that Ludovieus Mercatus, a Spanish physician, who wrote a book on hereditary diseases, was of opinion that the insanity appeared in every other, or every third, individual in lineal descent. But it is not so extraordinary as it seems; for we have a familiar physiological instance of the same thing when a daughter of a house transmits to her son any of the special masculine qualities of her family, which of necessity cannot be developed in her body, or when a son of the house transmits to his daughter any of the special feminine qualities of his family. In these cases the special sexual qualities must have been latent in the intermediate generation. Other qualities, healthy and morbid, that are not bound to sex may in like manner be latent in a generation, if they meet not in the circumstances of the individual's life with the conditions fitted to stimulate them into active display.

In the pathological action of the law of variation or invention of which I have spoken we have an explanation of the *de novo* production of a predisposition to insanity, which must manifestly have taken place once, and which takes place now from time to time. Were all madness swept from the face of the earth tomorrow, past all doubt men would breed it afresh before tomorrow's tomorrow. Two subjects concerning which information may be set down as wanting, and which urgently need exact investigation at the present time, are (a) The different antecedent conditions of the generation of a predisposition to insanity; and (b) The different signs, mental and bodily, by which such a predisposition betrays itself. Of the latter I shall treat in due course; respecting the first, when it comes to be studied seriously, I may note that besides the law of variation which is manifested in the results of the combinations of germ-elements, we shall have to take account—secondly, of the unquestionable influence of the particular mental and bodily state of one or both parents before and at the time of propagation; thirdly, of the important influence upon the child's constitution which is exerted for good or ill by the mental and bodily state of the mother during gestation; and, fourthly, of the influences brought to bear upon the child during the first years of growth and development of its susceptible nervous system. The neutralization of a tendency to insanity, through which it comes to pass that it sometimes becomes extinct, is due, first, to the favourable influence of a happy marriage, that is to say, one which is antagonistic, not consentient, to its development, and secondly, to the beneficial effect of conditions of life suited to check its development. There is yet a third weighty cause to be taken into account, namely, the natural tendency of the organism to revert to the sound type. Were it not for these hygienic agencies all the world must become mad sooner or later. But as a matter of fact, in the unceasing flow of the stream of life ill tendencies are being constantly formed and unformed, as chemical compounds are formed and unformed.

Those who have had much to do with the treatment of insane persons have not failed to note the marked mental peculiarities of their near relations in many instances, and to lament that they oftentimes show themselves more distrustful, more difficult to reason with, more impracticable, than the member of the family who is confessedly insane. In the first place, they have such an intimate radical sympathy of nature with those tendencies of character which have culminated in insanity in him, that they cannot sincerely see alienation which is patent to all the rest of the world: they will minimise bit by bit, finding reason or excuse for each strange act, feeling, or idea, until they have accounted for all the strangeness of it, and it only remains for the patient listener to confess that the palpable madness was after all very natural in him, and that their relative is not mad like other mad persons, or at any rate that what would be great madness in all the rest of the world is not madness in him. In the second place, as a consequence of their essential likeness and sympathy of nature, they will question, dispute, carp at every restraint which those under whose care he is may find it necessary to place upon him; notwithstanding that they may have been obliged to send him from home and to put him under control because he was an intolerable trouble or an actual menace and a danger, they will talk as if they would exact a mode of treatment which entirely ignored his insanity, and will end probably, if he does not get better, in the firm belief that his disease has been caused and kept in action by the improper treatment to which he has been subjected. The worst of them would risk the chance of his attendant being killed by a lunatic rather than suffer what they call his sensitive disposition to be hurt by the necessary means of control, and if such a catastrophe happened their genuine sympathies would be with him, not with the victim of his violence. Their intensely suspicious and distrustful natures, their tortuous habits of thought, their wiles and insincerities, their entire absorption in a narrow selfishness, mark a disposition which is incapable of coming into wholesome relations with mankind; it is of a character to lead to guile in social intercourse, to petty fraud in business, and, when the conditions of life are hard and tempt to evil-doing, even to crime, and which in any case is pretty sure to breed insanity or crime in the next generation. Moral feeling is based upon sympathy; to have it one must have imagination enough to realise the relations of others and to enter ideally into their feelings; whereas these persons have not the least capacity of going in feeling beyond the range of their family, unless it be to embrace a favourite cat or dog, and are governed by an intense and narrow family selfishness. They are capable sometimes of an extraordinary self-sacrifice for one another within that small circle, but they are completely shut up within it. Being in such slight and unstable relations with their kind, what wonder that a son or daughter who has descended from such an unsound stock and who most likely sucked in suspicion and egoism with the mother's milk, should get so far astray as to be loosened from wholesome bonds of social relation and to become insane or criminal!

Good moral feeling is to be looked upon as an essential part of a sound and rightly developed character in the present state of human evolution in civilised lands; its acquisition is the condition of development in the progress of *humanization*. Whosoever is destitute of it is to that extent a defective being; he marks the beginning of race-degeneracy; and if propitious influences do not chance to check or to neutralize the morbid tendency, his children will exhibit a further degree of degeneracy and be actual morbid varieties. Whether the particular outcome of the morbid strain shall be vice, or madness, or crime, will depend much on the circumstances of life, but there is no doubt in my mind that one way in which insanity is generated *de novo* is though the deterioration of nature which is shown in the absence of moral sense. It was the last acquisition in the progress of *humanization*, and its decay is the first sign of the commencement of human degeneracy. And as absence of moral sense in the generation may be followed by insanity in the next, so I have observed that, conversely, insanity in one generation sometimes leaves the evil legacy of a defective moral sense to the next. Any course of life then which persistently ignores the altruistic relations of an individual as a social unit, which is in truth a systematic negation of the moral law of human progress, deteriorates his higher nature, and so initiates a degeneracy which may issue in actual mental derangement in his posterity.

Morbid Heredity

—This is a subject respecting which it is not possible to get exact and trustworthy information. So strong is the feeling of disgrace attaching to the occurrence of insanity in a family, and so eager the desire to hide it, that persons who are not usually given to saying what is not true will disclaim or deny ostentatiously the existence of any hereditary taint, when it is known certainly to exist or is betrayed plainly by the features, manner, and thoughts of those who are denying it. Not even its prevalence in royal families has sufficed to make madness a fashionable disease. The main value of the many doubtful statistics which have been collected by authors in order to decide how large a part hereditary taint plays in the production of insanity is to prove that with the increase of opportunities of obtaining exact information the greater is the proportion of cases in which its influence is detected; the more careful and exact the researches the fuller is the stream of hereditary tendency which they disclose, Esquirol noted it in 150 our of 264 cases of his private patients; Burrows clearly ascertained that it existed in six-sevenths of the whole of his patients; on the other hand, there have been some authors who have brought the proportion down as low as one-tenth. Some years ago I made a tolerably precise examination of the family histories of fifty insane persons taken without any selection; there was a strongly marked predisposition in fourteen cases—that is in 1 in 3.57, and in ten more cases there was sufficient evidence of family degeneration to warrant more than a suspicion of inherited fault of organization. In about half the cases then was there reason to suspect morbid predisposition. I have recently inquired into the histories of fifty more cases, all ladies, the opportunities being such as could only occur in private medical practice, and with these results: that in twenty cases there was the distinct history of hereditary predisposition; in thirteen cases there was such evidence of it in the features of the malady as to beget the strongest suspicion of it; in seventeen cases there was no evidence whatever of it. In the second fifty cases my opportunities of getting information were more favourable in consequence of more frequent personal inter-course with the friends, and it sometimes happened that the information sought for was obtained quite accidentally after heredity had been denied. What is the exact proportion of cases in which some degree or kind of hereditary predisposition exists must needs be an unprofitable discussion in view of the difficulty and complexity of the inquiry; suffice it to say broadly that the most careful researches agree to fit it as certainly not lower than one-fourth, probably as high as one-half, possibly as high even as three-fourths.

Two weighty considerations have to be taken into account in relation to this question: first, that the native infirmity or taint may be small or great, showing itself in different degrees of intensity, so as on the one hand to take effect only when conspiring with more or less powerful exciting causes, or on the other hand to give rise to insanity even amidst the most favourable external circumstances; and, secondly, that not mental derangement only in the parents, but other forms of nervous disease in them, such as epilepsy, paroxysmal neuralgia, strong hysteria, dipsomania, spasmodic asthma, hypochondriasis, and that outcome of a sensitive and feeble nervous system, suicide, may predispose to mental derangement in the offspring, as, conversely, insanity in the parent may predispose to other forms of nervous disease in the offspring. We properly distinguish in our nomenclature the different nervous diseases which are met with in practice according to the broad outlines of their symptoms, but it frequently happens that they blend, combine, or replace one another in a way that confounds our distinctions, giving rise to hybrid varieties intermediate between those which are regarded as typical.

This mingling and transformation of neuroses, which is observed sometimes in the individual, is more plainly manifest when the history of the course of nervous disease is traced through generations; if instead of limiting attention to the individual we go on to scan and track the organic evolution and decay of a family—processes which are sometimes going on simultaneously in different members of it, one displaying the outcome of its morbid, another of its progressive tendencies—it is seen how close are the fundamental relations of certain nervous diseases and how artificial the distinctions between them sometimes appear. Epilepsy in the parent comes out perhaps as some form of insanity in the offspring, or insanity in the parent as epilepsy in the child. Estimating roughly the probable breeding results of a number of epileptic parents, one might say that they would be very likely to lose many children at an early age; that the chances were great that some children would be epileptic; and that there was almost as great a risk that some would become insane. Chorea or other convulsions in the child may be the consequence of great nervous excitability, natural or accidentally produced, in the mother. In families where there is a strong predisposition to insanity, one member shall sometimes suffer from one form of nervous disease, and another from another form: one perhaps has epilepsy, another is afflicted with a severe neuralgia or with hysteria, a third may commit suicide, a fourth becomes maniacal or melancholic, and it might even happen sometimes that a fifth evinced remarkable artistic talent. Neuralgic headaches or megrims, various spasmodic movements or *tics*, asthma and allied spasmodic troubles of breathing will oftentimes be discovered to own a neurotic inheritance or to found one. The neurotic diathesis is fundamental; its outcomes are various, and determined we know not how; but they may, I think, be either predominantly sensory, or motor, or trophic in character.

Were we only as exact as we could wish to be in our researches we ought then, in studying hereditary action and its issues, to mark the different roads. It is plain there may be (a) Heredity of the same form—that is, when a person suffers from the same kind of mental derangement as a parent had which he seldom does except in the cases of suicide and dipsomania; (b) Heredity of allied form, as when he suffers from another kind of mental derangement than that which his parent had—is maniacal, for example, when he or she was melancholic; and (c) Heredity with transformation of neurosis—when the ancestral malady was not mental derangement of any sort, but some other kind of nervous disease. Whatever the exact number of cases of mental disorder in which hereditary predisposition of some degree or kind, derived from the preceding or from a more remote generation, is positively ascertained, it may be asserted broadly that in the majority there has been a native instability or infirmity of nervous element in the individual whereby he has been unable to bear the too heavy burden of his life, and has broken down in mind. Complex and various as the constitutional idiosyncrasies of men notably are, it is obvious that statistics can never yield exact and conclusive information concerning the causation of insanity; here, as in so many other instances of their employment, their principal value is that they make known distinctly the existence of a certain *tendency*, so to speak, which, once we have fairly grasped it, furnishes a good starting-point for further and more rigorous researches: they indicate the direction which a more exact method of inquiry should take.

There is reason to think that an innate taint or infirmity of nerve-element may modify the manner in which other diseases commonly manifest themselves; for example, where it exists, gout flying about the body will occasion obscure nervous symptoms which puzzle the inexperienced practitioner, and it will sometimes issue in a downright attack of insanity, instead of showing itself by its ordinary inflammations. On the other hand, there is no doubt that a parental disease which does not affect specially the nervous system may notwithstanding be at the foundation of a delicate nervous constitution in the offspring: scrofula, phthisis, syphilis perhaps, gout and diabetes appear sometimes to play this part. On going through an idiot asylum the appearance of scrofula among its inmates is sufficiently striking; perhaps two-thirds, or even more, of all idiots are of the scrofulous constitution. Lugol, who wrote a treatise on scrofula, professes to have found insanity by no means uncommon amongst the parents of scrofulous and tuberculous persons, and in one chapter he treats of hereditary scrofula from paralytic, epileptic, and insane parents. In estimating the value of observations of this kind, however, we may easily be deceived unless we are careful to reflect that, independently of any special relation between the two diseases, the enfeebled nutrition of scrofula would be likely to light up any latent predisposition to insanity which there might be, and so might seem to have originated it when it was only a contributory factor, and, on the other hand, that insanity, and especially those forms of it in which nutrition was much affected, would foster the development of a predisposition to scrofula or phthisis.

Several writers on insanity have taken notice of a connection between it and phthisis which they have thought to be more than accidental. Schroeder van der Kolk was confident that a hereditary predisposition to phthisis might predispose to or develop into insanity, and, on the other hand, that insanity predisposed to phthisis. With phthisis, however, there commonly goes, as is well-known, a particularly eager, intense, impulsive, and sanguine temperament, which may breed a more insanely disposed temperament in the offspring, apart from any influence which the actual tubercular tendency may be supposed to have or to have not. I am the more apt to think this the explanation, because there is a third-rate artistic or poetic temperament, altogether wanting in sobriety, breadth, and repose, and manifesting itself in intense but narrow idealisms, of an extravagant or even grotesque character sometimes, or in caterwauling shrieks of emotional spasm, put forth as poetry, which closely resembles the phthisical temperament, and which is very likely to breed insanity. There is no question in my mind that insanity and phthisis are often met with as concomitant or sequent effects in the course of family decadence, whether they predispose to one another or not; they are two diseases through which a family stock that is undergoing degeneracy gradually becomes extinct, especially in those cases where the degeneracy is the outcome of breeding in and in until all variety and vigour have been bred out of the stock. When we are searching for the predisposing conditions or a morbid neurosis in a particular case, and fail to discover any history of antecedent insanity or epilepsy, we shall do well then to inquire whether phthisis is a family disease. It is alleged that as many as two-thirds of all idiots die of phthisis. According to Dr. Clouston's observations, made at the Morningside Asylum, tubercular deposit is twice as frequent in the bodies of those who die insane as it is in the bodies of those who die sane, and he professes to have found a distinctly greater frequency of hereditary predisposition to insanity among the tubercular than among the non-tubercular patients. There is not, I think, sufficient reason to suppose that the remarkable remission of the symptoms of insanity which undoubtedly takes place often during the exacerbation of phthisis in a patient who has the two diseases, with the active recurrence of the mental symptoms when the signs of phthisical activity abate, testifies to any special connection between them; for it appears to be no more than an instance of such abatement of mental symptoms as is observed when other acute disease befalls in an insane patient.

The late M. Morel of Rouen prosecuted some original and instructive researches into the formation of degenerate or morbid varieties of the human kind, showing the steps of the descent by which degeneracy increases through generations, and issues finally, if unchecked by counteracting influences, in the extinction of the family. When some of the unfavourable conditions of life which are believed to originate disease—such as the poisoned air of a marshy district, the unknown endemic causes of cretinism, the overcrowding and starvation of large cities, continued intemperance or excesses of any kind, frequent intermarriages in families—have engendered a morbid variety, it is the beginning of a calamity which may gather force through generations, until the degeneration has gone so far that the continuation of the species along that line is impossible. Insanity, of what form soever, whether mania, melancholia, moral insanity, dementia, may be looked upon then philosophically as a stage in the descent towards sterile idiocy; as might be proved experimentally by the intermarriage of insane persons for two or three generations, and as is proved undesignedly sometimes by the disastrous consequences of frequent intermarriages in foolish families. The history of one family which Morel investigated with great care may be quoted as an extreme example of the natural course of degeneration when it goes on unchecked through generations. Were it an invention only, it would be one of those inventions that teach excellent truth. It may be summed up thus:-

First Generation.—Immorality, depravity, alcoholic excesses, and great moral degradation in great-grandfather, who was killed in a tavern brawl.

Second Generation.—Hereditary drunkenness, maniacal attacks ending in general paralysis in the grandfather.

Third Generation.—Sobriety, but hypochondriacal tendencies,

153

delusions of persecution, and homicidal tendencies in the father.

Fourth Generation.—Defective intelligence. First attack of mania at sixteen years of age; stupidity and transition to complete idiocy. Probable extinction of the morbid line; for the generative functions were as little developed as those of a child of twelve years of age. He had two sisters, who were both defective physically and morally, and were classed as imbeciles. To make the proof of morbid heredity more striking, it may be added that the mother had an adulterous child while the father was confined in the asylum, and that this child did not exhibit any signs of degeneracy.

In this history of a family we have an instructive example of a retrograde movement of the human kind, ending in so wide a deviation from the normal type that sterility ensues; it is the opposite of that movement of progressive specialization and increasing complexity of relation with the external which mark advancing development. All the moral and intellectual acquisitions of culture which the race has been slowly putting on by organized inheritance of the accumulated experience of countless generations of men are rapidly put off in a few generations, until the lowest human and fundamental animal elements only are left in an abortive state: in place of sound and proper social elements which may take their part and discharge their function harmoniously in the special organism we have morbid elements fit only for excretion from it. The comparison of the social fabric with the bodily organism is well founded and instructive. As in bodily disease there is a retrograde metamorphosis of formative action whereby morbid elements are produced which cannot minister to healthy function, but will, if not got rid of, occasion disorder or death; so in the social fabric there is likewise retrograde metamorphosis whereby morbid varieties or degenerations of the human kind are produced, which, being antisocial, will, if not rendered innocuous by sequestration in it, or if not extruded violently from it, give rise to disorder incompatible with its stability. How exactly do the results of degeneracy accord with what was said concerning the aim of human progress and the fundamental meaning of insanity!

In the lowest forms of insanity and idiocy there are sometimes exhibited remarkable animal-like instincts and traits of character which may even go along with corresponding conformation of body: witness the stories told—I know not how truly—of idiot mothers who, after delivery, have gnawed through the umbilical cord; the idiot described by Pinel, who was much like a sheep in appearance, in habits, and in his cry; the idiot described by Dr. Mitchell, who presented a singular resemblance to a monkey in his features, in the conformation of his body and in his habits; the habit of rumination of food which has been observed in some insane persons and idiots and the savage fury and the bestialities exhibited by others:—all these testify to the brute brain within the man's, and may be looked upon as instances of partial reversion, proofs that the animal has not yet completely died out of him, faint echoes from a far distant past testifying to a kinship which he has almost outgrown. It may be thought a wild notion that man should even now display traces of his primeval kinship when countless ages have confessedly elapsed since he started on the track of his special development, but a little consideration will take from the strangeness of it. In the first place, long way as he is from the animals, he still passes in the course of his embryonic development through successive stages at which he resembles not a little the permanent conditions of certain classes of them; he may be said, in fact, to represent in succession a fish, a bird, a quadruped in his course before he becomes human; and these transitional phases are presumably to be interpreted as the abstract and brief chronicle of the successive throes or stages of evolution through which nature went before man was brought forth. Whether that be so or not, the metamorphoses are proofs at any rate that the foundations of his being are laid upon the same lines as those of the vertebrate animals, and that he has deep within him common qualities of nature which, when the higher qualities of his special nature are gone, will manifest themselves in animal-like traits of character. In the second place, let any one consider curiously the fundamental instincts of self-conservation and propagation, resolutely, laying bare their roots, taking note of their intimations in children long before their meaning is understood by them, and giving attention to their manifestations among all sorts and conditions of men, savage and civilised, he will not fail to perceive and confess how thoroughly animal is man at bottom. He will apprehend this the more clearly if he goes on to trace, as he may, the development of many of the highest qualities of human intelligence and feeling from their roots in these fundamental instincts. Our sympathies with other living things, our interests in their sufferings and doings, our success in understanding them and making ourselves understood by them, our power to train and use them for our services, would be impossible but for a common foundation of nature.

It has been a question whether a father or a mother was more likely to transmit an insane bias to the children. Esquirol found that it descended more often from the mother than from the father, and from the mother to the daughters more often than to the sons; and to this opinion Baillarger subscribes. From an elaborate report to the French Government by M. Béhic it would seem that it is most likely to pass from father to son and from mother to daughter; for out of 1,000 admissions of each sex into French asylums he found that 264 males and 266 females had suffered from hereditary predisposition; that of the 264 males 128 had inherited the disease from their fathers, 110 from their mothers, and 26 from both parents; and that of the 266 females, 100 had inherited from fathers, 130 from mothers, and 36 from both parents. It might be questioned whether the sex of the parent in itself has much directly to do with determining the line of descent to son or daughter; it is not perhaps that the male inherits preferentially from the male, and the female from the female, by virtue of sex, but that there is more insanity inherited from one or the other according as there are more male or female children among the offspring. If male children have preponderated in the family of the father who transmits the insanity to his children, and if he displays in marriage that superior potency in propagation by which his family tendency obtains and male children preponderate among this offspring, there will most likely be more cases of insanity descending from father to son, but if female children preponderate among his offspring, it is probable that there will be a stronger stream of descent from father to daughter. To get at real information we should have to go deeper and to discover the unknown causes which determine sex. It is hard to understand that a daughter who resembles an insane father in her whole temperament of body and mind more than a son does should be less likely than the son to inherit a morbid taint of character from him. Mr. Galton's first inquiries concerning hereditary genius led him to the conclusion that, contrary to common opinion, the female influence was inferior to the male in transmitting ability, but when he came to revise his data more closely, he saw reason to conclude that the influence of females is but little inferior to that of males in such transmission. It may be said with equal truth probably both of ability and insanity that while transmission to the same sex and transmission to the other sex are common enough, the relative frequency of their occurrence is yet uncertain.

Some writers subscribe to the plausible theory which has come down from antiquity, that madness, like other hereditary diseases, is most likely to be transmitted to the child which resembles most in features and disposition the insane parent, and that a person who has the misfortune to be so descended may therefore take comfort to himself if he is unlike that parent. However, the conclusion must not be made absolute; it does not follow that a child who resembles a parent in features shall have a similar disposition, since there is assuredly no constant relation between resemblance of features and of moral disposition; and of course it is not where the bodily features are alike, but where the mental disposition is of the same kind, that we should expct to observe such operation of the law of heredity. I have noticed too in some cases that a likeness to one parent or to his or her family type which comes out strongly at one period of life may wane gradually and be replaced by a greater likeness to the other parent or to his or her family type at a later period of life; the son who calls to mind his mother at twenty years old perhaps calls his father to mind at forty; and the daugher who was like her father at twenty puts on more of her mother's similitude at forty. It is plain then that a son or a daughter who had been unlike the insane parent might as time went on take up with the family resemblance a tendency to the parental disease. In any case there is no doubt that a child born after an outbreak of parental insanity is more likely to suffer from insanity than one that was born before the outbreak.

In considering the period of life at which a hereditary predisposition to insanity or any other such predisposition will show itself in actual disease, it should be borne in mind that certain organs or systems of organs are particularly active at certain ages, when they will naturally be more prone to fall into that disordered action to which they are intrinsically disposed. In like manner they may be less predisposed to one and more predisposed to another kind of morbid action when their decay and the decline of their functions begin in old age. In infancy, as Petit has pointed out, the lymphatic and the nervous systems predominate, for which reason scrofula and epilepsy are the hereditary diseases which then most show themselves. As years go on the muscular system undergoes great development, the sexual organs begin their function, and the whole vascular system is very active; wherefore inflammatory diseases are most apt to occur, pulmonary diseases to accompany or to follow the development of the chest, and nervous derangements of a hysterical or allied nature to attest the revolution which the development of the sexual organs produces in the entire economy. Before puberty nature's chief concern has been with physical development; but with the new desires and impulses which spring up after puberty, when the individual life begins to expand into social life, the mind undergoes a transformation, and the consequence is that hereditary insanity may declare itself; if not directly after puberty as the result of the natural physiological action becoming pathological, still in the years that immediately follow it, when the mind is most tried, being under a strain of energy in the novel adjustment to the conditions of active life, or when overworked in the subsequent years of eager competition during manhood. Many men break down too in these years from the enervating effects of sexual excesses upon an excitable and feeble nervous system, and of course women may break down under the trials of pregnancy and parturition. In later manhood rheumatism and gout attest, the former perhaps a muscular system which, having reached the prime of its energy, now discovers a strain of weakness or begins to decline; the latter, a decay of the powers of assimilation and nutrition which is not acknowledged prudently by giving them less to do. At a more advanced age still the abdomen seems to take up the tale: the energy of feeling and desire, which has its physiological source in the visceral organs and inspires vigorous self-assertion and practical will, abates gradually as they become dull and weary; the result being a tendency to sombre and floomy feelings which may pass into hypochondria and melancholia. Lastly in old age the tissues degenerate and the cerebral vessels give way in apoplexy; or the brain shrinks in decay and senile dementia ensures.

Consanguineous Marriages

—Whether these marriages breed degenerate offspring is a question which has been much disputed, some writers have impugned the general opinion that their effects are bad. It is a subject concerning which it is difficult to make exact inquiries, and impossible to arrive at trustworthy results; and Mr. G. Darwin, who undertook a series of painstaking inquiries lately, was obliged to abandon them without having reached conclusions which he could put forward with any confidence; so far as they went, however, his inquiries seemed to show that there was not good reason to declare that such marriages had any ill effect. Inasmuch as the wisdom of mankind is greater than the wisdom of any individual in any matter of common experience, where no special means of observation have been used, because the area thereof is so much greater, the numerous springs which feed it flowing into the common receptacle from all quarters and in all ages, I cannot help thinking that we ought justly to attach great weight to the prohibitions of intermarriages of near of kin which have been made by all sorts of peoples in all times and places: they are apparently an argument of the universal belief of their ill effects. Amongst the lower races the range of prohibition is much greater than in the civilised world, extending to the most distant relatives by blood. Certainly the popular conviction nowadays is that such intermarriages are more prone than not-akin marriages to breed idiocy, insanity, and deaf-mutism. Whosoever wishes to test the opinion with animals let him try experiments with a select breed of pigs, breeding in and in for several generations, and never crossing them with any strain from without, and he will find in full time, if his experiments coincide with mine accidentally made once, that his sows have no young or only two or three at a litter, and that they are very likely to savagely worry those which they have: that he must, if he would go on keeping pigs, cross or change his breed. For the last dozen years or so a record has been kept of the number of mares among racers which have proved barren or have prematurely slipped their foals; and it deserves notice, Mr. Darwin says, as showing how infertile these highly nurtured and closely interbred animals have become, that not far from one third of the mares fail to produce living foals.

Henry Maudsley had the singular good fortune to live in the golden age of Victorian affluence, an affluence characterized as much by material success as by a wealth of intellectual activity unmatched since the time of Isaac Newton. There was, paradoxically perhaps, an associated upsurge of social unrest and spiritual discontent: doubts were openly expressed by scholars as to the validity of Christian dogma, and scientists questioned the tenets of fundamentalism. The same iconoclasts showed that the earth had previously been inhabited by species of plants and animals long extinct, but whose remains, such as those of the huge dinosaurs, were to be found, even here in Britain.

Maudsley, probably the most outstanding philosopher-psychiatrist of the 19th century could not avoid being caught up in the momentous intellectual debates going on around him, even if he had wished to. Paramount amongst these philosophical preoccupations was that of Evolution, the theoretical explanation of man's origins, a theory which was patently at odds with the time-honoured story of his origins as told in *Genesis*.

Although the name of Charles Darwin is the one most closely associated with the theory of evolution, he was not, in fact, the first to have formulated comparable theories. Alfred Russel Wallace, for instance, had independently discovered the principal of natural selection before Darwin had published The Origin of Species in 1859; and both Wallace and Darwin had read and had been influenced by the work of Thomas Robert Malthus, an English political economist who specialized in population studies.

There was at least one important difference between the evolutionary theories of Wallace and Darwin: whereas the former postulated that the human mind could not have originated by evolutionary processes, the latter believed the very opposite. There can be no doubt from a study of Maudsley's own writings that he sided with Darwin, and in this respect he was supported by the evolutionary philosopher, Herbert Spencer, who in his *Principals of Psychology* put forward a thesis of the mind and its significance in evolutionary progress through differentiation.

Maudsley, himself primarily a psychiatrist, was nevertheless of sufficient standing among naturalists and philosophers alike for his views on evolution to be listened to with respect. Thus Darwin saw fit to quote Maudsley frequently in his writings, particularly in the *Descent of Man* and in the *Expression of the Emotions*. But Maudsley had the edge on his contemporaries just because he was a psychiatrist and had, therefore, a profound knowledge of mental illness. In this way he was capable of projecting evolutionary principles into the study of morbid as well as normal mental states and activities.

The influence of evolutionary principles is repeatedly exemplified in this chapter. For example, on p. 143* he writes, 'Beneath the family nature is the more general human nature, and beneath that again the still deeper lying and more general animal nature, which, long way as man is from his nearest of animal kin, has by no means worked out of him.' Again on p. 154 he describes how, 'In the lowest forms of insanity and idiocy there are sometimes exhibited remarkable animal-like instincts and traits or character which may even go along with corresponding conformation of body . . .; all these testify to the brute brain within the man's, and may be looked upon

---

* Page cross-references refer to this edition, not Maudsley's original.

as instances of partial reversion, proofs that the animal has not yet completely died out of him, faint echoes from a far distant past testifying to a kinship which he has almost outgrown.' He could not be more explicit than he is later in the same passage; 'he may be said, in fact, to represent in succession a fish, a bird, a quadruped in his course before he becomes human; and these transitional phases are presumably to be interpreted as the abstract and brief chronicle of the successive throes or stages of evolution through which nature went before man was brought forth.'

For Maudsley, the psychiatrist, the aetiology of mental disease was a besetting problem. He readily acknowledges its complexity on p. 139 when he writes, 'The causes of mental derangement . . . are so vague and general . . . that the knowledge of them (as they are described in books) yields us very little help when we are brought face to face with a concrete case and endeavour to gain a clear conception of its causation.' He develops his own thinking on the subject, however, as the chapter proceeds. On p. 140 for example, he writes, 'As the causation of insanity may thus reach back through a lifetime, and even have its roots far back in foregoing generations, it is easy to perceive how little is taught by specifying a single moral cause, such as grief, vanity, ambition, which may after all be, and often is, a prominent early symptom of the disease which, striking the attention of observers, gets credit for having caused it.' Or even more succinctly on p. 141 he writes: 'But when unfavourable action from without conspires with an infirmity of nature within, then the conditions of disorder are established, and the discord, which a madman is, is produced.' What, in effect, Maudsley is attempting to resolve is the selfsame nature-nurture controversy with which we continue to grapple even today. However, it is self-evident that the emphasis, according to Maudsley, is far more on nature than on nurture. He talks on p. 142 of 'a destiny made for each one by his inheritance; he is the necessary organic consequent of certain organic antecedents; and it is impossible he should escape the tyranny of his organisation.'

What, in fact, he is leading up to is his exposition of the theory of morbid heredity or degeneracy which in evolutional terms could be termed retrospective evolution. This Maudsley makes clear. He writes, p. 144 '. . . and to the evident fact that men in the long run advance by evolutional variations upon what they have inherited from their forefathers, or go back upon it by retrograde morbid varieties.'

Although it seems abundantly clear that Maudsley was committed to the theory of degeneration and hereditarianism in the aetiology of mental disease, it was not his own brain-child. It is imperative to look across the Channel, to France, to find the major expositors of the theory. It was J. E. D. Esquirol, a distinguished French psychiatrist, who in his *Mental Maladies*, published in 1838, first gave recognition to hereditary pathological predisposition. However, it fell to J. J. Moreau, a student of Esquirol, and B. A. Morel to develop the theory, although others such as Jules Baillarger and Ulysée Trélat added their quota.

It is agreed that in this context pride of place must go to Moreau and Morel. In 1857 Morel published *Treatise on the Physical, Intellectual, and Moral Degeneracy of the Human Race*, and in 1859 Moreau followed with his *Morbid Psychology and its Relationship to the Philosophy of History*. Of the two, Morel's contribution is considered to be the more important, and, indeed, it was hailed by a contemporary worker as the most influential psychiatric text of the nineteenth century.

Morel considered degeneracy to be a 'morbid deviation from the primitive human type,' and attributed the acquisition of 'taints, *inter alia*, to alcoholism and poor nutrition; 'taints' which in some sinister fashion could be transmitted from one generation to the next. He went further and claimed that in the course of three generations the 'tainted' families became sterile and so extinguished themselves.

As the doctrine of hereditarianism gained strength so more and more 'taints' were incorporated. Enormous importance was attributed to epilepsy, but not to the exclusion of chorea and hysteria. The net was eventually cast so wide as to include virtually everything that could be squeezed under the umbrella of 'general illnesses', ailments as diverse as tuberculosis, typhoid gever, scrofula, hypochondria and the like.

Maudsley 'sets forth at almost superfluous length' in this chapter that he is as one with his French colleagues in his advocacy of Morbid Heredity. It is possible that he went even further in his search for 'taints'.

To take two examples: the first is on p. 149 where he writes: '. . . and, secondly, that not mental derangement only in the parents, but other forms of nervous disease in them, such as epilepsy, paroxysmal neuralgia, strong hysteria, dipsomania, spasmodic asthma, hypochondriasis, and suicide . . . may predispose to mental derangement in the offspring . . .'; the second example appears on p. 150 and refers to the relevance of epilepsy in the genesis of insanity. Maudsley writes: 'Epilepsy in the parent comes out perhaps as some form of insanity in the offspring, or insanity in the parent as epilepsy in the child.'

In spite of some of the patent absurdities of hereditary degeneration as the explanation of the causation of mental disease, it continued to hold sway until well into the 20th century. Perhaps the reason, or reasons, for the disinclination to modify, let alone destroy, the theory lay in the attempt, as Morel himself puts it in his treatise, 'to link mental alienation to general medicine more strongly than has been done until now.' In this context it is of vital importance to appreciate that in the France of Napoleon III, psychiatrists, alienists as they were significantly called, were unpopular not only with their medical colleagues, but were anathema to State and Church (Morel was a devout Catholic). They were virtually isolated and this all-embracing theory of degeneracy could be seen as an attempt to curry favour with their antagonists and so join the mainstream of French medicine and in so doing gain acceptance by the establishment of Church and State.

The eventual break-up of the theory in the 20th century might conceivably be attributed to the emergency of psychoanalytic postulations as to the aetiology of mental disorder. More important is the tragic and indisputable fact which emerged during the First World War, namely, that young men of impeccable character and of seemingly untainted heredity broke down in their thousands into mental wrecks after a few months, or even weeks in the trenches. In hereditary terms, therefore, 'Rien n'est parfait' least of all man.

H. R. Rollin

REFERENCES

Baillarger, J. (1844). Recherches statistiques sur l'hérédité de la folie, *Annales Médico-psychologiques,* **3**.

Esquirol, J. F. D. (1845). *Mental Maladies: A treatise on Insanity*, transl. E. K. Hunt, Lea and Blanchard, Philadelphia.

Moreau, (de Tours), J. J. (1852). De la Prédisposition héréditaire, *Annales Medico-psychologiques,* **4**, 451.

Morel, B. A. (1860). *Traité des Maladies Mentales*, Masson, Paris.

Trélat, U. (1856). Des causes de la folie. *Annales Médico-psychologiques,* **2**.
* Page cross-references refer to this edition, not Mandsley's original.

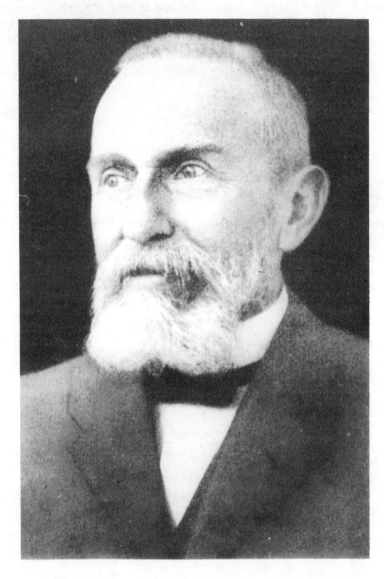

Bleuler

9

The Fundamental Symptoms of Dementia Praecox or the Group of Schizophrenias
Eugen Bleuler, 1911

SYMPTOMATOLOGY

Introduction

Certain symptoms of schizophrenia are present in every case and at every period of the illness even though, as with every other disease symptom, they must have attained a certain degree of intensity before they can be recognized with any certainty. Here, of course, we are discussing only the large symptom-complexes as a whole. For example, the peculiar association disturbance is always present, but not each and every aspect of it. Sometimes the anomalies of association may manifest themselves in "blocking," or in the splitting of ideas; at other times in different schizophrenic symptoms.

Besides these specific permanent or fundamental symptoms, we can find a host of other, more accessory manifestations such as delusions, hallucinations or catatonic symptoms. These may be completely lacking during certain periods, or even throughout the entire course of the disease; at other times, they alone may permanently determine the clinical picture.

As far as we know, the fundamental symptoms are characteristic of schizophrenia, while the accessory symptoms may also appear in other types of illness. Nevertheless, even in such cases close scrutiny often reveals peculiarities of genesis or manifestation of a symptom, which are only found in schizophrenia. We can expect that gradually we will come to recognize the characteristic features in a great number of these accessory symptoms.

A description of the symptoms can be based only on clear-cut cases. But it is extremely important to recognize that they exist in varying degrees and shadings on the entire scale from pathological to normal; also the milder cases, latent schizophrenics with far less manifest symptoms, are many times more common than the overt, manifest cases. Furthermore, in view of the fluctuating character which distinguishes the clinical picture of schizophrenia, it is not to be expected that we shall be able to demonstrate each and every symptom at each and every moment of the disease.

The Fundamental Symptoms

The fundamental symptoms consist of disturbances of association and affectivity, the predilection for fantasy as against reality, and the inclination to divorce oneself from reality (autism). Furthermore, we can add the absence of those very symptoms which play such a great role in certain other diseases such as primary disturbances of perception, orientation and memory, etc.

A The Simple Functions

1 The altered simple functions

Association

In this malady the associations lose their continuity. Of the thousands of associative threads which guide our thinking, this disease seems to interrupt, quite haphazardly, sometimes such single threads, sometimes a whole group, and sometimes even large segments of them. In this way, thinking becomes illogical and often bizarre. Furthermore, the associations tend to proceed along new lines, of which so far the following are known to us: two ideas, fortuitously encountered, are combined into one thought, the logical form being determined by incidental circumstances. Clang-associations receive unusual significance, as do indirect associations. Two or more ideas are condensed into a single one. The tendency to stereotype produces the inclination to cling to one idea to which the patient then returns again and again. Generally, there is a marked dearth of ideas to the point of monoideism. Frequently some idea will dominate the train of thought in the form of blocking, "naming," or echopraxia. In the various types of schizophrenia, distractibility does not seem to be disturbed in a uniform manner. A high degree of associational disturbance usually results in states of confusion.

As to the time element in associations, we know of two disturbances peculiar to schizophrenia—pressure of thoughts, that is, a pathologically increased flow of ideas, and the particularly characteristic "blocking."

A young schizophrenic who had first appeared as either paranoid or hebephrenic and then some years later became markedly catatonic, wrote the following spontaneously:

The Golden Age of Horticulture

"At the time of the new moon, Venus stands in Egypt's August-sky and illuminates with her rays the commercial ports of Suez, Cairo, and Alexandria. In this historically famous city of the Califs, there is a museum of Assyrian monuments from Macedonia. There flourish plantain trees, bananas, corn-cobs, oats, clover and barley, also figs, lemons, oranges, and olives. Olive-oil is an Arabian liquor-sauce which the Afghans, Moors and Moslems use in ostrich-farming. The Indian plantain-tree is the whiskey of the Parsees and Arabs. The Parsee or Caucasian possesses as much influence over his elephant as does the Moor over his dromedary. The camel is the sport of Jews and Arabs. Barley, rice, and sugar-cane called artichoke, grow remarkably well in India. The Brahmins live as castes in Beluchistan. The Circassians occupy Manchuria in China. China is the Eldorado of the Pawnees."

A hebephrenic patient, ill for fifteen years but still able to work and still full of ambitions, gave me the following oral answer to the question, "Who was Epaminondas?"

"Epaminondas was one of those who are especially powerful on land and on sea. He led mighty fleet manoeuvres and open sea-battles against Pelopidas, but in the second Punic War he was defeated by the sinking of an armed frigate. With his ships he wandered from Athens to Hain Mamre, brought Caledonian grapes and pomegranates there, and conquered the Beduins. He besieged the Acropolis with gun-boats and had the Persian garrisons put to the stake as living torches. The succeeding Pope Gregory VII . . . eh . . . Nero, followed his example and because of him all the Athenians, all the Roman-Germanic-Celtic tribes who did not favor the priests, were burned by the Druids on Corpus Christi Day as a sacrifice to the Sun-God, Baal. That is the Stone Age. Spearheads made of bronze."

These two performances indicate a moderate degree of schizophrenic association disturbance. Though they stem from two patients whose clinical picture is diametrically different, yet they are amazingly similar. In these patients, the most important determinant of the associations is completely lacking—the concept of purpose. The first patient apparently desires to describe oriental gardens, as such an odd idea for a plain, simple clerk who had never left his native land but idled in a hospital ward for years. The second patient formally adheres to the question put to him, but in fact never speaks of Epaminondas; actually he covers a much larger group of ideas.

This means that thoughts are subordinated to some sort of general idea, but they are not related and directed by any unifying concept of purpose or goal. It looks as though ideas of a certain category (in the first case pertaining to the Orient, in the second, to data of ancient history) were thrown into one pot, mixed, and subsequently picked out at random, and linked with each other by mere grammatical form or other auxiliary images. Still, certain sequences of the ideas are more closely linked to each other by some sort of common threat which, however, proves too loose to provide a logically useful connection. (Fleet-manoeuvres—sea-battle—armed frigate; Acropolis—Persian garrison—burning—living torches,—Nero; priests—Druids—Corpus Christi Day—Sun-God Baal, etc.)

In analyzing the disturbances of association, we must realize the influences which actually guide our thinking. Associations formed in terms of habit, similarity, subordination, causality, etc., of course will never generate truly fertile thoughts. Only the goal-directed concept can weld the links of the associative chain into logical thought. However, what we mean by a goal-directed concept is not just one single idea, but an infinitely complicated hierarchy of ideas. If we work out a particular theme, the first goal is to give permanent formulation to a part-idea for which, usually, a sentence will serve as a symbol. A further, more generalized goal is the construction of a paragraph which again will be subordinated to a chapter and so forth.

Not only our goal-concept, but also the supposedly simpler, subordinate ideas with which we ordinarily operate, are composed of numerous elements which change according to context. The idea of water is quite different depending on whether it refers to chemistry, physiology, navigation, landscape, inundation, or source of power. Each of these special ideas becomes connected with the other ideas by a quite different set of threads. No healthy person thinks of crystal water when his house is being swept away by a flood; nor will he think of water as a medium of transportation when he is thirsty.

Naturally, even the most limited idea of water is composed of various concepts such as fluid, evaporable, cold, colorless, etc. But in the normal mind only those part concepts dominate the picture that belong to a given frame of reference. The others exist only potentially, or at least retreat into the background so that we cannot even demonstrate their influence.

The direction of our associations is determined not by any single force but by an almost infinite number of influences. In the thought processes of schizophrenia, however, all the associative threads indicated here, whether singly or in haphazard groupings, may remain totally ineffective.

A few more examples may illustrate this:

"Dear Mother: Today I am feeling better than yesterday. I really don't feel much like writing. But I love to write to you. After all, I can tackle it twice. Yesterday, Sunday, I would have been so happy if you and Louise and I could have gone to the park. One has such a lovely view from Stephan's Castle. Actually, it is very lovely in Burgholzli. Louise wrote Burgholzli on her two last letters, I mean to say on the envelopes, no, the 'couverts' which I received. However, I have written Burgholzli in the spot where I put the date. There are also patients in Burgholzli who call it 'Holzliburg.' Others talk of a factory. One may also regard it as a health-resort.

"I am writing on paper. The pen which I am using is from a factory called 'Perry & Co.' This factory is in England. I assume this. Behind the name of Perry & Co. the city of London is inscribed; but not the city. The city of London is in England. I know this from my school-days. Then, I always liked geography. My last teacher in that subject was Professor August A. He was a man with black eyes. I also like black eyes. There are also blue and gray eyes and other sorts, too. I have heard it said that snakes have green eyes. All people have eyes. There are some, too, who are blind. These blind people are led about by a boy. It must be very terrible not to be able to see. There are people who can't see and, in addition, can't hear. I know some who hear too much. One can hear too much. There are many sick people in Burgholzli; they are called patients. One of them I like a great deal. His name is E. Sch. He taught me that in Burgholzli there are many kinds, patients, inmates, attendants. Then there are some who are not here at all They are all peculiar people. . . ."

A non-schizophrenic informant would tell us what in his immediate environment affected him; what may have made him feel comfortable or uncomfortable; or, perhaps, something that might interest his reader. There is complete absence of any such purpose here. The common denominator of all of the patient's ideas rests in the fact that they are present in his awareness, but not because they have any close relation to him. In this respect, the thinking is even more scattered than that of "Horticulture," or of "Epaminondas." On the other hand, it is better co-ordinated as to details. Whereas in the other examples coherence of details was the exception, and only referred to small groups, in this letter we do not find any sudden breaks. In this respect, the "laws of association" remain in force. In an experimental set-up which would exclude the idea of a main purpose, these associations would even have to be considered perfectly valid: London—geography-lesson—geography-teacher—his black eyes— gray eyes—green snake-eyes—human eyes—blind people— their companions—horrible fate, etc. Although nearly all the ideas expressed are correct, nevertheless the letter is meaningless. The patient has the goal of writing, but nothing to write about.

A hebephrenic wishes to sign her name "B. Graf" in the customary position at the end of a letter. She writes "Gra;" then another word beginning with "Gr" comes to her mind; whereupon she changes the "a" to "o," affixes "s," and then repeats the Word "Gross" twice over. Thus, the whole complex of concepts which was at the root of the purpose of signing her name, has all at once become completely ineffective, with the exception of the first two letters, "Gr." In this way the patients may lose themselves in the most irrelevant side-associations, and a uniform chain of thought does not come about. This symptom has also been called "Vorbeidenken" (a sort of non-sequitur thinking, skimming past things).

To the question: "What was your father?" a patient answers "Johann Friedrich." He understood that the question concerned his father but the inquiry about his father's occupation did not influence his retort; instead, he answered the unasked question as to his father's name. If such cases are investigated more closely, we usually find that the patient grasped the question as such but that the corresponding concepts were never elaborated in his mind.

Another hebephrenic writes: "The mountains which are outlined in the swellings of the oxygen are beautiful." This is a description of a walk the patient had taken in which chemical terms do not fit. Obviously, something about "fresh-air" floated into his mind because in the next sentence the patient begins very abruptly to talk about his health.

A similar example: "Are you very unhappy?"—"No".—"Is something weighing heavily on your mind?"—"Yes. Iron is heavy." —"Heavy" is here suddenly conceived in its physical sense.

In some cases, all the threads between thoughts are torn. Unless new paths are found, we have stupor or blocking. Frequently the patient drops a thought in an entirely matter-of-course way, only to proceed to quite a different one that has no recognizable associative connection with the previous one.

In the following fragment of an "Autobiography" the sudden leaps are marked by the symbol (*). Part of these "cesuras" are explicable by environmental influences and points of contact (distractibility).

"One must have arisen sufficiently early and then there is usually the necessary 'appetite' present. 'L'appétit vient en mangeant,' says the Frenchman. *With time and years the individual becomes so lazy in public life that he is not even capable of writing any more. On such a sheet of paper, one can squeeze many letters if one is careful not to transgress by one 'square shoe.' * In such fine weather one should be able to take a walk in the woods. Naturally, not alone, but with a girl. * At the end of a year one always renders the annual accounting.* The sun is now in the sky yet it is not yet 10 o'clock. In Burgholzli, too? I don't know since I have no watch with me as I used to have! Après le manger, On va p. . . . ! There are also plenty of entertainments for people who do not and never did belong to this hospital. In Switzerland it is not permitted to do mischief with human flesh!! * Le foin, hay, L'herbe grass, mordre- bite, etc. etc. etc. and so on! R. K. In any event, much 'merchandise' comes to Burgholzli from Zurich. Otherwise we would not have to stay in 'bed' until it may please this or that person to 'tell' who is to blame that one is no longer permitted to go about freely. O . . . * 1000 hundredweights. * Appendage to acorns!!!

In the usual speech and writing, this peculiar disconnecting of associative threads is often combined with other disturbances, so that it is quite difficult to find a pure sample. In acute states, this anomaly can go so far that it becomes an exception if a sequence of thoughts can be traced along its many links. This has been termed "dissociated thinking" or "incoherence"; the external disease picture can be labeled "confusion." Sometimes, however, only the patient's manner of expression is obscure so that logical transitions may still be assumed to exist.

All the indicated disturbances may range from a maximum which corresponds to complete confusion, to a minimum which may be hardly noticeable. Not every thought-association in a schizophrenic is of this kind. Whereas in the severe cases, false associations are actually dominant, in cases of "cured" or latent dementia praecox only patient and persistent observations reveal even a single such error in thinking.

The emergence of new ideas becomes most apparent in question and answer interviews and in association experiments in which the patient must respond to a stimulus-word with the first word or idea which comes to his mind. Thus, a patient stares at a candle and replies to the question what he sees: "There is a candle; eternal light: * Barbara v. R. in S. * Something right behind. Barbels (a kind of viol), yes, they are found in the Rhine." On ordering the patient to go to work, one might receive the following answer: "Why do you let it drop? * The sun is in the sky. * Why do you let it drop?" (No one had dropped anything.) Aside from breaks in thought, marked with the symbol (*), it is apparent that even the first sentence has no connection with the order given the patient. This is quite usual; often a reply to a question is only a formal retort, but its content has nothing to do with the question posed.

"That is the little Jew's clock in regard to Daniel" is given in response instead of a greeting. In the above-mentioned "Autobiography" we find: "In any event, much merchandise is sent to Burgholzli from Zurich. Otherwise we would not have to stay in bed." The new idea of "staying in bed" is introduced formally as proof of the preceding idea.

At this point, we can sum up the discussion as follows:

In the normal thinking process, the numerous actual and latent images combine to determine each association. In schizophrenia, however, single images or whole combinations may be rendered ineffective, in an apparently haphazard fashion. Instead, thinking operates with ideas and concepts which have no, or a completely insufficient, connection with the main idea and should therefore be excluded from the thought-process. The result is that thinking becomes confused, bizarre, incorrect, abrupt. Sometimes, all the associative threads fail and the thought chain is totally interrupted; after such "blocking," ideas may emerge which have no recognizable connection with preceding ones.

The emergence of an idea without any connection with a previous train of thought, or without any external stimulus, is (in spite of Swoboda) so foreign to normal psychology that one is obliged to look even in the patient's seemingly most far-fetched ideas, for the associative path originating in a previous concept or in an external stimulus. In this way, it may be possible in some, though not in all cases, to demonstrate the connecting links. Still, in a sufficient number of cases, we will succeed in pointing out several of the main directions along which the derailment of thoughts took place.

Even where only a part of the associative threads is interrupted, other influences, which under normal circumstances are not noticeable, become operative in the place of logical directives. As far as we know, they are for the most part the very same directives which determine the emergence of new connections after the total break in thought: connections with accidentally aroused ideas, condensations, clang-associations intermediate associations, and perseveration of ideas (stereotypy). All these thought-connections are not foreign to the normal psyche either. But they occur only exceptionally and incidentally, whereas in schizophrenia they are exaggerated to the point of caricature and often actually dominate the thought-process.

Most frequently, we can observe how *two ideas without any intrinsic relation with each other, preoccupying the patient simultaneously are simply being connected.* The logical form of the connection will depend on the accompanying circumstances. If one asks the patient a question, he responds with any idea which he may have at the moment. If he looks for a reason, such ideas are simply causally connected. If he has a pathologically exaggerated self-consciousness, or if he feels slighted, he will refer the new ideas directly to himself in accordance with the affective valence of these complexes.

Occasionally the two thoughts originate in the external circumstances or in the train of thought itself:

"How are you?" "Bad," (with a smiling face). "You look very well; everything going all right?" (patting the patient on the back). "No, I have a pain in my back," (pointing out the place where she was patted). "Why are you laughing?" "Because you are clearing out the chest of drawers." "But you already laughed before that." "Because the things were still in it."

Most commonly, thought-connections are made with things which are of emotional concern to the patient.

In the hearing of a catatonic, something was said about a fish-market. She begins to repeat, "Yes, I am also a shark-fish." Thus she employs an entirely peculiar and impossible clang association; impossible, that is, for every other waking human being except a schizophrenic. The association "fish-market—shark-fish" is used in order to express the idea that she is someone very bad; yet she ignores the complete impossibility of the reality of her identification.

A patient varied the stereotyped phrase, "I don't feel good," used by her over a span of thirty years, by way of substituting various dialect expressions for "good," also using the English word "well." One day she took the word "well" and changed it to say, "I don't feel velo" (velo-bicycle).

The *condensations*, that is, the contractions of many ideas into one, are in principle not different from the accidental associative connections. A catatonic associates to the word, "sail," "steam-sail," combining in the two ideas, "steam-boat" and "sail-boat." In the construction of delusions and symbols, condensation is an outstanding component and the cause of a number of portemanteau words: "sadsome" for sad and lonesome, or, to use a German example *"trauram"* for *"traurig"* and *"grausam."*

Not infrequently the tendency towards stereotypy is a further cause for the derailment of the patient's associational activity. The patients are caught in and remain fixed to the same circle of ideas, the same words, the same sentence structures, or, at any rate, return to them again and again without any logical need.

The stereotypies can remain fixed for long periods. In a few cases, we noted that after four weeks the same answer was given to 40 per cent of the stimulus-words as was given on the first occasion. A patient reacted to the word, "so," with the incomprehensible "that is a canal;" it then was found that on a previous day she had given the very same sentence in response to "sea." The same patient associated: to "count"—"that is to eat," and later, "country"—"that is to eat a great deal." There again we have the same fixation on the assonance of the words.

In the pseudo-flight of ideas of the acute confused schizophrenic the consistent return to what was said before, is a common occurrence. The tendency toward stereotypy, combined with a lack of purposeful goal in their thinking, leads on the one hand to *"Klebedenken"* (adhesive, sticky type of thinking), to a kind of *perseveration*, and on the other hand to a general impoverishment of thought. The patients then always talk about the same topic (monoideismus) and are incapable of interesting themselves in anything else.

It may be due to purposelessness and stereotypy of ideas, that the patient is really unable to pursue a thought to its conclusion; a senseless compulsion to associate may replace thinking proper. Thus, a hebephrenic was unable to tear himself away from the concepts "love" and "have;" and for a long time kept spontaneously associating such chains as the following: "love, theft, gift, lady, have, love, theft, gift, lady, love, theft, taken back, taken back, taken back, taken back, have . . ."

In this manner patients get entangled in long enumerations which clearly betray the schizophrenic character of their associative disturbances.

In association experiments it is not at all a rare occurrence that patients begin to name whatever they see, so that they respond, for example, to the different stimulus-words by enumerating all the furniture in the room. They do this even when they have understood the point of the experiment perfectly and want to get away from this idea.

This symptom has an external, and at times also an inner similarity to what Sommer has called *naming* and *touching*. In many patients, and especially in those who are somewhat confused, the only recognizable association to impressions coming from the external world, consists in naming them: "mirror," "table"; or they are rendered by sentences: "This is a barometer. This is a gas-lamp. These are coats." This sort of "naming" does not only appear in response to visual impressions. For example, I take a patient by the hand; and she says, "the hand"; or asked to do something, she designates it by some catch-word: "into the garden," "to undress." In a quite analogous way hallucinating patients will often "name" their activities: "Now he is sitting down"; "Now he wants to write"; "Now he is writing." The transition from the writing of letters simply enumerating things or events around them to this "naming" is very fluid. The patient who described what was written on his steel-pen is not so very far removed from the "naming" patient. Also to this group belongs the patient who, on seeing somebody approaching carrying a lantern, remarked: "I declare that this is a lantern." Common to all is the fastening upon a sense impression because of the lack of a goal-concept. The patients link up and tack on ideas to any and all possible ones whether they come from within or without. The idea with which they link, and the direction which this process takes, is variable and, as far as the associative activity is concerned, determined by accident, exactly as in the case of our letterwriting patient.

If a given conception involves motor-elements, then the only recognizable association can be that the corresponding idea is acted out. The patient acts out, imitates, copies what he hears and sees: *echopraxia* and *echolalia*. In fact, I cannot separate "naming" and "echopraxia," at least not as a matter of principle. Every idea or concept has a motor element; in the actions he sees performed before his very eyes, in the words he hears spoken, this component is quite obvious in the healthy person. If there are no reasons for drawing on other associations, it is very understandable that such motor components will not be inhibited or repressed. Therefore we include here such occurrences as the following: a patient cracked the glass-panel out of a door; another patient proceeds to creep in and out of the hole thus made. He keeps it up continuously without knowing why he is doing so.

* * * *

The most extraordinary formal element of schizophrenic thought processes is that termed "blocking." The associative activity often seems to come to an abrupt and complete stand-still. When it is again resumed, ideas emerge which have no or at least very insufficient connection with what went on before.

While conversing with a patient, one does not note anything abnormal in the temporal aspect of his chain of ideas. Statement and counter-statement, question and answer follow one another as in any normal conversation. But all of a sudden, in the middle of a sentence or in passing to a new idea, the patient stops and cannot continue any further. Often he is able to overcome the obstacle by repeating the attempt. Another time, he succeeds only in thinking in a new direction. Frequently, the blocking cannot be overcome for quite a long interval; in such cases it can spread over the entire psyche, the patient remaining silent and motionless and also more or less without thoughts.

This concept of blocking we owe to Kraepelin. It is of fundamental significance in the symptomatology and diagnosis of schizophrenia. We meet it again in the motor sphere—in actions, in remembering, and even in the field of perception.

The "blocking" of the train of thought is perceived by the patients themselves who usually describe it under various names. Mostly, but not always, they find it a condition that is quite unpleasant. An intelligent catatonic woman had to sit still for hours at a time, "in order to find her thoughts again." Another patient could find nothing to say about it than, "I can sometimes speak and sometimes not." Another patient feels as if "he died away" (Abraham). Still another complains of "obstacles to thinking," or "a tightness in his head as if my head were drawn together." Yet another describes it "as if someone drew a rubber sack over him." A peasant woman expresses it as "if something was being pressed against her face and chest, it is just as if my mouth was being held closed, as if someone said 'keep your mouth shut!' " In this last example, there is also blocking of the motor functions of speaking which a patient of Rust described with the words "that his powers of speech were being withheld from him." It is something quite common to find that the blocking is attributed to foreign influence. Thus, while one of our patients was asked to sing songs, he was suddenly unable to continue. The "voices" told him, "See, you have again forgotten." But these "voices" were those very agents who, according to the patient, provoked his lapse of memory.

Jung heard from one of his patients the best term for designating the phenomenon; subjectively she experienced it as "thought-deprivation." The term is so apt that many schizophrenics know instantly what is meant by it. If a patient immediately answers with a "Yes" to the question, "Do you experience thought-deprivation?" and then goes on to describe what he understands by this expression, one can very well make the diagnosis of schizophrenia with a considerable degree of certainty. At least, we have not found any exception to this conclusion as yet. Even patients who have used different descriptive words for the concept of "blocking" know what is meant by "thought-deprivation." A patient promptly responded to Jung's question as to whether he suffered from deprivation of his thoughts with: "So you call it thought-deprivation, up to now I have always called it 'thought-obstruction.' " Kraepelin's patient expressed it similarly as "withdrawal of the thoughts."

The disturbances of association, as described, are characteristic for schizophrenia.

Affectivity

In the outspoken forms of schizophrenia, the "emotional deterioration" stands in the forefront of the clinical picture. It has been known since the early years of modern psychiatry that an "acute curable" psychosis became "chronic" when the affects began to disappear. Many schizophrenics in the later stages cease to show any affect for years and even decades at a time. They sit about the institutions to which they are confined with expressionless faces, hunched-up, the image of indifference. They permit themselves to be dressed and undressed like automatons, to be led from their customary place of inactivity to the mess-hall, and back again without expressing any sign of satisfaction or dissatisfaction. They do not even seem to react to injuries inflicted on them by other patients.

Even in the less severe forms of the illness, indifference seems to be the external sign of their state; and indifference to everything—to friends and relations, to vocation or enjoyment, to duties or rights, to good fortune or to bad. "I don't care the least, one way or another," is what a patient of Binswanger said. Generally the defect shows itself most strikingly in relation to the most vital of the patient's interests and it does not make any difference whether or not their comprehension requires complicated thinking. A mother may show right at the beginning of her illness that she is indifferent to the weal and woes of her children; yet she may employ not only the words of a normally feeling mother but really understand everything that is good or bad for a child. She may, as the occasion requires (e.g., when she uses it for an excuse to try and obtain her release from the hospital), discuss the matter quite competently. It is a matter of indifference for such a patient whether her family or herself are going to wreck and ruin. The sense of self-preservation is often reduced to zero. The patients do not bother any more about whether they starve or not, whether they lie on a snowbank or on a red-hot oven. During a fire in the hospital, a number of patients had to be led out of the threatened ward; they themselves would never have moved from their places; they would have allowed themselves to be suffocated or burnt without showing an affective response. Illnesses, threats of every possible evil will not disturb the peace of many a schizophrenic. What happens to others is of course of no concern at all to them. In a ward one patient kills another; his ward-mates do not find it necessary to call the attendant. A student almost choked the life out of his mother; he cannot understand why such a fuss is made over "a few harsh words!" A patient writes home for the first time after a month-and-a-half in the institution; but aside from a few irrelevant and insignificant phrases, he can only ask how the cat is getting along.

Schizophrenics can write whole autobiographies without manifesting the least bit of emotion. They will describe their suffering and their actions as if it were a theme in physics. A Croatian woman, who could speak only her native tongue, manages to wander off to Zurich; remains in the hospital for months without being able to make herself understood since she pays no attention to gestures, although she is of lively temperament. Finally a country-woman of hers speaks to her. The patient answers the questions but does not show the least affect. A hebephrenic talks about his father's death: "Since I was at home at that time, I went to the funeral and was happy, however, that it was not I who was being buried; I am buried alive now." Generally, it is very striking how many patients, particularly the older ones, reveal the same indifference to their own delusions, with which, however, they are constantly preoccupied.

During a lengthy clinical presentation a paranoid complains constantly about his persecutions but sits very calmly and non-chalantly as he tells his story. Asked if he thought his hallucinations were real, he answers with a shrug of his shoulders: "Perhaps they are pathological, perhaps they are real." The question very obviously does not interest him. It is common knowledge that older paranoids relate with the greatest calmness how they were flayed and burnt during the night; how their bowels were torn out. A hebephrenic comes to the doctor to ask him, please, not to kill her. Although she really believes that it is a matter of life and death, she remains completely affectless.

Often we do note significant "basic moods," so that one cannot really speak of an all-pervading indifference in these patients. The mood may be euphoric, sad, or anxious. We see the transitions from a euphoric mood to indifference or a mixture of both in the very frequent emotional states of hebephrenics who show what is called a "callous indifference," or what the French call *"je'm'en-fichisme,"* and the English, "I don't give a damn!" The patients are then, if not happy, at least quite pleased with themselves and the world. Unpleasant occurrences are not felt as disagreeable. On such occasions their answers become quite insolent. This reaction is facilitated because their inaccurate associations supply them with very appropriate material. Also, other moods express themselves in a similar way. For twenty years one of our patients was known as "the good-natured mad-woman" because she presented her senseless complaints with so much laughter and bonhomie.

In those acute episodes of this disease that were formerly called mania and melancholia, the affect is of course not lacking but it takes on a special coloring or tone which often in itself permits the diagnosis of the disease. In place of the clear, deeply felt affect of the manic-depressive psychosis, we have the impression of emotionality which does not go very deep at all. Above all, however, consistency of affective manifestation is absent. The words which are supposed to express pain or pleasure, the tone of voice, the gestures do not seem consistent or appropriate to the patient's total attitude. The mimic lacks unity—the wrinkled forehead, for example, expresses something like surprise; the eyes with their little crows feet give the impression of laughter and the corners of the mouth may be drooping as if in sorrow. Often the facial expression seems exaggerated and highly melodramatic. The stiffness or awkwardness of movements are very striking in these cases. Both complaints and jubilation become monotonous.

It is easier to sense these phenomena than to describe them. What can best be emphasized in the presentation is the lack of adaptability to changing thought content, the deficiency in the capacity for modulation. The affective mood of the manic schizophrenic hardly follows or does not follow at all the changing content of thought. The true manic, just like the normal individual, accompanies the emotional nuances of his thoughts with the appropriate qualitative and quantitative modifications of affective manifestations; the definitely schizophrenic patient shows little or none of such modulations, whether he is making a witticism or complaining about his incarceration, or telling us his life-story. A catatonic patient complained that her husband was in prison. I assured her that he was free upon which she answered, "Is he, that's fine." Yet she made this answer in as unchanged, complaining a tone as if I had confirmed her husband's imprisonment.

Such an attitude is only apparently different from indifference. Whatever affect there is, it certainly is not a reaction to a thought, but rather some abnormal basic state of affectivity, a different adjustment of the affective zero-point. Patients with other types of psychosis will react according to their concepts with vacillations either upward or downward from this affective zero-point; not so the schizophrenic.

In acute stages, rapid alteration of affective expression may occur even without any basic, continuing mood, within a brief space of time, e.g. during a clinical presentation. Because of some haphazard, accidental association, the patient will switch in one second from exaggerated, intense, angry agitation with cursing, screaming, jumping about, to an exaggeratedly erotic, happy mood, only to become tearful and sad a few minutes later. In these cases the entire personality seems to change with the affect. In contrast to the above discussed fixation of certain components of a previous affective expression, we find here that previous affects do not seem to operate as far as they normally would. Quite suddenly, there will appear a completely new emotional register. This kind of quick reversal and emotional rigidity differentiates these cases easily from the organic types.

Even when the affects change, they usually do so more slowly than in the healthy. The affects seem often to lag behind the ideas. During an interview, a female patient was repeatedly shown the picture of a child. It took one-quarter of an hour for the corresponding sorrowful affect to appear. Also, during celebrations one can observe how much longer it takes the schizophrenic to get into the party mood than it does the healthy person. Although anger and fury tend to linger on, they may set in as abruptly in the normal as in the schizophrenic. One cannot regard this as special lability of the patients. However, there undoubtedly is a pathological lingering of affect in the usual tendency of schizophrenics to persist in their anger or even increase it for long periods, even though the reason for this emotion no longer exists.

From all of this we must draw the conclusion that the lability of the schizophrenic represents an unessential phenomenon.

Even when cerebral atrophy sets in, the affects often still make their appearance, with the result that some of these disturbed individuals differ little from the usual cases of senility, "who can cry and laugh whenever they so desire." I observed a catatonic for ten years who, except for the very earliest period of her illness, had only hurled insults at me and had sat with her tongue protruding from the corner of her mouth, in a demonstratively negativistic attitude. When I visited the hospital ten years after having left I saw her again and she rushed to greet me and threw her arms around me as if I were an old friend. A paranoid patient, whom I had known to be emotionally indifferent for thirty years, had an apoplectic attack. As she was attracting flies with sweets, I asked her once jokingly whether the flies would not eat her up too. She fell in with the joke: "There are big, big ones which want to eat me." She laughed at the first half of the sentence, but with the second half she was so overcome that she burst out crying (as do true senile cases) being overwhelmed by the idea of being eaten.

Thus there can be no doubt at all that the psyche's capacity to produce affects has not disappeared in schizophrenia. Therefore, it should be no cause for surprise to find one or the other affect still well preserved even in the severe cases. But the specific nature of the affect we find is largely determined by "accident." Still, there are certain emotions which have a better chance of being encountered than others.

As we saw above, we were often able to reveal erotic strivings (in the subtle sense). Quite frequently, when we are able to follow up the patient's day-dreams, we find most delicate feelings in the very patient who displayed nothing but violence and filth to the world.

Even in advanced cases, instead of interest we meet its equivalent—curiosity. Patients who apparently were not the least concerned with anything around them, always seemed to be able to manage things in such a way that, should a door open, they would be able to look through it or overhear a conversation, or get a glance at a book lying open. They will do this even at a time when they appear too torpid even to touch what they consider peculiar. In cases institutionalized for a long time we observe a certain growing attachment to the hospital. Schizophrenics who have worked in a hospital for many years develop a kind of affection for the institution. They show an interest in the management of the farm, and occasionally even spontaneously contribute something to it. They might show homesickness for the institution after they have been discharged. Just as often, however, we find that these hard-working patients perform their daily stint like veritable automatons unperturbed by rain or snow, heat or frost.

It is in the range of irritability, anger, and even fury, that we find most frequently preservation of the affects. Many institutionalized patients show reaction only in this way. The attendant personnel is always in danger of being insulted or attacked while carrying out the ordinarily, daily routine care, even when bringing the patients their food. Between such extreme and nowadays rare cases, and just the ordinary irritability, there is every degree of gradation.

In hospitals and institutions, this irritability in connection with the delusional system and negativism of the patients is particularly difficult to manage. The "persecuted" are dissatisfied with their environment, considering it the source of the persecution. Other patients, who believe that all their desires have been fulfilled, are disturbed by their environment in their happy dreams—reason enough for anger and fury. Thus, anger is the usual reaction of many patients to their hallucinations, and, what is very significant, even when their "voices" do not have anything especially unpleasant to say.

Quite frequently one finds that parental love is the only affective element that is preserved apart from the patient's irritability. Mothers, in particular, often remain truly concerned about the well-being of their children; whereas they may not care about anything else, not even about their own physical health. Such patients will show real joy when their children visit them or when they receive good news of their children. A woman patient, who had been ill for some thirty years and who for a long time had been in an advanced hallucinatory condition, tried to convince her physician, whom she had singled out for her son-in-law, that her disease had not been inherited by her daughter.

Also, the feeling of sympathy for others is not always extinguished. Often patients can very well sympathize with another's situation or condition, especially in institutions where the majority know each other quite well. A hebephrenic, whose very speech was confusion, held the cigar-holder to the mouth of another patient suffering from muscular atrophy who could no longer hold the cigar between his own lips. He did this with a patience and indefatigability of which no normal person would ever be capable. It sometimes happens that such schizophrenic Samaritans succeed in feeding an abstentious patient who could not be fed by anyone else.

It is indeed striking how early those feelings that regulate social intercourse among people are blunted. It hardly makes any difference to the patient whether he is addressing a person in authority or someone more humbly-placed, whether a man or a woman. Often there is not a trace of modesty left, even in patients who are otherwise relatively not too deteriorated. They will confess or relate all sorts of misdeeds which they themselves recognize as such. They will expound on their sexual experiences in the vilest terms. They will masturbate openly. A patient, an intelligent high school student, writes to his mother as follows: "Dear Mother, come to see me as soon as possible. I must know how old you were the night my father made me."

Yet the strong emotionality exhibited in petty matters can be in marked contrast to the severe defects described above. A hebephrenic who worked for a time in our office, strutted around carefully togged out, manicured and pomaded and did not in the least seem to mind the teasing which he was subjected to by another uncouth employee. Yet when his mother wrote, asking him to come home to see his dying father, he sent her a few words of "consolation" but did not go home. Two female patients eat their own excrement. One of them, an old maid, is still very reluctant and coy about revealing her age; the other, a painter, took the greatest delight in the pretty colours of her "odd food."

The ethical qualities of the schizophrenics are of great variety. By and large, the patients appear as much blunted in this direction as in others. Since most of them are not very active, few of them become criminals. Occasionally one does become a thief or a swindler subsequent to the outbreak of his illness. It is then impossible to say whether a previously inhibited tendency has made its appearance or whether the disease itself produced the criminal behavior. Thus, as far as morality is concerned, one can trust schizophrenics just as little or as much as one can normal persons. The situation is far worse with regard to their unpredictability. But on the whole it can be said that there is less lying, stealing, swindling and slandering among the patients than among the healthy. In milder cases there appears quite often a very painstaking conscientiousness and scrupulousness. Of course, the assaults committed as results of delusions have nothing to do with the question of ethics, since from the patients' point of view they are merely justifiable acts of self-defense.

Thus the character of the schizophrenic is as manifold as that of the normal. Nevertheless, the indifference, the tendency to withdraw, the inaccessibility to influence, the moodiness and the irritability—all these peculiarities are recurring characteristics which doubtlessly invest all the advanced cases with a certain common external appearance. In spite of all difficulties some are able to maintain a likeable, even loveable, character until quite late in the course of the disease. Others become monsters of the most vengeful, cruel, deceitful type, given to every sort of excesses. The disease can transform a congenitally bad person into a harmless one by the very loss of energy and activity, but apparently it cannot make him better.

Patients with schizophrenia react differently to their affective disturbances. The majority are not aware of them and consider their reaction as normal. The more intelligent, however, may reason about it quite acutely. At the beginning they sense the emotional emptiness as rather painful, so that they may easily be mistaken for melancholics. One of our catatonics considered himself as "insensibilized;" one of Jung's patients could not pray any more because of "hardening of her feelings." Later, they tend to displace the changes in themselves to the outer world which itself becomes hollow, empty, strange, because of these affective changes. Often the element of strangeness has a touch of the uncanny and hostile.

Others, as for example Aschaffenburg's patient, express it in a very characteristic way. After a mild attack of the illness she felt herself subjectively decidedly better than she had been before her illness. Previously whenever it was necessary to lend a hand with family matters, concerns and chores, she felt compelled by her moral feelings to sacrifice her rest and her health; after her illness she was able to live for herself without twinges of conscience. Some hebephrenics exhibit their indifference quite consciously.

Occasionally, a patient will maintain that he has a marked and powerful affect, whereas the observer can note none or another type of affect than that which the patient professes to feel. Whether the patient means something other than we do in his use of terms or whether the phenomenon can be explained by the psychic splitting, I must leave to future research.

Especially conspicuous in schizophrenics is the frequently encounterd parathymia. The patients are able to react to sad news with cheerfulness or even with laughter. These patients will often become sad or, even more frequently, irritated by events to which others would react with indifference or with pleasure. A mere "how-do-you-do" can upset them. Many times they will attach erotic feelings to someone or something which does not at all appear to be suitable. A patient states that her bath water was poisoned, that it had a very bitter taste, and she accompanies her words with a coy erotic giggle. Other patients are in love with a ward-mate with complete disregard of sex, ugliness, or even repulsiveness. They will relate laughingly their torturing hallucinations, or portray themselves with a cheerful mien as unfortunate creatures. A particularly frequent form of parathymia is represented by unprovoked or inappropriate bursts of laughter. The dysfunction of affect may manifest itself in the quantitative relation of the feelings to each other. Thus a patient of Masselon's broke out into loud laughter at the news of her brother's death, because she was so pleased at receiving letters with black borders; but the loss of the brother did not seem to arouse any feeling.

Parathymia can never really be differentiated from paramimia. One of our catatonics appeared melancholic on admission, yet soon after said that she had enjoyed the admission-formalities and that the physician's handshake, for instance, appeared to her as something holy. Another female catatonic patient approached one of the women attendants whom she liked and told her in the friendliest manner and in her sweetest tone of voice: "I really would like to slap your face, people like you are usually called s. o. b.'s." A third patient danced about and hummed a popular song but maintained throughout an expression of distress and a heart-breaking tone of voice.

The above-mentioned lack of essential unity in expression can lead to a sort of paramimia. A woman patient complained bitterly about her "voices" and body-hallucinations; her mouth and her forehead manifested disgust, but her eyes expressed happy eroticism. After a few minutes the mouth also assumed the expression of happiness while her forehead continued to appear gloomy and wrinkled. She herself stated that the feelings which she described as uncomfortable, in certain respect were also pleasant. Thus each and every component of an expressive attitude (including voice, posture, movement of hands, feet, etc.) may be dissociated and react in contradiction to the others.

Ambivalence

The tendency of the schizophrenic psyche to endow the most diverse psychisms with both a positive and negative indicator at one and the same time is not always quite explicit. Yet, after sufficiently long observation, one will find it to be present even in the mild cases. It is such an immediate consequence of the schizophrenic association disturbance that its complete absence appears highly improbable. It is for this reason that we include it among the fundamental symptoms.

The very same concept can be accompanied simultaneously by pleasant and unpleasant feelings (*affective ambivalence*): the husband both loves and hates his wife. The patient's hallucinations reveal to the mother the "longed-for" death of the child by the unloved husband. She breaks out in endless sobbing and moaning. She suffers the most intense anxiety that they are going to shoot her and yet she constantly begs the attendant to shoot her. She claims there is a black man outside her room. Then she breaks into a startling confusion of tearful demands, complaints and violence, demanding that she be kept in the hospital and permitted to join the black man. She verbigerates, "You devil, you angel, you devil, you angel." (She is referring here to her lover.)

In *ambivalence of will* ("*Ambi-Tendenz*"), the patient wishes to eat and does not wish to eat. He starts to bring the spoon to his mouth dozens of times but never completes the act, or makes some other useless movement. He clamors for his release and then resists with much cursing when he is informed that he will be discharged from the institution. He demands work, only to become furious when something is given him to do, and cannot decide to do the work. One patient, during one of his first attacks of illness, was bitterly conscience-stricken because once, in his youth, he had committed fellatio on a young boy. Yet in later years he persistently, and with crude violence attempts to commit fellatio on other patients. The "voices" advise him to drown himself and in the very same sentence, much to his surprise they scornfully berate him for wishing to drown himself.

It is *intellectual ambivalence* when a patient says in the same breath: "I am Dr. H.; I am not Dr. H.;" or "I am a human being like yourself, even though I am not a human being". Quite frequently we hear such statements, and often indeed without the same words used in the second sentence being given another meaning than they had in the first.

A philosophically educated catatonic made the following observation himself: "When one expresses a thought, one always sees the counter-thought. This intensifies itself and becomes so rapid that one doesn't really know which was the first." A less sophisticated patient, whom I had made aware of the fact that in reply to a very friendly letter from his wife he had written her a farewell letter stated: "I could have just as well written another letter; to say good-bye or to say good-bye; it is all the same."

One can easily demonstrate that the patients do not note contradictions when we take their negative answers for positive ones. I asked a patient: "Do you hear 'voices'?" He definitely denied it. I continued: "What do they say to you?" "Oh, all sorts of things." He may even offer an example of what they say. More often it is obvious from the speech and behavior of the patients that they think a thought and its converse simultaneously, though it may not always be as conspicuous as in the following sentence: "She had no handkerchief; she choked it with the handkerchief." The expression of an idea by its opposite falls into the same category: a patient complains that the master-key to the wards was taken away from him, whereas he really wants that the key be given to him. In Schreber's "special language," "reward" means "punishment," and "poison" means "food," etc.

The three forms of ambivalence are not easily distinguished from one another as these examples illustrate. Affectivity and will are merely different facets of the same function; even the intellectual contradictions often cannot be separated from the affective. A mixture of megalomania with delusions of persecution and inferiority may result from wishes and fears, or from assertion and denial of one's own stature. The patient is especially powerful and at the same time powerless; the beloved or the protector becomes just as easily the persecutor without surrendering his previous role. It is more exceptional for the enemy to become the friend and ally. A Catholic paranoid patient had joined the Old-Catholic sect. He claimed to be persecuted by the Pope who nevertheless wanted to shower the patient with millions of dollars. Similarly, many patients complain about persecution but really believe that the persecution serves for their education, improvement, and as a preliminary step to their elevation to some higher rank or station.

Ambivalence shows every gradation down to negativism, particularly in the form of "Ambitendenz." We will see later that this is of significance in the structure of delusions.

The intact simple functions

In contrast to the organic psychoses, we find in schizophrenia, at least with our present methods of examination, that sensation, memory, consciousness and motility are not directly disturbed. A very far advanced disease process may perhaps alter even these functions; but in those patients in whom such disturbances do appear we cannot differentiate these changes from the secondary alterations which are seen at times. The anomalies we know in those areas are all secondary, and thus merely accidental phenomena. Although at times they may dominate the whole clinical picture (as for example, the hallucinations), they are to be classified as "accessory" symptoms.

In the literature we find much discussion of alterations in these functions. They are based for the most part on the misconception of the patients' negativism, indifference, and reluctance to think, and above all on their random responses. These and similar sources of error led Masselon (457, p. 115) to say that the patients are rarely able to give the year, month or day, and often do not even know the season of the year. The physician must always use indirect methods to obtain correct information concerning the actual knowledge that a patient may possess. Never must one conclude from merely negative answers that a patient does not know what is asked of him. The simple question concerning the year is very often answered incorrectly; whereas the same patient, when he has occasion to write a letter, shows himself fully oriented as to the date. A patient coming to us from prison does not "know" the year is 1899 but immediately afterwards admits that it was in 1897 that she went to prison and "remained there for two years."

Disturbances and defects are very often falsely diagnosed because the examiner and the patient do not really speak the same language. The patient takes symbolically what the physician understands in its literal sense. Thus a patient insisted that he could not see, that he was blind, while it was more than obvious that his eyesight was unimpaired. What he meant was that he did not perceive things "as reality." A female patient insisted with the greatest firmness, in answer to the question as to how long she had been in the hospital, that she had been there only three days, although she had given many proofs of her normal temporal orientation and had been in the institution for many weeks. This time-period of "three days" was for her identical with "my whole life." She herself was able to give the explanation: that the "first day" corresponded to the one in her earliest youth when she had been morally delinquent; the "second day" corresponded to that on which she had done the same thing as a grown-up young woman; the "third day" had not yet been brought to completion. This last idea was in unmistakable reference to the fact that she had transferred her love onto the resident physician. Just as often, we encounter the reverse phenomenon: a figurative phrase is taken in its literal sense by the patient.

It is especially important to know that these patients carry on a kind of "double-entry bookkeeping" in many of their relationships. They know the real state of affairs as well as the falsified one and will answer according to the circumstances with one kind or the other type of orientation—or both together. This last is especially frequent in misrecognizing people: the physician "is now here as Dr. N.," at other times he becomes the former lover.

The Compound Functions

The complex functions which result from the coordinated operations of the functions previously discussed, such as attention, intelligence, will, and action, are, of course, disturbed to the extent that the elementary (simple) functions on which they depend are altered. Only association and affectivity have to be considered here. However, schizophrenia is characterized by a very peculiar alteration of the relation between the patient's inner life and the external world. The inner life assumes pathological predominance (autism).

Relation to reality: Autism

The most severe schizophrenics, who have no more contact with the outside world, live in a world of their own. They have encased themselves with their desires and wishes (which they consider fulfilled) or occupy themselves with the trials and tribulations of their persecutory ideas; they have cut themselves off as much as possible from any contact with the external world.

This detachment from reality, together with the relative and absolute predominance of the inner life, we term autism.

In less severe cases, the affective and logical significance of reality is only somewhat damaged. The patients are still able to move about in the external world but neither evidence nor logic have any influence on their hopes and delusions. Everything which is in contradiction to their complexes simply does not exist for their thinking or feeling.

An intelligent lady who for many years was mistaken for a neurasthenic "had built a wall around herself so closely confining that she often felt as if she actually were in a chimney." An otherwise socially acceptable woman patient sings at a concert, but unfortunately once started she cannot stop. The audience begins to whistle and hoot and create a disturbance; she does not bother a bit, but continues singing and feels quite satisfied when she finally ends. A well-educated young woman, whose illness is hardly noticeable suddenly moves her bowels before a whole social gathering and cannot comprehend the embarrassment which she causes among her friends. During the course of about ten years, a patient gave me from time to time a note on which the same four words were always written and which signified that he had been unjustly incarcerated. It did not make any difference to him if he handed me a half-dozen of these notes at the same time. He did not understand the senselessness of his action when one discussed it with him. Withal, this patient showed good judgment about other patients and worked independently in his ward. Very frequently schizophrenics will give us numerous letters without expecting any answer; or they will ask us a dozen questions one after the other without even giving us time to answer. They predict an event for a certain day, but are so little bothered when the prophecy does not come to pass that they do not even seek to find explanations. Even where reality has apparently become identical with the patient's pathological creations, it will often be ignored.

The wishes and desires of many patients revolve around their release from the hospital. Yet they remain indifferent to the actual discharge. One of our patients who has a marked complex about children made an attempt to murder his wife because she only bore him four children in ten years. Yet he is quite indifferent to the children themselves. Other paitents are in love with someone. If this person is actually present, he makes no impression on them at all; if he dies, they do not care. One patient constantly begs to be given the key to the door of his ward. When it is finally given to him, he does not know what to do with it and returns it almost at once. He tries a thousand times each day to open the door. If it is left unlocked, he becomes embarrassed and does not know what to do. He continuously pursues the doctor at each of his visits with the words: "Please, Doctor." Asked what he desires, he appears surprised and has nothing further to say. A woman patient asked to see her doctor. When she was summoned to the interview, she at last was able after a few minutes of perplexity to make her wishes known by pointing to his wedding ring. For weeks on end, a mother exerts every means at her command to see her child. When permission is granted her, she prefers to have a glass of wine. For years a woman longs for a divorce from her husband. When at long last she gets her divorce, she refuses to believe in it at all, and becomes furious if she is not addressed by her husband's name. Many a patient consumes himself with anxiety over his imminent death but will not take the least precaution for his self-preservation and remains totally unmoved in the face of real danger to his life.

Autism is not always to be detected at the very first glance. Initially the behavior of many patients betrays nothing remarkable. It is only on prolonged observation that one sees how much they always seek their own way, and how very little they permit their environment to influence them. Even severe chronic patients show quite good contact with their environment with regard to indifferent, everyday affairs. They chatter, participate in games, seek out stimulation—but they are always selective. They keep their complexes to themselves, never saying a word about them and not wishing to have them touched upon in any way from the outside.

Thus the indifference of patients toward what would be considered their nearest and dearest interest becomes understandable. Other things are of far greater importance to them. They do not react any more to influences from the outside. They appear "stuporous" even where no other disturbance inhibits their will or actions. The external world must often appear to them as rather hostile since it tends to disturb them in their fantasies. However, there are also cases where the shutting off from the outside world is caused by contrary reasons. Particularly in the beginning of their illness, these patients quite consciously shun any contact with reality because their affects are so powerful that they must avoid everything which might arouse their emotions. The apathy toward the outer world is then a secondary one springing from a hypertrophied sensitivity.

Autism is also manifested by many patients externally. (Naturally, this is, as a rule, unintentional.) Not only do they not concern themselves with anything around them, but they sit around with faces constantly averted, looking at a blank wall; or they shut off their sensory portals by drawing a skirt or bed clothes over their heads. Indeed, formerly, when the patients were mostly abandoned to their own devices, they could often be found in bent-over, squatting positions, an indication that they were trying to restrict as much as possible of the sensory surface area of their skin.

Misunderstandings stemming from the autistic thought processes can hardly ever, or only with great difficulty, be corrected by the patients.

A hebephrenic lies on a bench in a thoroughly vile mood. As she catches sight of me, she attempts to sit up. I beg her not to disturb herself. She answers in an irritated tone that if she could sit up she would not be lying down, apparently imagining that I was reproaching her for lying on the bench. Several times, using different words, I repeat the suggestion that she remain lying quietly as she was. She merely becomes more and more irritated. Everything I say is interpreted falsely by her in the sense and direction of her autistic train of thought.

The autistic world has as much reality for the patient as the true one, but his is a different kind of reality. Frequently, they cannot keep the two kinds of reality separated from each other even though they can make the distinction in principle. A patient heard us speaking of a certain Dr. N. Immediately afterwards he asks whether it was a hallucination or whether we had spoken of a Dr. N.—Busch (doing reading experiments) has demonstrated the very poor ability of patients to differentiate between idea and perception.

The reality of the autistic world may also seem more valid than that of reality itself; the patients then hold their fantasy world for the real, reality for an illusion. They no longer believe in the evidence of their own senses. Schreber described his attendants as "miracled up, changeable individuals." The patient may be very aware that other people judge the environment differently. He also knows that he himself sees it in that form but it is not *real* to him. "They say, that you are the doctor, but I don't know it," or even, "But you are really Minister N." To a considerable extent, reality is transformed through illusions and largely replaced by hallucinations (twilight states, *Dämmerzustände*).

In the usual hallucinatory conditions, more validity is, as a rule, ascribed to the illusions; yet the patients continue to act and orient themselves in accordance with reality. Many of them, however, no longer act at all, not even in accordance with their autistic thinking. This may occur in stuporous conditions, or the autism itself may reach such a high degree of intensity, that the patients' actions lose all relation to the blocked-off reality. The sick person deals with the real world as little as the normal person deals with his dreams. Frequently both disturbances, the stuporous immobility and the exclusion of reality, occur simultaneously.

Patients who show no clouding of consciousness often appear much less autistic than they really are because they are able to suppress their autistic thoughts or, like certain hysterics, seem to be occupied with them only in a theoretical way, and ordinarily allow them only very little influence upon their actions. These patients rarely remain under our observation for very long because we are inclined to discharge them as improved or cured.

A complete and constant exclusion of the external world appears, if at all, only in the most severe degree of stupor. In milder cases the real and the autistic worlds exist not only side by side, but often become entangled with one another in the most illogical manner. The doctor is at one moment not only the hospital-physician and at another the shoemaker S., but he is both in the same thought-content of the patient. A patient who was still fairly well-mannered and capable of work, made herself a rag-doll which she considered to be the child of her imaginary lover. When this "lover" of hers made a trip to Berlin, she wanted to send "the child" after him, as a precautionary measure. But she first went to the police, to ask whether it would be considered as illegal to send "the child" as luggage instead of on a passenger ticket.

Wishes and fears constitute the contents of autistic thinking. In those rare cases where the contradictions to reality are not felt at all, it is the wishes alone which are involved; fears appear when the patient senses the obstacles to the fulfillment of his wishes. Even where no true delusions arise autism is demonstrable in the patients' inability to cope with reality, in their inappropriate reactions to outside influences (irritability), and in their lack of resistance to every and any idea and urge.

In the same way as autistic feeling is detached from reality, autistic thinking obeys its own special laws. To be sure, autistic thinking makes use of the customary logical connections insofar as they are suitable but it is in no way bound to such logical laws.

Autistic thinking is directed by affective needs; the patient thinks in symbols, in analogies, in fragmentary concepts, in accidental connections. Should the same patient turn back to reality he may be able to think sharply and logically.

Thus we have to distinguish between realistic and autistic thinking which exist side by side in the same patient. In realistic thinking the patient orients himself quite well in time and space. He adjusts his actions to reality insofar as they appear normal. The autistic thinking is the source of the delusions, of the crude offenses against logic and propriety, and all the other pathological symptoms. The two forms of thought are often fairly well separated so that the patient is able at times to think completely autistically and at other times completely normally. In other cases the two forms mix, going on to complete fusion, as we saw in the cases cited above.

The patient need not become conscious of the peculiarity, of the deviation of his autistic thinking from his previous realistic type of thinking. However, the more intelligent patients may for years gauge the difference. They experience the autistic state as painful; only rarely as pleasurable. They complain that reality seems different from what it was before. Things and people are no longer what they are supposed to be. They are changed, strange, no longer have any relationship to the patient. A released patient described it, "as if she were running around in an open grave, so strange did the world appear." Another "had started to think herself into an entirely different life. By comparison, everything was quite different; even her sweetheart was not the way she had imagined him." A still very intelligent woman patient considered it a change for the better that, at will, she could transpose herself into a state of the greatest (sexual and religious) bliss. She even wanted to give us instructions to enable us to do likewise.

Autism must not be confused with "the unconscious." Both autistic, and realistic thinking can be conscious as well as unconscious.

The Significance of Individual Symptoms for the Differential Diagnosis

With respect to intellectual symptoms, disturbances of perception, orientation, and memory, in the sense that they were previously defined, never belong to schizophrenia; whereas they prove the existence of some other psychosis, they do not exclude the possibility of schizophrenia. On the other hand, definite schizophrenic disturbances of association alone are sufficient for the diagnosis.

In healthy persons and other non-schizophrenics blockings are transitory phenomena for which there are always some definite reasons that can be discovered. In schizophrenics, the blocks mostly prove themselves insurmountable; their psychological roots are often not easily discerned, and they have a tendency to generalize themselves, i.e., they are also found outside their connection with the complexes. However, it is sometimes impossible to differentiate a hysterical blocking from a schizophrenic one at a given moment. Furthermore, one must not confuse the emotional stupor, which in imbeciles, particularly, may last for weeks, with the pathological symptom.

The systematic splitting, with reference to personality, for example, may be found in many other psychotic conditions; in hysteria they are even more marked than in schizophrenia (multiple personalities). Definite splitting, however, in the sense that various personality fragments exist side by side in a state of clear orientation as to environment, will only be found in our disease.

Autism in itself cannot be utilized for the diagnosis since it occurs in hysterical dream states, especially, and since it dominates also in some way the delusional ideas of the paretic. In the non-schizophrenic cases, the symptom has a somewhat different appearance, but it is difficult to describe that difference. Epileptics and organic cases simply withdraw into themselves when they assume attitudes which resemble autism, whereas the schizophrenics place themselves in conflict with and opposition to reality. Moreover, in non-schizophrenics, the isolation from the outside world is not as complete as in our patients; under certain circumstances, non-schizophrenics may not take an active interest in reality, but they immediately establish rapport with it when they are addressed, for example.

Obscurity of concepts is also a partial phenomenon of other diseases; however, if it has progressed so far that different persons or things are identified with each other in a state of clear consciousness, we must assume schizophrenia with certainty. Transitivism may also be observed in non-schizophrenics, but only when they are in a state of clouded consciousness. Isolated neologisms are of no significance from the standpoint of diagnosis (epilepsy), but if someone expresses an essential part of his thoughts in new words, he is schizophrenic. As a joke, a manic person may speak in a selfmade language, with no thought of making himself understood. The schizophrenic speaks his "artificial language" in the same way as we use our habitual idiom, but it does not matter to him whether or not he is understood.

The absence of ability for discussion is nowhere as conspicuous as in schizophrenics. Even when our patients agree to discuss their false notions, we regularly find alongside of correct and cleverly defended ideas others which are simply "so," as the patients like to say, and where entirely senseless deductions are made. The schizophrenic can split off facts which do not suit his affects; the obstinate person will just ignore them.

The expression of sudden ideas, especially when they are at the same time senseless or in contradiction to the rest of the personality, is a fairly reliable sign of schizophrenia.

The schizophrenic type of attention is often unmistakable; despite a complete lack of interest, the passive registration of external events functions perfectly. I have observed this phenomenon only in schizophrenia.

As for hallucination, it is important to note their preference for the auditory sphere and for body-sensations (cave: neuritic phenomena which can stimulate body hallucinations.) Where delusions of physical persecutions, and auditory hallucinations continually dominate the clinical picture, one can practically always conclude that one is dealing with schizophrenia. The phenomenon of thoughts being heard (*Gedankenlautwerden*) occurs only very rarely in other psychoses. The isolation of the hallucinations from the realistic content of consciousness is also characteristic.

Schizophrenic hallucinations surely have still other characteristic peculiarities. But I do not venture to elaborate on them here because we know too little about the other hallucinatory psychoses.

Delusions often characterize themselves as schizophrenic merely by their content. Their senseless, poorly thought out, and fragmentary quality cannot be mistaken. Yet similar delusional ideas often occur in organic diseases (e.g. the hypochondriacal delusions of a depressed paretic) but the differences are not easily described. It is most indicative of schizophrenia when the delusions are not at all developed, when they are in strongest contrast to the simplest reality, and yet are expressed during periods of apparently clear consciousness. When a person continually produces entirely illogical ideas of persecution in a state of full clarity of consciousness he is nearly always a schizophrenic; if the characteristic hallucinations are also present, the diagnosis is certain.

The delusion that everyone already knows what the patient is thinking is almost pathognomonic.

The schizophrenic para-functioning and a-functioning of affectivity are decisive signs of our psychosis if we succeed in differentiating them from other forms of indifference. Persistent indifference toward vital interests is schizophrenic, even though with respect to less important issues we may find a normal emotional response. Since there are different average levels of affectivity, it is important to be alert not so much for minor deviations of mood in the direction of indifference as for the lack of capacity to modulate these moods. If the patient remains quantitatively and qualitatively rigid with regard to the same feelings, even though he responds to ideas of varying values, it would indicate schizophrenia. In mild cases, however, this symptom may be absent, or it may acquire similarity to the indifference of hysterics.

An especially important and often very early sign is the unmotivated affect-less laughter. It is not easily mistaken for the laughter-spasms of nervous people.

As is well known, catatonic symptoms do not solely occur in schizophrenia. At least, it is still impossible to differentiate them always from similar conditions in organic psychoses. However, if they are very pronounced, and in the majority, schizophrenia is to be assumed.

Flexibilitas cerea (waxy catalepsy) is seen outside of catatonia in organic diseases. In addition, it occurs in epilepsy usually at the conclusion of attacks, occasionally in hysterics and perhaps in fever psychoses, certainly in the fever conditions of children. The rigid form of catalepsy is found more often in organic brain diseases of all kinds and in epilepsy. In such cases, however, the rigidity is generally independent of attempts at passive movements, whereas in the schizophrenic such attempts usually provoke or add to the muscle tone.

The other forms of command-automatism can probably occur in various states of non-schizophrenics, characterized by lack of will power; perhaps we can also find echopraxia, although in our cases it is extremely rare outside of schizophrenia. We encounter it occasionally in the form of echolalia in focal brain diseases, however, on a different psychological basis.

In practice, negativism cannot yet be separated from other forms of rejection. All kinds of healthy as well as sick persons become negativistic when they happen to be in a bad mood. If this mood is combined with obscure ideas concerning the environment as is so often the case with epileptics and organic patients, it can easily be mistaken for negativism. On the other hand, the simple resistance of anxious patients has rather the character of a gesture of flight and defense; it can be influenced by the physician's attitude and sometimes simply by friendly reassurance. These characteristics are absent in the schizophrenic who strikes us by contrast with his extraordinary indifference towards actual attacks made on his person. It is more difficult to distinguish negativism from a simple hostile attitude regarding the external world since hostile opposition towards the environment is one of the main roots of negativism. Negativism may also exist alongside, as well as independently, of such attitudes on the part of the patient; it is then often difficult to separate the two elements. Adamant and unreasonable negativism however, occurs very seldom in patients other than schizophrenics. Nevertheless, we must remember that even genuine negativism is not necessarily generalized and that it may manifest or conceal itself only under specific conditions or with respect to certain persons. Obstinacy, which also rests on a kind of exaggerated autism, differs from negativism in that the latter is a general symptom and that it remains entirely alien to normal feelings in most of its expressions.

Stereotypies are most common in schizophrenics, but they are not wholly absent in other types of patients and even in normal people. However, most catatonic stereotypies differ from the others in their senselessness and in their lack of correspondence with the patients' feelings and thoughts. Verbigeration is generally easily differentiated from poverty of ideas and perseveration (in organics), both of which may cause word repetition, if one only considers the possibility of these different symptoms. The stereotyped attitude of paretics is most commonly confused with catatonic symptoms.

When dealing with "mannerisms," one must also be alert for the exaggerated, the inappropriate, etc. To some degree, mannerisms are frequently present in healthy individuals as well as in the mentally ill. Once our attention is brought to bear on them, tics are usually easily differentiated. If the mannerisms are very pronounced, they constitute an important point of differentiation from other diseases.

Stupor which also occurs in organic brain diseases, in manic-depressive psychosis, epilepsy, and hysteria can as such only be utilized for the diagnosis, if the schizophrenic genesis of the stupor (blocking, autism, etc.) can either be proven of excluded. Furthermore, a stupor is probably always schizophrenic if the patient appears to be in a state of clear consciousness and carefully observes his environment. It is also important to keep in mind that Gross was unable to detect in his cases of catatonic stupor disturbances of comprehension or evidence of motor inhibitions.

In acute attacks of any kind the diagnosis is made on the basis of the presence of the specific schizophrenic symptoms. The experienced specialist can often make the diagnosis by evaluating solely the overall impression he receives from the patient; indeed, the disease is so common that he runs a very small risk if he uses some caution. However, by using such methods of diagnosis one deprives oneself of the opportunity to detect in time the more unusual states of agitation which do not yet fit into the framework of the diseases. Furthermore, complete certainty as to the diagnosis can only be gained by establishing proof of the existence of decisive symptoms. Up to now, I have observed exclusively in schizophrenia sudden remissions in the midst of an acute episode. During these remissions the patient behaves as if nothing unusual had happened in spite of the fact that his memory is intact. The clouded, mentally inert states (*Benommenbeit*) are naturally difficult to investigate. They are schizophrenic if we can prove that the degree of what we call "the clouded state" is out of any proportion to the actual obstruction of thinking, in so far as the patients still observe and register everything going on around them.

INTRODUCTION

Much has been written on the historical aspects of dementia praecox and schizophrenia and most of it by psychiatrists (Guiraud, 1968; Rieder, 1974; Scharfetter, 1975; Corbett, 1978; Raskin, 1975; Hoenig, 1983; Lantéri-Laura and Gros, 1982). The Morel–Kraepelin–Bleuler–Schneider genealogy is rehearsed *ad nauseam* although it is historically inaccurate (Midenet, 1972; Baruk, 1973).

We have inherited a view of the disease which remains descriptive and in the absence of biological markers tautological. The bequeathed concepts enshrine partially overlapping clusters of symptoms obtained from observing patient populations that are no more. The displacement undergone by the semiological boundaries of schizophrenia is therefore so marked that there may be little in common between Kraepelin's or Bleuler's old notions and the symptom constellation forced upon us by DSM III.

THE HISTORICAL MYTH

Bleuler has been regarded, like Pinel once was, as the initiator of a new tradition. He is seen as a humanitarian psychiatrist who broke away from the bad old days, psychologized madness and slayed the organicist dragon. If not releasing the madman from his chains at least he freed him from the inhuman psychiatry of the 19th century. However attractive this view may be it is anhistorical. Like Pinel a hundred years earlier, Bleuler is but the culmination of a historical process which, starting with Royer Collard, Moreau de Tours, Falret, Magnan, Brentano, Jackson and Freud, had been seeking ways of introducing psychological concepts into the definition of madness (Berrios, 1984). However poetic Bleuler's descriptions might be they are steeped in subjectivity. The schneiderian backlash put an end to his concept of schizophrenia.

THE BOOK

The excerpts reproduced here have been taken from a book published in 1911 but commissioned probably as early as 1906. It appeared as part of an impressive set of thirteen volumes edited by Gustav Aschaffenburg under the general title *Handbuch der Psychiatrie* and published by Franz Deuticke from Leipzig and Vienna. It is something of a historical problem to explain why other volumes, equally erudite and clinically fresh never made it. For example Aschaffenburg's two monographs on the *General Psychopathology* and on the *Classification of the Psychoses*, Stransky's on *Manic Depressive Insanity* and Redlich's on *Psychoses Related to Brain Disease* are supreme representatives of their genre. The only other volume more or less well known is Bonhöffer's *Exogenous Psychoses*.

Dementia praecox oder Gruppe der Schizophrenien was fourth in the section dedicated to 'Special Psychiatry'; with 420 pages it is one of the longest in the collection. Joseph Zinkin's 1950 English version is competent but his choice of some technical terms has been disputed (Gilman, 1983; Meduna and McCulloch, 1945). It was not Bleuler's first book nor indeed his first writing on dementia praecox. The main ideas in the book seem to have been the result of a collective intellectual effort in the Burghözli Hospital of the first decade of the 20th century (Bleuler, 1951). For example Jung's monograph (1907) on the *Psychology of Dementia Praecox* contains concepts which were to appear later in Bleuler's book (1911). The work atmosphere in this famous hospital seems to have been one of febrile enthusiasm, with dedicated residents doing two or more rounds a day, typing their own case notes in the evening and living an almost monastic life (Ellenberger, 1970).

Bleuler was one of the first asylum psychiatrists to apply Freudian concepts to the psychoses. The conflictive presence of Carl Gustav Jung, who had been working in the hospital since 1900, completes, with Freud and Bleuler, an important intellectual triangle whose relevance to the contents of the book has not yet been fully assessed.

He was born on 30 April 1857 in Zollikon, a small village near Zürich. Of peasant stock, his family seem to have been involved in the struggle for peasants' rights that culminated in the foundation of Zürich University in 1833 (Brill, 1939; Zilboorg, 1939; Various Authors, 1941; Klaesi, 1956; Ellenberger, 1970). It is said that the sight of professors of psychiatry imported from Germany (Griesinger was one of them) not understanding the local dialect of the patients inspired Bleuler to become a psychiatrist. Trained under Burckhardt and Schaerer at Waldau, Charcot and Magnan in Paris, the von Gudden Institute in Munich and then Forel at the Burghölzli, he became its director in 1898. He retired in 1927 and died on 15 July 1939. Abraham, Binswanger, Jung, Brill, Minkowski and many others went through is hands. Apart from the work on schizophrenia he published an important monograph on *Suggestibility, Affectivity and Paranoia* (1906), a psychiatric textbook (1916) and a large number of papers.

THE CONCEPTS

Bleuler's views on dementia praecox developed gradually but crystallized some time before the monograph was published (Bleuler, 1908; Bleuler and Jung, 1980).

The factors that shaped Bleuler's notion of schizophrenia are many: Kraepelin's definition (that Bleuler professed to continue), Associationism and Faculty Psychology, the psychodynamic Zeitgeist, his ample clinical experience and probably the nationalistic redefinition of swiss psychiatry vis-à-vis its German counterpart (Haenel, 1982). Very early Bleuler (1902) had acknowledged that both the concept and the description of dementia praecox stemmed from Kraepelin. In his monograph (1911) he went on to justify his preference for the word schizophrenia (which he had used for the first time in 1908) on the view that the old term had become too fatalistic and was often taken literally (i.e. as dementia affecting the young) (p. 4).

But as is often the case a change in name led to a change in the descriptive metaphor. The notion of 'Splitting' (Spaltung) was at the basis of the neologism. The view that mental functions could be split asunder was very popular during this period. The concepts of 'Intrapsychic ataxia' (Stransky, 1903), 'Discordance' (Chaslin, 1912) and 'Sejunction' (Wernicke, 1894) also carried a similar referent and shared a common conceptual pedigree: faculty psychology. Under the influence of Herbart a view of the mind as a harmonious set of functions had once again become popular (Jülicher, 1961). Any disharmony would create disorder and this led to madness (Berrios, 1985b).

Characteristically Kraepelin (1919) refrained from producing a speculative pathophysiology of dementia praecox; instead he offered a description, a natural history and a prognosis. To others the temptation to fill the gap between causes and symptoms remained irresistible and since the 1860s 'mediating hypotheses', both 'mechanistic' and 'experiential' had been tried. Amongst the former, speculative neurophysiology was a popular choice (Luys, 1876; Meynert 1884; Carpenter, 1879); amongst the latter the preference was for emotional experiences; these were made into symbolic representations of processes occurring beyond awareness and endowed with causal power. For good or evil psychodynamic notions of the latter type won the day. All symptoms of schizophrenia were 'psychologized' including forms of behaviour that until then had been considered as neurophysiological dysfunctions short-circuiting awareness. For example, the disorders of motility (stereotypies, echo phenomena) were no longer to be considered as a pathology of motor behaviour but of the will (Lagriffe, 1913). According to the new explanation the 'ideoemotional complex' became the real 'origin' of the movement. Casualties to this interpretation fell not only catatonic symptomatology but also the motor behaviour of encephalitis lethargica and Parkinson's disease (Berrios, 1987b).

Since from the historical viewpoint the concept of 'Spaltung' was not new (Scharfetter, 1975) it would be useful to understand its success in the hands of Bleuler. One reason may be that he offered it in the superior 'envelope' of his considerable knowledge and experience. In fact the clinical architecture of the book does not suffer if all reference to 'splitting' is deleted.

According to Bleuler there are fundamental and accessory symptoms. The former are caused by organic factors (e.g. toxins), the latter by psychological mechanisms and hence are understandable (Bleuler, 1984). This dichotomous way of analysing symptoms was developed by Monroe and Reynolds in the 1850s and taken up by Jackson and Ribot in the 1880s (Berrios, 1985a). In neurology it allowed the separation of symptoms into those caused by deficit and those resulting from disinhibited functions. Bleuler made it play a similar role: some symptoms resulted from organic deficit, others from psychological disorganization. Jung resorted to a similar model (Bleuler and Jung, 1908; Giraud, 1985).

Associationism and Faculty Psychology were equally important to the Bleulerian hypothesis. According to the ancient theory of Associationism, psychological functions (whether cognition, emotion or volition) can be analysed into units and have their combinatorial rules worked out. It had been in fluctuating vogue since the time of Hobbes and Locke (Warren, 1921; Hoeldtke, 1967). Popular again during the 18th century in the work of Condillac and Hartley, it underwent temporary eclipse during the rise of Faculty Psychology with Kant, Reid, Stewart and Hamilton (Albrecht, 1970; Brooks, 1976). Resuscitated again by the Mills, Herbart, Bain and Spencer and later Weber, Fechner, Donders and Wundt it reigned supreme during the second half of the 19th century. Psychophysics and experimental psychology would not have developed without the assistance of Association- ism (Boring, 1950). The concept of 'loosening of associations' results from the direct application of the associationistic metaphor. As thoughts become disconnected from one another chaos ensues. The bizarre and superficially incomprehensible nature of thought disorder is a manifestation of this pathology. Bleuler and Jung (1908) developed word association tests for the quantification of thought disorder in schizophrenia (Leys, 1985).

The 'loosening of associations' was considered by Bleuler to be 'toxic' in origin. The behavioural and experiential chaos that followed however he did not consider as entropic or meaningless; instead he allowed himself to become trapped in the Freudian web of total comprehensibility. Jaspers (1963) was rather critical of this view: 'in the most literal sense of the term they (Bleuler and Jung) have rediscovered the "meaning of madness" or at least they believe they have' (p. 410).

Bleuler's fundamental symptoms are too abstract and subjective in nature to allow operationalization and can be reduced *ad absurdum* with facility. And so they were by Minkowski (1927): 'in a number of respects I differ from Bleuler, particularly, under the influence of Bergson, I see the initial defect in schizophrenia not as a loosening of associations but as the loss of vital contact with reality' (p. 13).

Bleuler made use of the concept of 'complex' to explain the disturbance of emotions in the patient with schizophrenia; indeed it was once believed that Bleuler and Jung had created this notion; in fact the term had already been used by Breuer in 1895 (Laplanche and Pontalis, 1973). The introduction of 'complexes' as explanations created some debate. Hesnard (1914) was sympathetic but Kraepelin remains sceptical: 'Bleuler brings forward the view that in such states it is usually a case of contact with the "complexes", the sensitive traumata of life. I have not been able to convince myself of that. . .' (p. 35). Kurt Schneider (1959) for all his a-theoretical pretensions wrote: 'The everyday reactions of schizophrenics are often quite normal outwardly, provided the daily circumstances and conversation do not touch upon the particular psychotic content (complexes)' (p. 127).

It is in relation to the 'complex' that Bleuler's interest in Freudian ideas becomes particularly important as the explanatory force of this concept can only operate in the presence of psychodynamic machinery: it requires an inner space in which to reside an energy to be released; all this Bleuler obtained from the Freudian model (Proceedings, 1965; Ellenberger, 1970). Early on he had written a favourable review of Freud's *Studies on Hysteria* (Bleuler, 1896) and in 1900, soon after the publication of the *Interpretation of Dreams* he had asked Jung to read and comment upon the book in the weekly seminar at the Burghölzli. It is said that this was Jung's first contact with Freudian ideas.

From then on Bleuler and Jung endeavoured to understand psychotic behaviour in psychodynamic terms. But differences of interpretation soon began to appear as evidenced by the divergent views expressed in their joint paper on 'Complexes and causes of dementia praecox' (Bleuler and Jung, 1908). Whilst Bleuler stated that the complexes are not the cause of the illness but only modulate its manifestations, Jung went as far as saying that 'the complex not only determines the content of the symptom but also its cause' (Giraud, 1985). Bleuler's interest in psychoanalysis seems to have been selective and it is known that he refused to joint the International Psychoanalytic Association (Ellenberger, 1970).

His separation from Jung seems to have been a disagreeable affair. The ambitious and difficult personality of the latter caused increasing conflict after 1907. Often overtly aggressive towards Bleuler and frustrated by his failure to get a chair in Zürich, Jung abandoned the hospital in 1909 to dedicate himself to private practice (Ellenberger, 1970).

THE FUNDAMENTAL SYMPTOMS

The excerpts presented here also include Bleuler's description of the fundamental symptoms (Grundsymptome), both 'simple' and 'compound'. The former he defines as alterations of 'simple functions' (einfachen Funktionen). The term 'simple' already in psychiatric use during his period (e.g. 'simple dementia' in Diem, 1903) he leaves undefined. Bleuler's simple 'functions' ('Assoziationen, Affektivität und Ambivalenz') name mental states belonging to different levels of psychological organization: 'associations' are hypothetical constructs that explain how thoughts are glued together; 'affectivity' names a traditional mental faculty and 'ambivalence' a particular pathological state affecting all three faculties. This confusion is Bleuler's own and does not originate from the continental psychology of the period (Ziehen, 1909; Höffding, 1892; Klemm, 1911). He seems to have been one of the first psychiatrists to use the term 'Affektivität' in a very wide sense to designate: 'not only affects in the proper sense, but the slight feelings or feeling-tones of pleasure and unpleasure in every possible circumstance' (p. 6). Jung became particularly interested in this concept and in his 1908 monograph made it central to his 'psychological' account of dementia praecox.

Bleuler's favourite psychopathological mechanisms remained 'Splitting' (Spaltung) and 'Indifference' (Gleichgültigkeit). The former he made responsible for both the production of 'Association' disturbances and of 'Ambivalence'; the latter for the pathology of 'Affectivity' (Bleuler, 1911, p. 32). The status of these mechanisms is unclear and they seem to be but hypothetical constructs whose ghostly existence can be ascertained only by observing their behavioural manifestations.

The second set of fundamental symptoms Bleuler called 'Compound' functions (zusammengesetzten Funktionen) and includes autism, attention, will, person, schizophrenic dementia and activity and behaviour. At this stage all attempts at psychological classification are abandoned and the disorders become itemized descriptions.

DIFFERENTIAL DIAGNOSIS

Bleuler expressed clear preference for the presence of fundamental symptoms as indications of disease. But he warned about their marked variation in severity and the need to exercise a high level of suspicion in their identification. This was bound to affect the specificity of the diagnosis and cause an inordinate increase in false positives. This results in a pliable and overwide concept of schizophrenia. Bleuler was aware of this but did not mind. In his 'Lehrbuch' (1916) under the heading 'what is included under the term' (p. 436) he listed in fact most of the psychoses. This state of affairs was noticed by his contemporaries. Trénel (1912), in the first important French review of the 1911 monograph stated that Bleuler had: 'forced diseases which are absolutely different into a vast synthesis. . .in terms of what is currently known about psychology Bleuler has abused psychological analysis to the detriment of clinical observation. . .it seems as if he intended to outline a condition but only managed to outline a group ("genre") of conditions'. . . (furthermore) his coining a new name has simply been an exercise in: 'replacing a word with aetiological pretentions (dementia praecox) by another with psychopathological pretentions' (schizophrenia) (pp. 382–383). This attitude of rejection was widespread in France (Claude et al., 1924).

THE AFTERMATH

Bleuler's book has been influential. Apart from its obvious qualities—erudition, clinical richness, and theoretical competence—the timing of its publication was right. It suggested itself as a convenient compromise to a psychiatric community loyal to the old neuropsychiatry and yet genuinely interested in the new psychodynamic movement. The book contains the best of asylum psychiatry but also incorporates the new psychogenetic views. It made most symptoms 'understandable' (Jaspers, 1963) and offered an optimistic prognosis for the disease. Bleuler realized this and wrote at least two papers on early discharge from hospital (Bleuler, 1905, 1914). He also emphasized the role of environmental variables: 'but nowhere as much as in schizophrenia are all symptoms to be evaluated in terms of their entire psychic environment' (Bleuler, 1916; p. 438).

Another reason for the book's success may have been the fact that Bleuler's earlier publications created a sense of anticipation. In addition the book was always well sponsored not least by the laudable and persistent preoccupation with schizophrenia that has inspired the Burghölzli Hospital ever since.

The book was widely quoted both on the Continent and in the USA (where it was particularly influential). Rather surprisingly therefore the English translation took a long time to appear. Into French it was never fully rendered although Henry Ey translated fragments which, as he said, brought him into close contact with the essence of madness. The Spanish translation (1960) is but a rendition of the English one. There do not seem to exist complete translations in other languages.

Whatever the language, Bleuler's great book will have an assured existence, not so much for its theoretical speculations but for the beauty and rare quality of its clinical descriptions.

G. E. Berrios

REFERENCES

Albrecht, F. M. (1970). A reappraisal of faculty psychology, *J. Hist. Behav. Sci.* **6**, 36–40.
Baruk, H. (1973). Descriptive psychopathology: conceptual and historical aspects, *Psychological Medicine,* **14**, 303–313.
Berrios, G. E. (1985a). Positive and negative symptoms and Jackson: a conceptual history, *Arch. Gen. Psychiat.,* **42**, 95–97.
Berrios, G. E. (1985b). The psychopathology of affectivity: conceptual and historical aspects, *Psychological Medicine,* **15**, 745–756.
Berrios, G. E. (1987a). History of the functional psychoses, *British Medical Bulletin* (in press).
Berrios, G. E. (1987b). History of the psychiatric aspects of Parkinson's Disease, *J. Neurol Neurosurg Psychiat* (in press).
Bleuler, E. (1896). Review of 'Studies on Hysteria', *Münchener medizinische Wschr,* **43**, 524–525.
Bleuler, E. (1902). Dementia Praecox, *J. Mental Path.,* **3**, 113–120.
Bleuler, E. (1905). Frühe Entlassungen, *Psychiat. Neurol. Wschr,* **6**, 441–449.
Bleuler, E. (1906). *Affectivität, Suggestibilität, Paranoia,* Carl Marhold, Halle.

Bleuler, E. (1908). Die Prognose der Dementia praecox (Schizophreniegruppe), *Allg. Z. Psychiat.*, **65**, 436–464.

Bleuler, E. (1911). *Dementia praecox oder Gruppe der Schizophrenien*, Franz Deuticke, Leipzig.

Bleuler, E. (1914). Frühe Entlassungen, *Wien. med. Wschr*, **64**, 2499–2504.

Bleuler, E. (1916). *Lehrbuch der Psychiatrie*, Springer, Berlin.

Bleuler, E. and Jung, C. G. (1908). Komplexe und Krankheitsursache bei Dementia praecox, *Zentralblatt Nervenkrankheiten*, **31**, 220–227.

Bleuler, M. (1951). Geschichte des Burghölzlis und der psychiatrischen Universitäts-klinik. In *Zürcher Spitalgeschichte*, edited by Regierungsrat des Kantons Zürich, pp. 317–425.

Bleuler, M. (1984). Eugen Bleuler and Schizophrenia, *Brit. J. Psychiat.*, **144**, 327–328.

Boring, E. G. (1950). *A History of Experimental Psychology*, Appleton-Century-Crofts, New York.

Brill, A. A. (1939). In memoriam: Eugen Bleuler, *Amer. J. Psychiat.*, **96**, 513–516.

Brooks, G. P. (1976). The faculty psychology of Thomas Reid, *J. Hist. Behav. Sci.*, **12**, 65–77.

Carpenter, W. B. (1879). *Mental Physiology*, Kegan Paul, London.

Chaslin, P. (1912). *Eléments de Sémiologie et Clinique Mentales*, Asselin et Houzeau, Paris.

Claude, H., Borel, A. and Robin, G. (1924). Démence précoce, schizomanie et schizophrénie, *LEncephale*, **19**, 145–151.

Corbett, L. (1978). Clinical differentiation of the schizophrenic and affective disorders: a comparison of the bleulerian and phenomenological approaches to diagnosis. In *Psychiatric Diagnosis: Exploration of Biological Predictors*, H. S. Akiskal and W. L. Webb (Eds), Spectrum Publications, London.

Diem, O. (1903). Die einfach demente Form der Dementia praecox, *Arciv. für Psychiatrie und nerven Krankheiten*, **37**, 111–187.

Ellenberger, H. F. (1970). *The Discovery of the Unconscious. The History and Evolution of Dynamic Psychiatry*, Allen Lane, The Penguin Press, London.

Gilman, S. L. (1983). Why is schizophrenia 'bizarre': an historical essay in the vocabulary of psychiatry. *J. Hist. Behav. Sci.*, **19**, 127–135.

Giraud, J. M. (1985). C. G. Jung et les schizophrénies: étude chronologique (1903–1957), *L'Information Psychiatrique*, **61**, 1079–1085.

Giraud, P. (1968). Origine et évolution de la notion de la schizophrénie, *Confrontation Psychiatrique*, **2**, 9–29.

Haenel, T. (1982). *Zur Geschichte dr Psychiatrie. Gedanken zur allgemeinen und Basler Psychiatriegeschichte*, Birkhäuser, Basel.

Hesnard, A. (1914). Les théories psychologiques et métapsychiatriques de la démence précoe, *Journal de Psychologie*, **9**, 37–70.

Hoeldtke, R. (1967). The history of associationism and british medical psychology, *Medical History*, **11**, 46–64.

Hoenig, J. (1983). The concept of schizophrenia Kraepelin-Bleuler-Schneider, *Brit. J. Psychiat.*, **142**, 547–556.

Höffding, H. (1892). *Outlines of Psychology* (transl. M. E. Lowndes), MacMillan, London.

Jaspers, K. (1963). *General Psychopathology* (transl. J. Hoenig and M. W. Hamilton), Manchester University Press, Manchester.

Jülicher, L. (1961). *Die Psychologie J F Herbarts und ihre Bedeutung für die Psychiatrie des 19ten Jahrhunderts*, Rheinische Friedrich Wilhelms Universität, Bonn.

Jung, C. G. (1907). *Uber die Psychologie der Dementia praecox: Ein Versuch*, Carl Marhold, Halle.

Klaesi, J. (1956). Eugen Bleuler. In *Grosse Nervenärtze*, K. Kolle (Ed.), vol. I, Thieme, Stuttgart, pp. 7–16.

Klemm, O. (1911). *Geschichte der Psychologie*, Teubner, Leipzig.

Kraepelin, E. (1919). *Dementia praecox and paraphrenia* (transl. R. M. Barclay), E. and S. Livingstone, Edinburgh.

Lagriffe, L. (1913). Les troubles du mouvement dans la démence précoce, *Annales Médico-Psychologiques*, **71**, 136–148.

Lanteri-Laura, G. and Gros, M. (1982). Historique de la schizophrénie, *Encycl. Méd Chir., Psychiatrie, 37281 C10, 9*, Paris.

Laplanche, J. and Pontalis, J-B. (1973). *The Language of Psychoanalysis*, Hogarth Press, London.

Leys, R. (1985). Meyer, Jung, and the limits of association. *Bull. Hist. Med.* **59**, 345–360.

Luys, J. (1876). *Le Cerveau*, Germer Baillière, Paris.

Meduna, L. J. and McCulloch, W. S. (1945). The modern concept of Schizophrenia, *The Medical Clinics of North America*, **8**, 147–164.

Meynert, T. (1884). *Psychiatrie, Klinik der Erkrankungen des Vorderhirns*, Braumüller, Wien.

Midenet, M. (1972). La conception de la schizophrénie dans la psychiatrie allemande des années 1920 à 1933, *L'Encephale*, **61**, 333–349.

Minkowski, E. (1927). *La Schizophrénie: Psychopathologie des Schizoides et des Schizophrénes*, Payot, Paris.

Proceedings (1965). Les suites d'un débat historique: Eugen Bleuler-Sigmund Freud, *Bull. Soc. Suisse Psychanal.*, no. 2.

Raskin, D. E. (1975). Bleuler and Schizophrenia, *Brit. J. Psychiat.*, **127**, 231–234.

Rieder, R. O. (1974). The origins of our confession about schizophrenia, *Psychiatry*, **37**, 197–208.

Scharfetterm C, (1975). The historical development of the concept of schizophrenia. In *Studies of Schizophrenia*, M. H. Lader (Ed.), British Journal Special Publication No. 10, Headley Brothers Ltd, Chichester pp 5–9.

Schneider, K. (1959). *Clinical Psychopathology* (translated by Hamilton, M. W. and Anderson, E. W.), Grune and Stratton, New York.

Stransky, E. (1903). Zur Kenntnis gewisser erworbener Blödsinnsformen (zugleich ein Beitrag zur Lehre von der Dementia praecox), *Jb Psychiat Neurol*, **24**, 1–149.

Trénel, M. (1912). The démence précoce ou schizophrénie d'après la conception de Bleuler, *Revue Neurologique*, **6**, 372–383.

Various Authors (1941). Zum Andenken an Eugen Bleuler, *Schweizerisches Archiv für Neurologie und Psychiatrie*, **46**, 1–32.

Warren, H. C. (1921). *History of Association Psychology*, Charles Scribner's Sons, New York.

Wernicke, C. (1894). *Grundriss der Psychiatrie*, Thieme, Leipzig.

Zilboog, G. (1939). Eugen Bleuler, *Psychoanalytic Quarterly*, **7**, 382–384.

Ziehen, T. (1909). *Introduction to Physiological Psychology* (transl. C. C. Van Liew and O. W. Beyer), Allen and Unwin, London.

10

Demonstration Of Treponema pallidum *In The Brain In Cases Of General Paralysis*

Hideyo Noguchi MD and J.W. Moore MD
1913

In the present communication we wish to report the results of examinations for *Treponema pallidum* on seventy paretic brains. One of us (Noguchi) succeeded in finding the pallidum in twelve out of the seventy specimens.*

The relationship of paresis to syphilis has, for years, been one of the foremost topics of medical interest, especially to psychiatrists. Since 1857 when attention was first called† to the frequency of syphilis in the history of patients with paresis, the etiological importance of the former disease has steadily gained recognition until now probably the majority of writers agree with Kraepelin‡ that "We can to-day declare with the greatest certainty that syphilitic infection is an essential for the later appearance of paresis." Many, however, including a man of such enormous experience as Nonne, still refuse to concede that syphilis is more than an extremely common causative factor. Nonne§ says, "At the outset I desire to make it clear that progressive paralysis is not a specific syphilitic disease of the brain."

Among those who hold "without syphilis, no paresis," there are some who contend that paresis is nothing more nor less than a particular form of tertiary syphilis. Kraepelin objects to this view on two principal grounds,—the distinctly greater interval between

---

* The findings were confirmed later by Dr. Moore as well as by others, among whom we may mention Dr. Flexner and Dr. Dunlap. We take pleasure in expressing our gratitude to Dr. G.A. Smith, Superintendent of the Central Islip State Hospital, for the material studied.
† Esmarch, F., und Jessen, W., *Allg. Ztschr. f. Psychiat.*, 1857, xiv, 20.
‡ Kraepelin, E., Psychiatrie, Leipzig, 1904,ii.
§ Nonne, M., Syphilis und Nervensystem, Berlin, 1902.

syphilitic infection and paresis as compared with that in cerebral syphilis and the refractoriness of paresis to antisyphilitic treatment. This author, however, in commenting on the hitherto vain attempts to find *Treponema pallidum* in the tissues and body fluids of paresis, remarks, "This does not mean that the spirochæta is never present in the body of the paretic. It may have assumed forms so far unknown to us or have located in places where it has not yet been sought or where it is hard to find."

Of late years a few cases have been reported in which the findings of paresis occurred along with those of cerebral syphilis. Sträussler* has recently added two cases of this combination to several he had already reported. Ranke† and others have demonstrated *Spirochæta pallida* in the pia and vessel sheaths in congenitally syphilitic brains. In this country Dunlap, of the New York State Psychiatric Institute, has also shown the organisms in a case of cerebral syphilis. Dunlap has long been of the opinion that, although tertiary syphilis of the brain and general paralysis are quite distinct and seldom, if ever, occur together, they are but different manifestations of the same process.

The failure up to the present time to discover *Treponema pallidum* in the affected nervous system has doubtless added to the general conception that paresis, although of syphilitic origin, can exist without the pallidum playing an active part in the progressive processes. This assumption is valid, of course, only when we grant that *Treponema pallidum* can infallibly be demonstrated by the microscopical techniques hitherto employed. But, as will be seen presently, this is far from being the case. Besides, the individual experience on the part of the examiner has much to do with whether the organisms are viewed or remain undetected, especially in a tissue in which so many tortuous fibers are present as in the brain.

These facts, coupled with the very significant serological similarities between syphilis and paresis, and the fact that the trypanosome can be found in the brain in sleeping-sickness,—a disease in many respects similar to paresis,—led the writers to believe that further search for the syphilitic organism, either in granular or in spirochætal form,‡ in paresis was warranted. To this end, tissues were taken from seventy paretic brains in the possession of the pathologi-

* Sträussler, *Ztschr. f. d. ges. Neurol. u. Psychiat., Orig.*, 1912, xii, 365.
† Ranke, *Ztschr. f. d. Erforsch. u. Behandl. d. jugendl. Schwachsinns*, 1909, ii, 32,81,211.
‡ Noguchi, H., *Jour, A. Med. Assn.*, 1912, lix, 1236.

cal service of the Central Islip State Hospital and stained with the Levaditi silver method modified in certain respects to produce an elective stain for the pallidum. The specimens in most of the cases were taken from the first right frontal gyrus; in some, from the left hemispere or gyrus rectus.

The syphilitic organisms were found in twelve cases which were examples of undoubted general paralysis. The cases in which the pallida were found showed the classical physical signs. The postmortem findings in the brain in every case were definitely those of general paralysis. Ten were men and two were women. Seven were of the cerebral type, and five of the tabetic. In several instances the patients had been picked up on the street in a confused state and had no idea of the duration of the condition. In the seven cases in which the onset could be satisfactorily determined, the average duration was seventeen months, the longest thirty months, and the shortest five months. The majority were much below the average duration, as estimated by various authors, which varies from twenty-four to thirty-two months. It is possible, then, that we are more apt to find the spirochæta in those cases which run a fairly rapid course. The age varied from thirty-three to sixty years, with an average of forty-four years. Brief abstracts of the case records follow.

J.C. (103), age fifty years; duration of disease unknown. He was committed from the workhouse. There was much confusion; he was disoriented and his memory was extremely poor. The knee-jerks were unequal and exaggerated; the pupils sluggish and unequal. His speech was distorted, and there were marked tremors. Convulsions occurred. Death occurred after seven months in the hospital.

C.M. (106), age thirty-nine years; duration unknown, but probably about four months. Syphilis ten years previously. When he was admitted he was depressed and apprehensive; he had hallucinations of hearing; he was disoriented, and his memory was very poor, with spells of marked confusion. The knee-jerks were normal, the pupils sluggish. There were ataxia, distorted speech, course tremors, and convulsions. He died after eleven months in the hospital.

F.B. (113), age thirty-six years; duration before admission, fourteen months. Syphilis was denied. On admission he was dull, silly, mildly restless, and had occasional hallucinations. His memory showed marked discrepancies. The knee-jerks were absent, and the pupils slow to light and unequal. His speech was distorted, and he had convulsions. Later he developed a silly elation and deteriorated progressively. Death occurred after fourteen months in the hospital. The total duration of the disease was thirty months.

S.V. (131), colored, age thirty-seven years; the duration of the disease before admission is unknown. Syphilis eight years previously. He was euphoric, his memory was very poor, and he was disoriented. The knee-jerks were much diminished, the pupils slightly slow, his speech ataxic, and there were coarse tremors. Later he devloped typical expansive ideas and became very ataxic. Death occurred after twenty-seven months in the hospital.

J.D. (138), age thirty-three years; duration before admission, five months. He was admitted in an hallucinatory depression with nihilistic ideas and a history of a probable attempt at suicide. A complete mental status was impossible. The knee-jerks were exaggerated; pupils unequal, Argyll-Robertson sign present; there were marked tremors. The spinal fluid showed marked lymphocytosis. Death occurred after ten months in the hospital.

F.M. (169), age fifty-five years; duration of disease unknown. He was picked up on the street in a confused condition. He had absurd hypochondriacal ideas; "his insides were falling out," etc. He was disoriented and his memory was very poor. The knee-jerks were exaggerated, and the pupils sluggish. There were marked tremors, unsteadiness, and Romberg's sign. His speech was not seriously affected. Depression continued, and he insisted that he could not breathe or urinate, and that parts of him were dead. He died after four months in the hospital. The spinal fluid showed positive lymphocytosis and a positive Wassermann-Noguchi reaction.

E.W. (170), age forty-four years; duration unknown. He had had syphilis. The psychosis was a simple deterioration with marked confusion and disorientation but no delusions. He was silly, his memory was poor, and there were occasional attacks of excitement. The knee-jerks were diminished, and the pupils slightly slow. The speech showed extreme ataxia. Romberg's sign was present, and tremors were prominent. There were frequent convulsions. Death occurred after two months in the hospital.

E.R. (230), age forty-eight years; duration unknown. When admitted she was much demented, confused, completely disoriented, and her memory was poor. Her mood was one of silly elation. The knee-jerks were exaggerated, the pupillary reaction slow and of narrow range. There was marked distortion of speech and writing. There were coarse tremors and increasing ataxia. The spinal fluid showed marked pleocytosis. Death occurred after six months in the hospital.

M.M. (235), age forty-two years; duration uncertain. She had been blind from optic atrophy for two years before admission and had experienced occasional visual hallucinations, but definite mental symptoms seem to have begun only a few weeks before commitment, when she began to show a change of disposition and became forgetful. Syphilis probably occurred twenty years previously. Her husband was a paretic. On admission she was excited, resisting, and obscene. She seemed clear and gave correct answers in the orientation test but her memory showed marked discrepancies in time relations. The knee-jerks were absent, the pupils rigid, her speech drawling and distorted, no tremors, and only slight ataxia. The spinal fluid showed extreme lymphocytosis. She quieted down and during the next two years showed a gradual deterioration without any particular mental trend. Ataxia increased steadily; she had occasional apoplectic attacks and convulsions. Death occurred after two years in the hospital.

G.F. (236), age sixty years; duration before admission, one month. He became gradually childish, forgetful, and irritable. When admitted he was disoriented, and his memory was poor. The knee-jerks were absent, and the pupils unequal and slow; he speech was slurring and distorted. There were marked tremors and Romberg's sign. He deteriorated rapidly and died after four months in the hospital.

M.D. (242), age thirty-seven years; duration eight months. The onset seemed to date from an injury to the head. There was a probable history of syphilis. He was depressed, confused, and had attempted suicide. His memory was poor, and he was much demented. The knee-jerks were exaggerated; and the pupils unequal and Argyll-Robertson sign present; his speech was ataxic. There were tremors and occasional convulsions. He died after four months in the hospital. The total duration of the disease was one year.

F.B. (299) (figure I), age fifty-eight years; duration before admission, one month. There was a probable history of syphilis. He was depressed and whining, and had typical paretic ideas, such as that his bowels never moved, and that he had an incurable disease. He would point to a leg or an arm and say, "See, it's all dead, all gone,—there's no hope." His orientation and memory showed marked defects. The knee-jerks were slightly exaggerated, the pupils slow, his speech was distorted, and tremors were excessive. the spinal fluid showed pronounced lymphocytosis and a positive Wassermann-Noguchi reaction. Death occurred after eleven months in the hospital.

Naturally the first question that arises is. Are these not cases of cerebral syphilis in the narrower sense? In reply to this we can but review briefly the differential points. They all showed, in their clinical course, a diffuse, progressive deterioration in all the mental fields, and not the *demence lacunaire* so often observed in syphilitic brain disease. There were no cranial symptoms or other focal manifestations. These points are admittedly not convincing, for it is possible for an old syphilitic endarteritic-meningitic condition to simulate paresis so closely as to be indistinguishable by its clinical features from the latter disease. It is upon the post-mortem findings that the diagnosis must depend. Anatomically the brains of our cases showed the usual pial thickening, more marked over the frontal convexity. In two it was also prominent over the gyri recti, cerebellum, and cisterna, but id did not assume the degree of meningitis usually seen in syphilis of the base. In one case (235) there was an old hemorrhagic membrane beneath the dura; in another (131) there was a marked preponderance of the paretic process in the right hemisphere, but these conditions were not represented clinically and the findings were otherwise typical. In the microscopic examination the meningeal process in all cases was diffuse, being more marked in the frontal region. The vessel

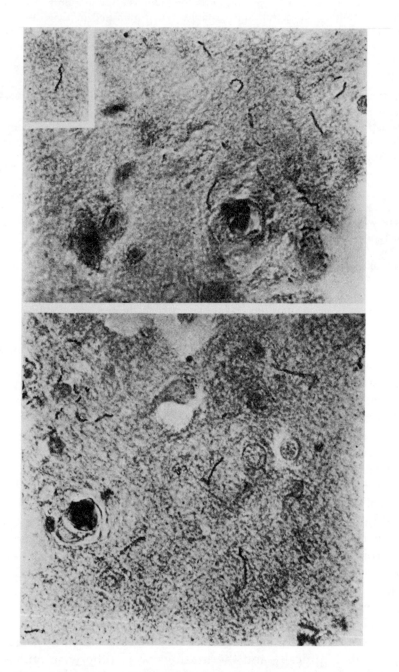

Fig. I *Treponema pallidum* in the cortical layer of the right frontal area of the brain (case 299). Stained, with slight modification, by Levaditi's method. × 1100.

infiltration was also diffuse and found at all depths of the cortex and in the marrow. Plasma cells were, in each case, numerous and usually outnumbered the lymphocytes. Red cells were always present. The nerve cell alterations and changes in the neuroglia do not present differential characteristcs and will not be enumerated. With regard to the vessels, a number of our cases, as in all general paralysis material, showed endarteritic changes. In six there was definite thickening of the vessel walls of the type described as syphilitic. In no instance did the intimal proliferation embarrass the lumen to any extent. In the remaining cases the vessels appeared normal. It seems hardly possible that the presence of the spirochætæ could be traced to the luetic endarteritis, since they were not found associated, at least with those vessels which are visible with the Levaditi stain. In none of the cases were there softenings, and no gummata were found either in gross or microscopically.

The spirochætæ were found in all layers of the cortex with the exception of the outer, or neuroglia layer. One was located at the border of this layer, but not within it. A few were found subcortically. In all instances they seemed to have wandered into the nerve tissue. They were not found in the vessel sheaths and seldom in close proximity to the larger vessels. There seems to be no ratio between the number of spirochætæ and the severity of the paretic process, although the case in which they were most numerous showed excessive paretic changes.

Whether or not, by improving the technique, *Treponema pallidum* can be demonstrated in a much higher percentage of paretic cases will be determined by further investigations.

Of all forms of brain disease with unsoundness of mind, general paralysis is, perhaps, the most interesting scientifically. It always has distinctive and marked bodily as well as mental symptoms and its course, termination and pathology can be predicted. It has been, and is now, being studied with unusual keenness in all civilized countries. Many of us regard it as being one of the chief keys of our future knowledge of brain and mental disease as its first description by Bayle, a French physician, in 1822, was the starting point of the modern clinical study of unsoundness of mind as a brain disease, thus exploding the older spiritual and metaphysical themes of the disease.

(T.S. Clouston, 1911)

Although syphilis had been a scourge in Europe since it had appeared in epidemic form at the end of the 15th century, over three centuries were to elapse before two French physicians—Bayle in 1822 and Calmeil in 1826—drew attention to a characteristic disease state which Calmeil named general paralysis of the insane. It was to be nearly a century later that the syphilitic aetiology of the condition was to be finally established by Noguchi and Moore when they discovered the spirochaete in the brain substance of general paralytics.

Despite a search for historical precedents, no really satisfactory accounts of the disease had appeared prior to Bayle and Calmeil. From then onwards, both the literature and the disease itself increased in a manner which suggested that a new epidemic disease had arisen. The number of patients admitted to mental hospitals throughout Europe and North America threatened to swamp the facilities; in some asylums as many as a quarter of the beds were filled by patients suffering from general paralysis. In 1874, the percentage of cases in British asylums was 14.1 for males and 3.2 for females.

By this time, the clinical characteristics of the condition had become firmly established but the aetiology was a different matter. There were two schools of thought, the first favouring a syphilitic aetiology, the second contesting this view but offering no real substitute.

Julius Mickle in his book *General Paralysis of the Insane*, which went into two editions (1880 and 1886), typifies the writing of the period. In the second edition, 450 pages of text were devoted to descriptions of the clinical and pathological findings, eight pages to therapy and hygiene. Even by 1903, William Osler was writing in his *Principles and Practice of Medicine*, the foremost medical textbook of its day in the English language:

Para or Metasyphilitic Affections—certain disorders not actually syphilitic yet so closely connected that a large proportion of the cases have had the disease, are termed by Fournier, parasyphilitic. These affections are not exclusively and necessarily caused by syphilis and they are not influenced by specific treatments. The chief of them are locomotor ataxia, dementia paralytica, certain types of epilepsy and, we may add, arterio-sclerosis.

If Osler could write in this way, it was apparent that by then the clinical approach had reached a dead-end. An etiological and therapeutic ignorance, as has been so often the case in medicine, led to some astonishing statements from even the most respected physicians. Thus Henry Maudsley considered sexual excess to be an exciting cause of the disease, indeed, in Mickle's words 'a very fertile cause of general paralysis'. Maudsley wrote of 'that quiet, steady continuance of excess for months or years by married people which was apt to be thought no vice or harm at all'. Krafft-Ebing believed, with other experienced physicians such as Guislain and Voisin, that the excessive use of tobacco might, at times, produce general paralysis; he described two men who developed the disease as a result of the excessive use of Virginia cigars (10–20 daily).

Happily, although the clinical seam was apparently exhausted, the application of the new scientific knowledge and techniques brought rapid advances in syphilology. Haensell, in 1881, managed to transmit syphilis to the rabbit. Twenty-two years later, Metchnikoff and Roux produced infection in primates.

The most important event, however, was the discovery by Schaudinn and Hoffman in 1905 of a spiral organism in fluid from chancres and from the enlarged inguinal glands. The organism was at first named the *Spirochaeta pallida* but later became the *Treponema pallidum*. New discoveries followed in rapid succession, a veritable explosion of knowledge. Perhaps the most important was the Wassermann Test, introduced in 1906, a specific test for syphilitic antibodies which gave positive results in blood and C.S.F. in 90 per cent of cases of general paralysis. Finally, as a result of Quincke's pioneering work on lumbar puncture, access to the C.S.F. resulted in new and particularly valuable diagnostic aids. The scene was set for the identification of the spirochaete in the Central Nervous System.

Neuropathology in the last two decades of the 19th century, in line with other laboratory sciences, had seen the introduction of new staining and cutting techniques, better microscopes and an increasing appreciation of the minute anatomy of the brain. Frederick Mott, who became Director of the Central Laboratory and Pathologist to the London County Asylums in 1895, published a monumental volume, *Syphilis of the Central Nervous System*, in 1910. In 1899, together with Manson, he had investigated several cases of trypanosomiasis which had come to England from the Congo, so that when a devastating epidemic arose in the new British Protectorate of Uganda, Mott was asked to become a member of the Sleeping Sickness Commission set up, at Government request, by the Royal Society.

Mott was immediately struck by the similarities between syphilis and trypanosomiasis, both being diseases 'characterised by inoculation, a period of incubation, affection of nearest lymphatic glands, followed by generalisation in the lymph due to escape of the trypanosomes from the blood stream into the lymph spaces of the tissues, where they set up a similar tissue reaction'. The two diseases were also similar in that the nervous system became affected, although Mott pointed out that while trypanosomiasis leads eventually to invasion of the nervous system, 'in syphilis not more than 5 per cent to 10 per cent even if untreated result in invasion of the Nervous System'.

In a study of the comparative neuropathology of trypanosome and spirochaete infections, Mott described the intense perivascular infiltration with lymphocytes and plasma cells in the nervous tissue, as well as the gliosis of the white matter which were seen in both conditions, but pointed out that neuronal degeneration did not occur in sleeping sickness.

Nevertheless, this striking resemblance between the brains of patients dying with acute general paralysis, brain syphilis and sleeping sickness did not answer two important questions which have puzzled us to this day: the first concerns the long delay in many cases between infection and general paralysis, and the second is why only 5 to 10 per cent of syphilitic individuals eventually developed general paralysis.

Despite Mott's great experience of genral paralysis and his conviction that it was the result of syphilitic infection, the final proof and the end of nearly a century of controversy could only come with the demonstration of the spirochaete in the brain. That was done by Noguchi and Moore in 1913. J.W. Moore, working at the Central Islip State Hospital in New York, was convinced that general paralysis was quite distinct from brain syphilis. He, nevertheless,undertook a search for the spirochaete using the Levaditi silver stain. Uncertain of his findings, Moore sent a duplicate set of slides to Noguchi, then working at the Rockefeller Institute, with the results outlined in their joint paper, results which put an end to a century of speculation and which now provided a sound basis for a rational therapy. Few remember Moore's part in the discovery, rather it is Noguchi who will always be associated with the detection of the spirochaete in the brain of general paralytics.

Hideyo Noguchi was born in 1876. He qualified at Tokyo University at a time when German medicine, with its scientific methods and its systematic and thorough approach to the study of disease, was the dominant influence in the Japanese medical schools. At the age of 25, Noguchi travelled to America to take up a post as Assistant Lecturer in Pathology in Philadelphia and from then onwards was to remain in the States, working for most of his career at the Rockefeller Institute. There he had become interested in the serology of syphilis and then in the study of all types of treponema. He investigated Weils disease and introduced the term leptospira, travelling to Cenral America in order to study yellow fever, thought by many to be a spirochaetal disease allied to what was then called infectious jaundice. Noguchi, in a long series of experiments, believed he had isolated the organism responsible for yellow fever and gave it the name *leptospira icteroides* produced a vaccine, an antiserum and even transmitted the organism from guinea pig to guinea pig via the mosquito vector of yellow fever. Alas, other workers, particularly British scientists working in the Gold Coast, could not confirm these findings. He therefore decided to travel to Accra in order to study African yellow fever in a part of the world formerly known as the white man's grave. Soon after starting work in Accra, Noguchi contracted yellow fever and died in 1928, at the age of 52. It is somewhat ironic that considering the importance of Noguchi's discoveries in so many tropical diseases, he is today probably best remembered for the identification of the spirochaete in the brains of general paralytics.

Following Noguchi and Moore's paper, other workers began a more intensive search for the spirochaete and Mott, amongst others, was eventually able to identify the organism in 60 per cent of cases of untreated paralytics. Special techniques and a prolonged search of the material was necessary. It was noted that the early acute cases were more likely to be positive than the chronic cases and that the percentage declined in proportion to the length of hospitalization.

Jahnel (1930), probably the most experienced investigator in the field, had pointed out that the spirochaete could be detected in 50 per cent of cases using an emulsion of the brain and the hanging drop technique but in only 25 per cent of stained sections. He had also noticed that the spirochaete seemed to increase periodically and at times almost disappeared—a phenomenon possibly accounting for the disparate findings.

Jahnel also recognized three types of distribution of spirochaetes. First, when the organisms were fairly evenly scattered through the cortex, a second when they occurred in swarms, dense circumscribed colonies being found in the cortex, and a third when the spirochaetes were clustered about the blood vessels.

The introduction of malaria therapy was also a potent stimulus to the neuropathological study of general paralysis. Jahnel and Weichbrod (1921) studied the destructive effects of high temperature on spirochaetes and showed that in rabbits with scrotal chancres, the spirochaetes completely disappeared after the animal had been subjected to recurrent pyrexia and found that the spirochaete fails to multiply at temperatures of 40–41°C. Examination of the brains of malaria treated patients who had died from intercurrent disease during a phase of remission, revealed an arrest in the histopathological process. Sträussler and Koskinas (1925) reported that a clinical remission was associated with regression and arrest of the pathological process.

Geary (1929), who worked in the laboratory Mott had once directed, examined the brains of 16 cases treated with malaria, 10 of whom showed definite improvement in the neuropathological appearances. No spirochaetes were found in 15 of the brains, suggesting that the pyrexia had caused the destruction of the spirochaetes. Geary concluded that although his cases had died from the disease, itself, 3 months to $2\frac{1}{2}$ years after treatment, nevertheless there was evidence, particularly regarding the vascular lesions, to suggest an improvement in the pathological process.

TREATMENT

After Noguchi and Moore, the question of the aetiology of general paralysis seems to have been settled; now efforts could be concentrated on treatment. In 1919 a new pentavalent arsenical, tryparsamide, was synthesized and although relatively useless in the early stages of syphilis, proved successful in producing remissions in up to 30 per cent of cases of general paralysis. Bismuth was introduced in 1921 and became an accepted adjunct to arsenical treatment, this chemotherapy continuing until the advent fo penicillin in 1943.

The toxic effects of these heavy metals was a serious problem, blindness a heavy price to pay for taking them. The search for less dangerous substances or for other methods of treatment, continued over the first two decades of the 20th century, eventually being rewarded by the discovery of malaria therapy.

For over three centuries heat had been used in the treatment of syphilis, the sweating treatment consisting of the patient being enclosed in a chamber which was heated up from below and in which the patient remained for between 15 and 60 minutes, depending on his ability to tolerate the heat. He was then put in a warm bed and allowed to sweat for the next hour. Six to nine treatments were given every two to three days. References abound to this treatment in the general literature of the 16th and early 17th centuries. Gradually, its popularity declined and mercury remained the standard anti-syphilitic for nearly 400 years until it was replaced by the arsenicals.

General paralysis remained incurable, the asylums filled with these dilapidated caricatures of humanity. However, a young Austrian psychiatrist, Julius Wagner-Jauregg, had become interested in the effect of intercurrent infections upon psychotic individuals (Schönbauer and Jantsch, 1950). He had had two women patients, one developing erysipelas and the other typhoid, who had shown a remision of their psychosis following recovery from their infections. Wagner-Jauregg read widely on the topic, discovering a formidable, even if anecdotal, literature.

In 1887, Wagner-Jauregg proposed that incurable psychotics be injected with erysipelas or malaria, a proposal which he, himself, put promptly into effect. Using streptococci, then tuberculin and, later, typoid vaccine as febrogenic agents, he had soon treated a heterogenous group of psychotics on whose progress he reported over the years. The results were encouraging, particularly in that most resistant condition, general paralysis.

It was not, however, until the First World War that Wagner-Jauregg was presented with the opportunity to use malaria, a technique which he had suggested almost thirty years previously. In 1917, Dr Fuchs, one of his assistants, told his Professor that he had a soldier under his care who had been serving on the Macedonian front, where malaria was rife, and who now showed signs of having developed the condition. Should he prescribe Quinine? In Wagner-Jauregg's own words: 'Da Kam mir wie der Blitz de Gedanke, mit dem Blut dieses Malarikers Paralytiker zu impfen. Ich sagte: "Nein" und erklarte Fuchs, dass ich mit dem Blut dieses Malarikers zwei Paralytiker impfen werde. Das geschah an 14 Juni 1917'. Blood was taken from the soldier and transferred by scarification to two general paralytics who had been selected for the experiment. Seven further cases were infected and of the nine, six improved, of whom three were, apparently, cured.

Despite the scepticism of the medical profession, malaria therapy soon became established as the principal treatment for general paralysis: Wagner-Jauregg received the Nobel Prize in 1927 and died, full of honours, at the age of 83 in September 1940.

In England, a special malaria therapy centre was set up at Horton Hospital in 1925, later to be called the Mott Clinic (Nicol, 1956). By 1956, over 3000 paralytics had received malaria therapy. Then, in 1943, penicillin was first used in the treatment of all forms of syphilis, proving remarkably effective and sounding the death knell of malaria therapy. For a time, the two treatments were combined but not for long, a cure, penicillin, had arrived at last.

Is it a consequence of penicillin treatment that the disease has become a rarity or has there been a natural decline in its frequency; has the spirochaete abandoned the nervous system to the slow viruses now so fashionably implicated in the aetiology of schizophrenia? Hare (1959), has suggested that a mutant neurotropic strain of spirochaete arose somewhere in Northern France toward the end of the 18th century, spread by venereal infection, affecting different countries at different times and filling the mental hospitals with cases of general paralysis. Slowly over the next 150 years, changes occurred in the sex ratio, the clinical picture, the mutability rate and in its prevalence. Its rarity today is such as to indicate a change in the disease, itself, rather than a magical effect of penicillin therapy.

Does the history of general paralysis illustrate, as Hare suggests, the mutability of disease? Is its history a preview of what is to come with the HTLV III virus—a new neurotropic virus, possibly arising in Africa and spreading worldwide, with profound systemic effects and sinister long-term neuropsychiatric implications? Psychiatry may well find itself as much concerned in the future with the effects of this new virus as it had in the past with general paralysis and other parasyphilitic disorders.

Denis Leigh

REFERENCES

Clouston, T.S. (1911). *Unsoundness of Mind*, Methuen and Co., London.

Geary, C. (1929). *Observations upon the Histopathology of General Paralysis Treated with Malaria and Relapsing Fever in The Mott Memorial*, H.K. Lewis & Co. Ltd, London, pp. 201–230.

Hare, E.H. (1959). The origin and spread of dementia paralytica, *J.Ment.Sci.***105**, 594–626.

Jahnel, F. (1930). Pathologische Anatomie Der Progressive Paralyse, in *Handbuch Der Geisteskrankheiten*, Vol.II, Julius Springer Verlag, Berlin, pp. 417–569.

Mickle, W.M. (1886). *General Paralysis of the Insane*, 2nd edn, H.K. Lewis & Co.Ltd., London.

Mott, F.W. (1910). *A System of Syphilis*, vol.IV, *Syphilis of the Nervous System*, Henry Frowde, Hodder & Stoughton, London.

Mott, F.W. (1915). The diagnosis and treatment of parenchymatous syphilis, *J. Ment.Sci.*, **61**, 175–197.

Nicol, W.D. (1956). General paralysis of the insane, *Brit.J.Ven.Dis.*, **XXXII**. 9–16.

Osler, W. (1903). *The Principles and Practice of Medicine*, D. Appleton & Co., New York.

Schönbauer, L. and Jantsch, M. (1950). *Julius Wagner-Jauregg Lebenserrinerungen*, Springer Verlag, Wien.

11
Dementia Praecox and Paraphrenia (1919) and Introductory Lectures on Clinical Psychiatry (1906) III Dementia Praecox
E. Kraepelin

DEMENTIA PRAECOX

Dementia praecox* consists of a series of states, the common characteristic of which is a peculiar destruction of the internal connections of the psychic personality. The effects of this injury predominate in the emotional and volitional spheres of mental life. To begin with, the assertion that this is a distinct disease has met with repeated and decided opposition, which has found its strongest expression in the writings of Marandon de Montyel and of Serbsky.† But even though in many details there are profound differences of opinion, still the conviction seems to be more and more gaining ground that dementia praecox on the whole represents a well characterised form of disease, and that we are justified in regarding the majority at least of the clinical pictures which are brought together here as the expression of a single morbid process, though outwardly they often diverge very far from one another.

---

* Finzi e Vedrani, Rivista sperim, de freniatria, xxv, 1899; Christian, Ann. medico-psychol. 1899, 1, 43; Trömner, Das Jùgendirresein (Dementia præcox), 1909; Sérieux, Gaz. hebdomad. Mars 1901; Revue de psychiatrie, Juin 1902; Jahrmarker, Zur Frage der Dementia præcox, 1902; Meeus, de la démence précoce chez lez jeunes gens. 1902; Masselon, Psychologie des Démences précoces; de la démence précoce. 1904; Stransky, Centralblatt für Nervenheilkunde xxvii. 1; Über die dementia præcox, 1909; Bernstein, Allg. Zeitschr. f. Psychiatrie, lx. 554; Deny et Roy, la démence précoce. 1903; Pighini, Rivista sperimentale di freniatria, xxxiv. 3; Hoche, Deutsche Klinik von Leyden-Klemperer, vi. 2, 197; Hecht, American Journal of nervous and mental diseases, 1905; 689; Evensen, Dementia præcox. 1904; Rizor, Archiv f. Psychiatrie, xliii. 760; Wieg. Wickenthal, Zur Klinik der Dementia præcox. 1908; Bleuler-Jahrmärker, Allgem. Zeitschr f. Psychiatrie, lxv. 429; Bleuler Dementia præcox oder Gruppe der Schizophrenien, Aschaffenburgs Ilandbuch der Psychiatrie, 1911 (Literatur) Deny et Lhermitte, Traité international de psychologie pathologique, ii, 439, 1911.
† Serbsky, Annales médico-psychologiques 1903, 2. 379; Marandon de Montyel, ebenda 1905, 2, 246; Soutzo, ebenda 1907, i. 243.

The objections have been directed even more against the name than against the clinical conception. I got the starting point of the line of thought which in 1896 led to dementia praecox being regarded as a distinct disease, on the one hand from the overpowering impression of the states of dementia quite similar to each other which developed from the most varied initial clinical symptoms, on the other hand from the experience connected with the observations of Hecker that these peculiar dementias seemed to stand in near relation to the period of youth. As there was no clinical recognition of it, the first thing to be done for the preliminary marking off of the newly circumscribed territory was to choose a name which would express both these points of view. The name "dementia praecox," which had already been used by Morel* and later by Pick (1891), seemed to me to answer this purpose sufficiently, till a profounder understanding would provide an appropriate name.

It has since been found that the assumptions upon which the name chosen rested are at least doubtful. As will have to be explained more in detail later, the possibility cannot in the present state of our knowledge be disputed, that a certain number of cases of dementia praecox attain to complete and permanent recovery, and also the relations to the period of youth do not appear to be without exception. I certainly consider that the facts are not by any means sufficiently cleared up yet in either direction. If therefore the name which is in dispute even though it has been already fairly generally adopted, is to be replaced by another it is to be hoped that it will not soon share the fate of so many names of the kind, and of dementia praecox itself in giving a view of the nature of the disease which will turn out to be doubtful or wrong.

From this point of view, as Wolff showed, a name that as far as possible said nothing would be preferable, as dysphrenia. The name proposed by Evensen "amblynoia," "amblythymia," further the "demenza primitiva" of the Italians, or the one preferred by Rieger, which meanwhile has certainly been already used in a narrower sense, "dementia simplex," might also be taken into consideration. Bernstein speaks of a "paratonia progressiva," a name that would suit only a part of the observed cases. Other investigators accentuate the peculiar disturbance of the inner psychic association in our patients and call the disease "dementia

---

* Morel, Traité des maladies mentales, 566, 1860.

dissociativa," "dissecans," "sejunctiva" or with Bleuler "schizo-phrenia." It remains to be seen how far one or other of these names will be adopted.

GENERAL PSYCHIC CLINICAL PICTURE

Now if we make a general survey of the psychic clinical picture of dementia praecox, as it has presented itself to us in the consideration of about a thousand cases which belong to the subject, there are apparently two principal groups of disorders which characterise the malady. On the one hand we observe a *weakening of those emotional activities which permanently form the mainsprings of volition.* In connection with this, mental activity and instinct for occupation become mute. The result of this part of the morbid process is emotional dullness, failure of mental activities, loss of mastery over volition, of endeavour, and of ability for independent action. The essence of personality is thereby destroyed, the best and most precious part of its being, as Griesinger once expressed it, torn from her. With the annihilation of personal will, the possibility of further development is lost, which is dependent wholly on the activity of volition. What remains is principally what has been previously learned in the domain of knowledge and practical work. But this also sooner or later goes to ruin unless the failing inner mainspring is replaced by outer stimulus which rouses to continual practice and so obviates the slow disappearance of ability. Whether and how far the malady directly injures the mental faculties apart from their gradual disappearance through disuse of mental function needs further inquiry. The rapidity with which deep-seated and perma-nent dementia sometimes develops in the domain of intellectual work makes the suggestion easy, that it also may itself be drawn by the disease into a sympathetic morbid state, even though it is invariably encroached on to a much less degree than emotion and volition. It is worthy of note in any case, that memory and acquired mental proficiency may occasionally be preserved in a surprising way when there is complete and final destruction of the personality itself.

The second group of disorders, which gives dementia praecox its peculiar stamp, has been examined in detail especially by Stransky.* It consists in the *loss of the inner unity* of the activities

---

* Stranksy, Jahrb, f. Psychiatrie, xxiv., 1903, 1; Wiener med. Presse 1905, 28.

of intellect, emotion, and volition in themselves and among one another. Stransky speaks of an annihilation of the "intrapsychic co-ordination," which is said to loosen or destroy the articulations of the "noopsyche" and the "thymopsyche" themselves as well as their mutual relations. This annihilation presents itself to us in the disorders of association described by Bleuler, in incoherence of the train of thought, in the sharp change of moods as well as in desultoriness and derailments in practical work. But further the near connection between thinking and feeling, between deliberation and emotional activity on the one hand, and practical work on the other is more or less lost. Emotions do not correspond to ideas. The patients laugh and weep without recognisable cause, without any relation to their circumstances and their experiences, smile while they narrate the tale of their attempts at suicide: they are very much pleased that they "chatter so foolishly," and must remain permanently in the institution; on the most insignificant occasions they fall into violent terror or outbursts of rage, and then immediately break out into a neighing laugh. It is just this disagreement between idea and emotion that gives their behaviour the stamp of "silliness." Stransky traces the soiling of the bed also to a morbid connection of this procedure with feelings of pleasure.

The work of the patients is not as in healthy people the expression of their view of life and temperament, it is not guided by the elaboration of perceptions, by deliberation and moods, but it is the incalculable result of chance external influences, and of impulses, cross impulses, and contrary impulses, rising similarly by chance internally. A patient sang as he jumped into the Neckar; others burn or scatter their money, try to cut the throat of a beloved child, or with pitiful screaming maltreat themselves in the most regardless way. The phenomena of paramimia belong to this group also, the side activities, as well as the oddities which result from them, but especially do the disorders of inner speech find their place here, which may likewise be understood from the point of view of a relaxation of the relations between idea and actual speech. By this destruction of inner concatenation and causation the whole of active life receives the stamp of the incalculable, the incomprehensible, and the distorted.

As it seems to me, there exists an inner connection between the two groups of disorders, which are here distinguished. What fashions our experiences into a firmly mortised building, in which each part must fit the other and subordinate itself to the general plan, are general conceptions and ideas. The even calm of our temper, the swift victory over sudden shocks, are guaranteed by the higher general emotions; on the one hand they work by acting as a check, and on the other hand they give to the background of our mood a definite colouring even when no emotional stimuli are caused by special internal or external experiences. Lastly, the inner unity of our will is conditioned by the general trend of volition which is always alive in us, and which is the product of our racial and personal development. We may therefore expect that a weakening or annihilation of the influence which general conceptions, higher emotions, and the permanent general trend of volition exercise on our thinking, feeling, and acting, must draw after it that inner *disintegration*, those "schizophrenic" disorders, which we meet with in dementia praecox. It seems to me that the disorders observed in the patients and the complaints to which they give utterance, point exactly to injury to the general scheme of our psychic development, as it fixes the substance of our personality. The general trend of volition and also the higher emotions might form the first point of attack. But further the instrument of general conceptions with its regulating influence on the train of thought would then also become worthless, if the will were not longer capable of using it. Weygandt speaks, obviously following a similar line of thought, of an "apperceptive dementia" in as far as the injured "active apperception" signifies the dominion of volition over the formation and the course of psychic processes.

* * * *

INTRODUCTORY LECTURES ON CLINICAL PSYCHIATRY: III DEMENTIA PRAECOX

Gentlemen,—You have before you to-day a strongly-built and well-nourished man, aged twenty-one, who entered the hospital a few weeks ago. He sits quietly looking in front of him, and does not raise his eyes when he is spoken to, but evidently understands all our questions very well, for he answers quite relevantly, though slowly and often only after repeated questioning. From his brief remarks, made in a low tone, we gather that he thinks he is ill, without getting any more precise information about the nature of the illness and its symptoms. The patient attributes his malady to the onanism he has practised since he was ten years old. He thinks that he has thus incurred the guilt of a sin against the sixth commandment, has very much reduced his power of working, has made himself feel languid and miserable, and has become a hypochondriac. Thus, as the result of reading certain books, he imagined that he had a rupture and suffered from wasting of the spinal cord, neither of which was the case. He would not associate with his comrades any longer, because he thought they saw the results of his vice and made fun of him. The patient makes all these statements in an indifferent tone, without looking up or troubling about his surroundings. His expression betrays no emotion; he only laughs for a moment now and then. There is occasional wrinkling of the forehead or facial spasm. Round the mouth and nose a fine, changing twitching is constantly observed.

The patient gives us a correct account of his past experiences. His knowledge speaks for the high degree of his education; indeed, he was ready to enter the University a year ago. He also knows where he is and how long he has been here, but he is only very imperfectly acquainted with the names of the people round him, and says that he has never asked about them. He can only give a very meagre account of the general events of the last year. In answer to our questions, he declares that he is ready to remain in the hospital for the present. He would certainly prefer it if he could enter a profession, but he cannot say what he would like to take up. No physical disturbances can be definitely made out, except exaggerated knee-jerks.

At first sight, perhaps the patient reminds you of the states of depression which we have learned to recognise in former lectures. But on closer examination you will easily understand that, in spite of certain isolated points of resemblance, we have to deal here with a disease having features of quite another kind. The patient makes his statements slowly and in monosyllables, not because his wish to answer meets with overpowering hindrances, but because he feels no desire to speak at all. He certainly hears and understands what is said to him very well, but he does not take the trouble to attend to it. He pays no heed, and answers whatever occurs to him without thinking. No visible effort of the will is to be noticed. All his movements are languid and expressionless, but are made without hindrance or trouble. There is no sign of emotional dejection, such as one would expect from the nature of his talk, and the patient remains quite dull throughout, experiencing neither fear nor hope nor desires. He is not at all deeply affected by what goes on before him, although he understands it without actual difficulty. It is all the same to him who appears or disappears, where he is, or who talks to him and takes care of him, and he does not even once ask their names.

This peculiar and fundamental want of any *strong feeling of the impressions of life*, with unimpaired ability to understand and to remember, is really the diagnostic symptom of the disease we have before us. It becomes still plainer if we observe the patient for a time, and see that, in spite of his good education, he lies in bed for weeks and months, or sits about without feeling the slightest need of occupation. He broods, staring in front of him with expressionless features, over which a vacant smile occasionally plays, or at the best turns over the leaves of a book for a moment, apparently speechless, and not troubling about anything. Even when he has visitors, he sits without showing any interest, does not ask about what is happening at home, hardly even greets his parents, and goes back indifferently to the ward. He can hardly be induced to write a letter, and says that he has nothing to write about. But he occasionally composes a letter to the doctor, expressing all kinds of distorted, half-formed ideas, with a peculiar and silly play on words, in very fair style, but with little connection. He begs for "a little more *allegro* in the treatment," and "liberationary movement with a view to the widening of the horizon," will "*ergo* extort some wit in lectures," and "*nota bene* for God's sake only does not wish to be combined with the club of the harmless." "Professional work is the balm of life."

These scraps of writing, as well as his statements that he is pondering over the world or putting himself together a moral philosophy, leave no doubt that, besides the emotional barrenness, there is also a high degree of *weakness* of *judgment* and *flightiness*, although the pure memory has suffered little, if at all. We have a *mental and emotional infirmity* to deal with, which reminds us only outwardly of the states of depression previously described. This infirmity is the incurable outcome of a very common history of disease, to which we will provisionally give the name of *Dementia Praecox*.

The development of the illness has been quite gradual. Our patient, whose parents suffered transitorily from "dejection," did not go to school till he was seven years old, as he was a delicate child and spoke badly, but when he did he learned quite well. He was considered to be a reserved and stubborn child. Having practised onanism at a very early age, he became more and more solitary in the last few years, and thought that he was laughed at by his brothers and sisters, and shut out from society because of his ugliness. For this reason he could not bear a looking-glass in his room. After passing the written examination on leaving school, a year ago, he gave up the *viva voce*, because he could not work any longer. He cried a great deal, masturbated much, ran about aimlessly, played in a senseless way on the piano, and began to write observations " 'On the Nerve-play of Life,' which he cannot get on with." He was incapable of any kind of work, even physical, felt "done for," asked for a revolver, ate Swedish matches to destroy himself, and lost all affection for his family. From time to time he became excited and troublesome, and shouted out of the window at night. In the hospital, too, a state of excitement lasting for several days was observed, in which he chattered in a confused way, made faces, ran about at full speed, wrote disconnected scraps of composition, and crossed and recrossed them with flourishes and unmeaning combinations of letters. After this a state of tranquillity ensued, in which he could give absolutely no account of his extraordinary behaviour.*

Besides the mental and emotional weakness, we meet with other very significant features in the case before us. The first of these is the silly, vacant *laugh*, which is constantly observed in dementia praecox. There is no joyous humour corresponding to this laugh; indeed, some patients complain that they cannot help laughing, without feeling at all inclined to laugh. Other important symptoms are *making faces* or grimacing, and the fine muscular twitching in the face which is also very characteristic of dementia praecox. Then we must notice the tendency to peculiar, distorted turns of speech—*senseless playing with syllables and words*—as it often assumes very extraordinary forms in this disease. Lastly, I may call

---

* The patient afterwards returned to the care of his family unchanged. He has now been in an asylum again for three and a half years, dull and demented.

your attention to the fact that, when you offer him your hand, the patient does not grasp it, but only *stretches his own hand out stiffly to meet it.* Here we have the first sign of a disturbance which is often developed in dementia praecox in the most astounding way.

As the illness-developed quite gradually, it is hardly possible to fix on any particular point of time as the beginning. In such cases, the change which is taking place is easily referred to some culpable looseness of morality, which it is sought to combat by educational means. Onanism in particular, which is very common in our patients, is usually held to be the source of the disease, so that cases of this kind were formerly spoken of as the insanity of onanism. I am nevertheless inclined to see in onanism a symptom, rather than the cause, of the disease. We often see the whole striking degree of onanism, and we also know degenerate onanists who present quite different symptoms. Hence there cannot well be any question of a regular causal connection between onanism and dementia praecox. Besides, the disease is just as common among women, in whom the weakening effet of onanism must be much slighter. Lastly, it is to be observed that the disease often sets in quite suddenly, another circumstance not exactly adapted to confirm the supposition of its onanistic origin.

Dementia praecox often begins with a state of depression, which at first may easily be confused with the kinds of depression already described. As an example of this, I will show you a day-labourer, aged twenty-two, who first came into the hospital three years ago. He belongs, it is said, to a healthy family, and did well at school. A few weeks before his admission he had some attacks of apprehension, and then became disturbed, ill-balanced and absent-minded, stared in front of him, spoke in a confused way, and expressed vague ideas of sin and persecution. On admission, he gave hesitating, broken answers, did sums and obeyed orders, but did not know where he was. He hardly spoke at all of his own accord, or at most muttered a few almost incomprehensible words: there was war; he could not eat, lived by the word of God; there was a raven at the window that wished to eat his flesh, and so on. Although he understood what was said to him quite well, and even let his attention be easily diverted, he did not trouble at all about his surroundings, had no desire to make himself clear about his position, and expressed neither apprehension nor desires. He generally lay in bed with a rigid, vacant expression, but often got up to kneel down or go about slowly. All his movements showed a certain constraint and want of freedom. His limbs remained for some time in the position in which you placed them. If you raised your arms quickly in front of him, he imitated the movement, and he also clapped his hands when it was done before him. These phenomena called respectively *flexibilitas cerea*, "*waxen flexibility*," a catalepsy in the one case, and *echopraxis* in the other, are familiar to us from experiments in hypnotism. They are always symptoms of a peculiar disturbance of volition, of which we include the various manifestations under the name of *automatic obedience*. Inequality of the pupils is also to be noticed in our patient, and I must mention the occurrence of an attack of unconsciousness, with twitching in the arms.

The patient's condition improved in the course of the next few months. He became clearer, his behaviour was more natural, and he had a distinct feeling of illness, but he remained strikingly apathetic and devoid of ideas. Nevertheless, he found employment outside, and only came back to the hospital a year ago. He had thrown himself in front of a train, losing his right foot and breaking his left arm. This time he was collected and clean about his surroundings, and showed considerable knowledge of geography and arithmetic, but spoke to none of his own accord, and lay in bed dully, with a vacant expression, without occupying himself or paying attention to what went on around him. He alleged as the reason for his attempted suicide that he was ill; his brain had burst out a year before. Since then he could not think by himself; others knew his thoughts, spoke about them, and heard if he read the newspaper.

The patient is still in the same condition to-day. He stares apathetically in front of him, does not glance round at his surroundings, although they are strange to him, and does not look up when he is spoken to. Yet it is possible to get a few relevant answers by questioning him urgently. He knows where he is, can tell the year and month and the names of the doctors, does simple sums, and can repeat the names of some towns and rivers, but at the same time he calls himself Wilhelm Rex, the son of the German Emperor. He does not worry about his position, and says he is willing to stay here, as his brain is injured and the veins are burst. The waxen flexibility and echopraxis can still be made out clearly. When told to give his hand, he stretches it out stiffly, without grasping.

---

* The patient has now spent five years in a nursing asylum, and has become quite affected and demented.

234

You will understand at once that we have a *state of dementia* before us, in which the faculty of comprehension and the recollection of knowledge previously acquired are much less affected than the judgment, and especially than the emotional impulses and the acts of volition which stand in closest relation to those impulses. The disease thus delineated agrees to a great extent with the case which was last described, in spite of the different development of the illness. The complete loss of mental activity, and of interest in particular, and the failure of every impulse to energy, are such characteristic and fundamental indications that they give a very definite stamp to the condition in both cases. Together with the weakness of judgment, they are invariable and permanent fundamental features of dementia praecox, accompanying the whole evolution of the disease. Compared with these, all other disturbances, however prominent they may be in individual cases, must be regarded as merely transitory, and therefore not absolutely diagnostic, features. This holds good, for instance, of delusions and hallucinations, which are very frequently present, but may be developed in very different degrees or be altogether absent, or disappear, without the fundamental features of the disease or its course and issue being in any way affected. Yet we may consider it a rule that states of depression which are accompanied *at the very beginning* by vivid hallucinations or confused delusions usually form the prelude to dementia praecox. Fluctuations in spirits are always only of a fugitive kind in this disease, and therefore cannot be made use of for the diagnosis. At the very onset, indeed, we often observe states of lively apprehension or sad depression, but generally we can soon satisfy ourselves that the affections of the emotions really disappear very quickly, even when the external signs of them continue for some time longer.

Looking at the strongly-built postman, aged thirty-five, who stands before you now, you will hardly believe that a few days ago this man not only tried to make away with himself, but also wished to persuade his wife to die with him. He had been cut down insensible from the water-pipe a few days before. The patient is pale, and his general nutrition is much impaired. He is quite collected, knows where he is, understands his position, and gives relevant and connected answers to questions. He says that he has been ill for five weeks. He suffered from headaches, and thought that his comrades talked about little failings of which he had been guilty in former places. He heard someone say, "We'll catch you; we'll pull your little shirt off." There was also a great

235

deal that he did not understand; there was telephoning into his ear. Then he hanged himself because of the voices. Later on he began to work again, but was still apprehensive. He was afraid he had passed false money and would go to prison for it, was confused in his head, and asked his wife to shoot herself with him, as she would be left in misfortune if he went to prison. He could not sleep or eat, and kept on reproaching himself. He saw a head, of which he was afraid at first, on the ceiling; then, with his eyes shut, he saw two tables, of which one was split, and on them a house with windows and an arch.

The patient relates all these experiences smilingly and with an affected way of speaking. He gives no further thought to his attempted suicide, or to his having been brought to the asylum. He offers his hand in a stiff, spread-out way, shows well-marked catalepsy and echopraxis, which also takes the form of echolalia, when he repeats words shouted to him immediately, sometimes distorting them. For the first part of his stay in the asylum he lay in bed almost all day, often with his eyes closed and without moving, not even stirring when he was spoken to or even pricked with a needle. As he sometimes related, he heard voices which said all manner of things before him or called them to him. He told in a whisper how he had seen a blue heart up above, and behind it quivering sunshine and another blue heart, "a little woman's heart." He also saw flashes of lightning and a comet with a long tail. The sun rose on the wrong side.

It is also to be noticed that for the last few days the patient has suddenly refused to eat, without any cause, so that it has been necessary to feed him artificially. He declined the suggestion that he should write to his wife, on the ground that he had more important things to do. He did not wish for a visit from her: "it would really not be worth while." When told to show his tongue, he opened his mouth, but rolled back his tongue with all his strength against his soft palate. Once, for a short time, he suddenly became blindly violent against his surroundings, without being able to give any account of his reasons afterwards. The only physical symptom worth noticing is a great increase in the knee-jerks.

It cannot have escaped you that the same fundamental symptoms of emotional dullness, absence of independent impulses of the will, and increased susceptibility of the will to influence, which have already struck us in the cases previously described, are to be found again in this description. And there are just as many details, such as the hallucinations and the extraordinary way of giving the hand, to support the conclusion that the present case is also one of dementia praecox, which we drew from the emotional dulness and the automatic obedience. Finally, we must take a number of disturbances, which we shall have to consider more exactly at the earliest opportunity—the patient's senseless resistance to receiving food, to showing his tongue, and to writing letters, and also his stuporose behaviour—in the same sense. We therefore come to the conclusion that in reality the case now before us most probably belongs to the same disease as the two cases previously described.

In those cases, however, we had to deal with diseases of several years' standing, which had resulted in a condition of incurable mental infirmity. Experience shows that this is by far the most frequent result of dementia praecox. The importance of our diagnosis would therefore consist in this: that we are now able, at the very beginning of the illness, to predict its resulting in a characteristic state of feebleness, in the same way as we arrived at certain probable conclusions about the further course of the disease in circular stupor. The prognosis, however, is really by no means simple. Whether dementia praecox is susceptible of a complete and permanent recovery answering to the strict demands of science is still very doubtful, if not impossible to decide. But improvements are not at all unusual, which in practice may be considered equivalent to cures. In these cases the patients suffer a certain impairment of their mental and emotional activity and of their power of action, and other slight remains of the symptoms of the disease may perhaps be recognized, yet they may be fully capable of filling their old place in simple relations. It is a more serious matter that in most of these cases the improvement is only *temporary*, and that such patients are in great danger of relapsing sooner or later, without any particular cause, and then generally suffer more serious injury from their illness. We had to record such an improvement in our second case, though it is true that it did not go very far. It was followed by a relapse. In the case of our third patient also we may hope for the disappearance of the present symptoms, but we must be prepared for their return in an even more serious form.*

---

* The patient, having made an extraordinary recovery physically, but with no proper understanding of his ailment, was discharged from the asylum after he had been there for three months. He has now been at home for four years and nine months, apparently cured.

INTRODUCTION

Emil Kraepelin (1856–1926) is now justly regarded as the foremost representative of the classical tradition in German clinical psychiatry. His major contributions were in the field of classification and diagnosis; in which nosological principles, insistence on the identity of causal factors, and course and outcome as the criteria of a mental disorder featured most prominently. Before Kraepelin introduced his great synthesizing concepts of dementia praecox and manic depressive psychosis, existing classifications were in confusion. In this area alone, his legacy surpassed in scope, permanence and heuristic value that of any of his predecessors and virtually all of his successors.

At a personal level, those who knew Kraepelin remarked on his pleasant responsive personality, his tactful ability to bring people together to work as an organised group, and of his gifts as a teacher. His scientific personality, on the other hand, was said to be detached and distant from the patient's inner life.

The essence of Kraepelin's method is conveyed by the preface to his *Lectures on Clinical Psychiatry* (Kraepelin, 1906):

> I have always kept the diagnostic point of view in the foreground, being convinced of its fundamental importance, not only to scientific ideas, but also as affecting the advice we shall have to give in our medical practice, and the methods of treatment to be adopted by us. In my opinion, what the student ought to learn in the hospital, besides the examination of patients, is not text-book knowledge, which he can acquire just as well, or better, at home, but how to turn his observations to account, and the careful judgement of any given case. These lectures, then, must not in any way be looked upon as a text-book of alienism. Their aim will be far better attained if they prove of some value as a guide to the clinical investigation of the insane.

As his writings demonstrate, careful observation and experimental method characterise him as one of the earliest and greatest advocates of clinical science in psychiatry.

Through the clinical study of the natural history of mental disorders, Kraepelin attempted to discover common features in these conditions which would be of value in assessing prognosis. On the basis of his work it became possible to classify mental disorders into three main classes: the organic psychoses, the endogenous psychoses without known structural pathology, and the deviations of personality and reactive states.

Kraepelin's far-reaching influence on the development of psychiatry was exerted mainly through the medium of his famous textbook, which Wundt had initially encouraged him to write. The *Kompendium der Psychiatrie* appeared in one volume for the first time in 1883 (Kraepelin, 1883). The

238

fourth edition (Kraepelin, 1893) was no longer a compendium but a *Lehrbuch*. It reached its classical form in 1899 (Kraepelin, 1899). The final, ninth edition appeared in two volumes in 1927 (Kraepelin and Lange, 1927). It is evident that over time many of Kraepelin's ideas required, and received, considerable subsequent revision. To his credit, he was always ready to be persuaded to modify his theoretical point of view, recognizing the manifest inadequacies of his, nevertheless, monumental achievement.

KRAEPELIN AND HIS CONTEMPORARIES: BIOGRAPHICAL BACKGROUND

Kraepelin was born at Neustrelitz, Mecklenburg, on February 15th 1856. He first entered the orbit of psychiatry as a medical student, when he submitted a competitive essay entitled *On the influence of acute diseases on the origin of mental diseases*. After graduating in medicine at Wurzburg in 1878, he worked briefly at a mental institution in Southern Germany, and then became an assistant to Gudden in Munich in 1878—the same year in which Charcot began his studies of hysteria at the Salpêtrière. In 1882 he moved to Leipzig, where he soon gave up neuro-anatomical studies with Flechsig in favour of psychological research with Erb and Wundt who played the major role in influencing his pupil towards an experimental orientation.

Following mental hospital appointments in München, Leubus and Dresden, Kraepelin became professor of psychiatry in Dorpat in 1886, in Heidelberg in 1890 and in München in 1904. In 1922 he retired from his chair so as to be able to devote himself entirely to the German Research Institute of Psychiatry, the Forschungsanstalt, which he founded in 1917.

Kraepelin travelled extensively to study mental disorder and administrative psychiatry in various parts of the world, and he is justifiably acknowledged to be one of the forerunners of what is now known as transcultural psychiatry. His work in criminology formed the basis of modern thinking on the relationship between psychiatric disorder and criminality. He also became famous for his practical work, e.g., a campaign against alcoholism, which was supported by Forel and Bleuler, among others.

CONCEPTS OF MENTAL DISORDER

In the middle of the 19th century Zeller and Griesinger had scorned attempts to subdivide the unitary psychosis—*die Einheitpsychose*. Towards the turn of the century, the prevailing views of determinism and causality were in the Platonic tradition. Mental disorders were generally held to consist of a finite number of disease entities, with distinct causes, psychological form, outcome, and cerebral pathology. In this philosophical climate, and as an accurate clinical observer, Kraepelin delineated syndromes which gained widespread and enduring recognition.

Criticism of Kraepelin's classification was in the Hippocratic tradition (e.g., Hoche, 1910). The dispute between Platonic and Hippocratic traditions centred on their differing concepts of disease entities; the former maintained that such things existed, the latter regarded them as abstactions. Jaspers pointed out that Kraepelin assumed that the same classification of patients would result regardless of whether aetiological, psychopathological or neuropathological criteria were used (Jaspers, 1959). He argued that no entities fulfilling these criteria had ever been found in psychiatry. Returning to the original question, whether or not there are only stages and variants of a single *Einheitspsychose* or a series of disease entities, Jaspers concluded: 'The latter view is right in so far that the idea of disease entities has become a fruitful orientation for the investigations of special psychiatry. The former view is right in so far that no actual disease entities exist in scientific psychiatry'. Late in his career, Kraepelin (1920) clearly acknowledged the complex causality of mental illnesses.

PRECURSORS OF DEMENTIA PRAECOX

In France, Pinel (1801) applied the term *la manie* to most patients; another large group of patients, also viewed as insane but not showing the same degree of affective excess, were said to have *la démence*, dementia, without a strong emotional component. In Britain, Haslam (1798) described what appeared to be similar patients who displayed a state which could not be termed maniacal or melancholic: a state of complete insanity, unaccompanied by 'furious or depressing passions'. These observations were corroborated elsewhere as the years passed.

A paranoid illness was described by Heinroth (1818); Laseague described *delire de persecution* in 1852; and in the same year Morel applied the term *démence précoce* to patients with intellectual deterioration, withdrawal and bizarre mannerisms, starting in adolescence (Morel, 1852). Similar patients were also described by Moreau.

In Germany in the 1860s, Snell was stimulated by the problem of monomania and tried to prove the existence of a third primary mental disease apart from melancholia and mania: primary insanity. Westphal, Hagen and Sander also worked with the concept of primary insanity, which finally gained acceptance in the form of Kraepelin's paranoia. Catatonia, stupor occurring in the absence of disease of the nervous system, was described as a separate disease by Kahlbaum (1874), who noted both its clinical features and its cyclic course. Hecker (1871), a student of Kahlbaum, published a monograph on hebephrenia, an illness which occurred in puberty and led to a 'silly' deterioration, that stressed its symptomatology and deteriorating course. Pick, in 1891, described a simplex syndrome, simple deterioration accompanied by a minimum of other symptoms, which remained after the two groups described by Hecker and Kahlbaum were separated from the broad category identified by Morel. Three years later, these three groupings were incorporated in Sommer's textbook.

DEMENTIA PRAECOX

The beginning of what we may view as the modern period comes with Kraepelin's delineation of the concept of dementia praecox. He initiated a detailed classification system for psychiatric disorders, and, by 1893, in the fourth edition of his textbook, he grouped *démence précoce*, hebephrenia, catatonia and dementia paranoides under 'psychological degeneration processes'. In this edition, Kraepelin used the term dementia praecox in a narrow sense to refer to patients who fitted Hecker's description of hebephrenia: paranoia and catatonia were seen as being distinct from this disorder. However, Kraepelin doubted the usefulness of the term dementia praecox: because, first, some patients attained complete and permanent recoveries; secondly, attention was drawn from the affective aspect of the disorder; and, last, not all cases began in adolescence.

The title of the chapter was changed to 'Dementia Praecox' in the fifth edition (Kraepelin, 1896). And the full concept of dementia praecox was first presented in a paper called 'The Diagnosis and Prognosis of Dementia Praecox', which Kraepelin delivered to the 29th Congress of South-Western German Psychiatry in Heidelberg on the 27th of November 1898.

In the eighth edition of his textbook Kraepelin (1913) defined dementia praecox as consisting of a series of clinical states which had as their common characteristics a peculiar destruction of the internal connections of the psychic personality with the most marked damage of the emotional life and of volition. Thus Kraepelin focused on both course and symptoms in defining the disorder, though it is often suggested that he emphasized the former rather than the latter.

In proposing a unitary concept of dementia praecox, Kraepelin had brought together disorders which had been described earlier in the century. He also recognized the clinical heterogeneity of patients given this diagnosis, and he subdivided dementia praecox into subtypes that depended on the prominence of particular symptoms. In early editions of his textbook, three subcategories were proposed: in the paranoid type, delusions were predominant; in the catatonic type, motor dysfunctions were most obvious; and in the hebephrenic type, emotional incongruity was the major feature. Following the proposals of Bleuler, Kraepelin later added a fourth subtype, simple, for which no single symptom was paramount.

Kraepelin's strength lay not in theory but in his clinical descriptions, and his writings are a lasting, rich descriptive account of the clinical features of dementia praecox. In the eighth edition of his textbook, for example, he grouped the symptoms of dementia praecox into 36 major categories, each of which contained hundreds of individual behaviours. Kraepelin made little effort to interrelate the symptoms: he stated only that they all reflected dementia and a loss of the usual unity among the functions: thinking, feeling, and acting. Kraepelin offered little speculation about the aetiology of dementia praecox: he believed the cause to be physiological (from 1896 he included it among the metabolic disorders) but recognized that empirical evidence was not available to support that hypothesis.

SUBSEQUENT DEVELOPMENTS

In contrast to Kraepelin's descriptive approach, Bleuler (1911) attempted both to define the core of these disorders (named by him, the schizophrenias), and to move away from what was regarded as Kraepelin's emphasis on prognosis in diagnosis. Kraepelin's work fostered a narrow definition of these disorders, with an emphasis on description, which has been refined and adopted by European psychiatry, most notably due to the work of Schneider (1957) on first rank symptoms. Bleuler's ideas, leading to a broader clinical concept of the schizophrenic disorders, with a strong theoretical emphasis, were taken up most enthusiastically in parts of the USA. There, Kasanin (1933) suggested the term schizo-affective psychosis to describe patients with dementia praecox with acute onset, and a combination of schizophrenic and affective symptoms, followed by relatively rapid recovery. Langfeldt (1937) later proposed the diagnosis schizophreniform psychosis for patients who recovered, who had an acute onset of disorder, the presence of precipitating stress, confusion, affective symptoms, and a family history of depression. A different pathway, leading to the influential concept of cycloid psychoses, was opened up by Schroeder (1926), Kleist (1921) and his pupils, and Leonhard (1959).

Currently, a large number of research diagnostic criteria for schizophrenic and other mental disorders are in use (Brockington et al., 1978). These tend to differ more in detail than in principle and are mostly based on a Kraepelinian model. The undoubted improvement in diagnostic reliability which may be achieved through the use of such criteria is offset by the questionable validity of the constructs thereby identified. Despite welcome advances in treatment methods and investigative techniques and the relatively recent introduction of diagnostic classifications in the form of the World Health Organization's (1978) International Classification of Diseases and the Diagnostic and Statistical Manual of the American Psychiatric Association (1980), the classification and diagnosis of functional psychoses, and especially the schizophrenias, remain in a disappointingly unsatisfactory state.

G. Wilkinson

REFERENCES

American Psychiatric Association (1980). *Diagnostic and Statistical Manual of Mental Disorders*, 3rd edn, American Psychiatric Association, Washington, D.C.

Bleuler, E. (1911). *Dementia Praecox or the Group of Schizophrenias* (transl. J. Zinkin, 1950), International Universities Press, New York.

Brockington, I. F., Kendell, R. E. and Leff, J. P. (1978). Definitions of schizophrenia: concordance and prediction of outcome. *Psychological Medicine*, **8**, 387–398.

Haslam, J. (1798). *Observations on Insanity: With Practical Remarks on the Disease, and an Account of the Morbid Appearances on Dissection*, Hatchard, London.

Hecker, E. (1871). Die Hebephrenie. *Archiv für Pathologische Anatomie und Physiologie und Klinische Medizin*, **52**, 394–429.

Heinroth, J. C. H. (1818). *Lehrbuch der Storungen des Seelenleben's oder der Seelenstorungen und ihrer Behandlung* vols 1 and 2, Vogel, Leipzig.

Hoche, A. (1910). Die Melancholiefrage. *Zentralblatt für Nervenheilkunde und Psychiatrie*, **21**, 193–203.

Jaspers, K. (1959). *Allgemeine Psychopathologie*, 7th edn (transl. J. Hoering and M. W. Hamilton, 1962), Manchester University Press, Manchester.

Kahlbaum, K. L. (1874). *Katatonie oder das Spannungsirresein*, Hirschwald, Berlin.

Kasanin, J. (1933). The acute schizoaffective psychoses. *American Journal of Psychiatry*, **13**, 97–123.

Kleist, K. (1921). Autochthonone Degenerationspsychosen. *Zeitschrift für die gesamte Neurologie-Psychiatrie*, **69**, 1.

Kraepelin, E. (1883). *Kompendium der Psychiatrie*, Abel, Leipzig.

Kraepelin, E. (1893). *Psychiatrie*, 4th edn, Meiner, Leipzig.

Kraepelin, E. (1896). *Psychiatrie*, 5th edn, Barth, Leipzig.

Kraepelin, E. (1899). *Psychiatrie*, 6th edn, Bart, Leipzig.

Kraepelin, E. (1906). *Lectures on Clinical Psychiatry* (authorized transl. from the 2nd German edition, revised and edited by T. Johnstone), 2nd English edn, Bailliére, Tindall and Cox, London.

Kraepelin, E. (1913). *Psychiatrie* 8th edn, vol. 3, Barth, Leipzig.

Kraepelin, E. (1920). Die Erscheinungsformen des Irreseins. *Zeitschrift für die gesamte Neurologie-Psychiatrie*, **62**, 1–29.

Kraepelin, E. and Lange, J. (1927). *Psychiatrie*, 9th edn, Bart, Leipzig.

Langfeldt, G. (1937). The prognosis in schizophrenia and the factors influencing the course of the disease. *Acta Psychiatrica et Neurologica Scandinavica*, suppl. 13.

Leonhard, K. (1959). *Anfteilung der Endogen Psychosen*, 2nd edn, Akademie Verlag, Berlin.

Morel, B. A. (1852). *Etudes Cliniques: Traité Théorique et Practique des Maladies Mentales*, Masson, Paris.

Pinel, P. (1801). *Traité Medico-philosophique sur Aliénation Mentale, ou la Manie*, Richard, Coville et Ravier, Paris.

Schneider, K. (1957). Primäre und Sekundäre Symptome bei der Schizophrenie. *Forschritte der Neurologie-Psychiatrie*, **25**, 487–490.

Schroeder, P. (1926). Uber Degenerationspsychosen (Metabolische Enkrankungen). *Zeitschrift für die gesamte Neurologe-Psychiatrie*, **105**, 539.

World Health Organization (1978). *Mental Disorders: Glossary and Guide to their Classification in Accordance with the Ninth Revision of the International Classification of Diseases*, World Health Organization, Geneva.

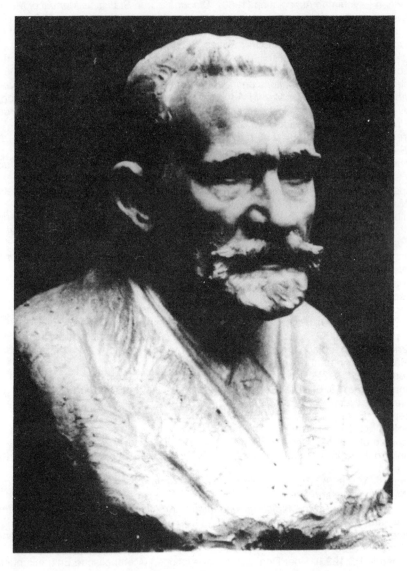

12

Manic Depressive Insanity and Paranoia (1921) and Introductory Lectures on Clinical Psychiatry (1906) I Melancholia
E. *Kraepelin*

MANIC-DEPRESSIVE INSANITY

Definition

Manic-depressive insanity, as it is to be described in this section, includes on the one hand the whole domain of so-called *periodic and circular insanity*, on the other hand *simple mania*, the greater part of the morbid states termed *melancholia* and also a not inconsiderable number of cases of *amentia*. Lastly, we include here certain slight and slightest colourings of *mood*, some of them periodic, some of them continuously morbid, which on the one hand are to be regarded as the rudiment of more severe disorders, on the other hand pass over without sharp boundary into the domain of *personal predisposition*. In the course of the years I have become more and more convinced that all the above-mentioned states only represent manifestations of a *single morbid process*. It is certainly possible that later a series of subordinate forms may be described, or even individual small groups again entirely separated off. But if this happens, then according to my view those symptoms will most certainly not be authoritative, which hitherto have usually been placed in the foreground.

What has brought me to this position is first the experience that notwithstanding manifold external differences certain *common fundamental features* yet recur in all the morbid states mentioned. Along with changing symptoms, which may appear temporarily or may be completely absent, we meet in all forms of manic-depressive insanity a quite definite, narrow group of disorders, though certainly of very varied character and composition. Without any one of them being absolutely characteristic of the malady, still in association they impress a uniform stamp on all the multiform clinical states. If one is conversant with them, one will in the great majority of cases be able to conclude in regard to any one of them that it belongs to the large group of forms of manic-depressive insanity by the peculiarity of the condition, and thus to gain a series of fixed points for the special clinical and prognostic significance of the case. Even a small part of the course of the disease usually enables us to arrive at this decision, just as in paralysis or dementia praecox the general psychic change often enough makes possible the diagnosis of the fundamental malady in its most different phases.

Of perhaps still greater significance than the classification of states by definite fundamental disorders is the experience that all the morbid forms brought together here as a clinical entity, *not only pass over the one into the other without recognisable boundaries, but that they may even replace each other in one and the same case.* On the one side, it is fundamentally and practically quite impossible to keep apart in any consistent way simple, periodic and circular cases; everywhere there are gradual transitions. But on the other side we see in the same patient not only mania and melancholia, but also states of the most profound confusion and perplexity, also well developed delusions, and lastly, the slightest fluctuations of mood alternating with each other. Moreover, permanent, one-sided colourings of mood very commonly form the background on which fully developed circumscribed attacks of manic-depressive insanity develop.

A further common bond which embraces all the morbid types brought together here and makes the keeping of them apart practically almost meaningless, is their *uniform prognosis.* There are indeed slight and severe attacks which may be of long or short duration, but they alternate irregularly in the same case. This difference is therefore of no use for the delimitation of different diseases. A grouping according to the frequency of the attacks might much rather be considered, which naturally would be extremely welcome to the physician. It appears, however, that here also we have not to do with fundamental differences, since in spite of certain general rules it has not been possible to separate out definite types from this point of view. On the contrary the universal experience is striking, that the attacks of manic-depressive insanity within the delimitation attempted here never lead to profound dementia, not even when they continue throughout life almost without interruption. Usually all morbid manifestations completely disappear; but where that is exceptionally not the case, only a rather slight, peculiar psychic weakness develops, which is just as common to the types here taken together as it is different from dementias in diseases of other kinds.

As a last support for the view here respresented of the unity of manic-depressive insanity the circumstance may be adduced, that the various forms which it comprehends may also apparently mutually replace one another in *heredity*. In members of the same family we frequently enough find side by side pronounced periodic or circular cases, occasionally isolated states of ill temper or confusion, lastly very slight, regular fluctuations of mood or permanent conspicuous colouration of disposition. From whatever point of view accordingly the manic-depressive morbid forms may be regarded, from that of aetiology or of clinical phenomena, the course or the issue—it is evident everywhere that here points of agreement exist, which make it possible to regard our domain as a unity and to delimit it from all the other morbid types hitherto discussed. Further experience must show whether and in what directions in this extensive domain smaller sub-groups can be separated from one another.

In the first place the difference of the states which usually make up the disease, presents itself as the most favourable ground of classification. As a rule the disease runs its course in isolated attacks more or less sharply defined from each other or from health, which are either like or unlike, or even very frequently are perfect antithesis. Accordingly we distinguish first of all *manic states* with the essential morbid symptoms of flight of ideas, exalted mood, and pressure of activity, and *melancholia or depressive states* with sad or anxious moodiness and also sluggishness of thought and action. These two opposed phases of the clinical state have given the disease its name. But besides them we observe also clinical *"mixed forms,"* in which the phenomena of mania and melancholia are combined with each other, so that states arise, which indeed are composed of the same morbid symptoms as these, but cannot without coercion be classified either with the one or with the other.

*   *   *   *

247

INTRODUCTORY LECTURES ON CLINICAL PSYCHIATRY: I MELANCHOLIA

Gentlemen,—After these introductory remarks, let us turn to the consideration of our patients. I will first place before you a farmer, aged fifty-nine, who was admitted to the hospital a year ago. The patient looks much older than he really is, principally owing to the loss of the teeth from his upper jaw. He not only understands our questions without any difficulty, but answers them relevantly and correctly; can tell where he is, and how long he has been here; knows the doctors, and can give the date and the day of the week. His expression is dejected. The corners of his mouth are rather drawn down, and his eyebrows drawn together. He usually stares in front of him, but he glances up when he is spoken to. On being questioned about his illness, he breaks into lamentations, saying that he did not tell the whole truth on his admission, but concealed the fact that he had fallen into sin in his youth and practised uncleanness with himself; everything he did was wrong. "I am so apprehensive, so wretched; I cannot lie still for anxiety. O God, if I had only not transgressed so grievously!" He has been ill for over a year, has had giddiness and headaches. It began with stomach-aches and head trouble, and he could not work any longer. "There was no impulse left." He can get no rest now, and fancies silly things, as if someone were in the room. Once it seemed to him that he had seen the Evil One: perhaps he would be carried off. So things seemed to him. As a boy, he had taken apples and nuts. "Conscience has said that that is not right; conscience has only awakened just now in my illness." He had also played with a cow, and by himself. "I reproach myself for that now." It seemed to him that he had fallen away from God and was now as free as a bird. His appetite is bad, and he has no stools. He cannot sleep. "If the mind does not sleep, all sorts of thoughts come." He has done silly things too. He fastened his neckerchief to strangle himself, but he was not really in earnest. Three sisters and a brother were ill too. The illnesses were not so bad; they soon recovered. "A brother has made away with himself through apprehension."

The patient tells us this in broken sentences, interrupted by wailing and groaning. In all other respects, he behaves naturally, does whatever he is told and only begs us not to let him be dragged away—" There is dreadful apprehension in my heart."

Except for a little trembling of the outspread fingers and slightly arhythmic action of the heart, we find no striking disturbances at the physical examination. As for the patient's former history, he is married and has four healthy children, while three are dead. The illness began gradually seven or eight months before his admission, without any assignable cause. Loss of appetite and dyspepsia appeared first, and then ideas of sin. His weight diminished a little after his admission, but has now slowly risen again 7 kilogrammes.

The most striking feature of this clinical picture is the *apprehensive depression*. At first sight, it resembles the anxieties of a healthy person, and the patient says that he was always rather apprehensive, and has only grown worse. But there is not the least external cause for the apprehension, and yet it has lasted for months, with increasing severity. This is the diagnostic sign of its morbidity. It is true that the patient himself refers to the sins of his youth as the cause of the apprehension, but it is clear that, even if they were ever really committed, they did not particularly disturb him before his illness; his conscience has only awakened now. His actions now appear to him in an entirely different and fatal light, and those morbid symptoms become prominent which are known as *"delusions of sin."* The patient's ideas that the Evil One was in the room, that he would be carried off, and that he had fallen away from God, must be regarded as a result of his apprehension. There is no question of real hallucinations in these statements; it only *seemed so* to the patient. He also has a strong feeling that some great change has come over him, and that he is "not the same as before." He is certainly not in a condition to form a correct conception of the morbidity of his ideas of sin and of his fears in detail.

We give the name of *melancholia* to this condition, in which we see the gradual development of a state of apprehensive depression, associated with more or less fully-developed delusions. The most common of these are ideas of sin, which generally have a religious colouring. Such are the ideas of having fallen away from God and being forsaken, or of being possessed by the devil. Hypochondriacal ideas—of never being well again, never having a stool again, etc.—are also far from uncommon. Together with these there is often apprehension of poverty, of having to starve, of being thrown into prison, of being brought before a court, or even of execution.

As a consequence of this mental unrest and these tormenting

ideas, the wish to have done with life develops almost invariably, and patients very often become suicidal. Our first patient only made a rather feeble attempt at suicide, but I will now show you a widow, aged fifty-four, who has made very serious efforts to take her own life. This patient has no insane history. She married at the age of thirty, and has four healthy children. She says that her husband died two years ago, and since then she has slept badly. Being obliged to sell her home at that time, because the inheritance was to be divided. she grew apprehensive, and thought that she would come to want, although, on quiet consideration, she saw that her fears were groundless. She complained of heat in her head and uneasiness at her heart, felt weak and excited, and was tired of life, especially in the morning. She says she could get no sleep at night, even with sleeping-powders. Suddenly the thought came to her, "What are you doing in the world now? Try to get out of it, so as to be at rest. It's no good any longer." Then she hung herself up behind the house with her handkerchief, and became unconscious, but her son cut her down and brought her to the hospital.

Here she was quite collected, and was orderly in thought and behaviour. She understood the morbidity of her condition, but feared that she would never be well again. She said she could not bear it any longer, and could not stay here; she was driven to despair. She was very fond of talking about her condition, and loudly lamented that she was so apprehensive, asking for a clergyman to come and drive out the Evil One. At this she was seized with violent trembling in her whole body, and declared that she had no peace; she could not rest, her heart beat so; her head was bursting, she could not live any longer; she wished to die at home; thoughts of suicide tormented her unceasingly. Her sleep and appetite were bad, but no other physical disturbance could be discovered. In the course of the first few months her mental condition improved fairly quickly, and, at the urgent desire of her relations, leave of absence was granted with the family of her daughter. But the apprehension and thoughts of suicide became so marked that she had to be brought back to the hospital within a fortnight. Here her condition is still improving, though very slowly and with many fluctuations. Her recovery has been much delayed by a carious affection of the right parietal bone and the left wrist, which necessitated repeated interference, but is now in a tolerably healthy condition.

This patient, too, is quite clear as to her surroundings, and gives connected information about her condition. She has no real delusions, apart from fear that she will never be well again. Indeed, we find that the real meaning of the whole picture of disease is only permanent *apprehensive depression*, with the same accompaniments as we see in mental agitation in the sane—i.e., loss of sleep and appetite, and failure of the general nutrition. The resemblance to anxiety in a sane person is all the greater because the depression has followed a painful external cause. But we can easily see that the severity, and more especially the duration of the emotional depression have gone beyond the limits of what is normal. The patient herself sees clearly enough that her apprehension is not justified by her real position in life, and that there is absolutely no reason why she should wish to die.

This sense of the morbid nature of the apprehension, or "insight into the disease," is not always present in melancholia. In those cases, more especially, in which there are marked *delusions* this important symptom may be altogether absent for a long time together. As an example, I will show you a widow, aged fifty-six, who nursed her son when he was ill of typhus two and a quarter years ago. She then had a feverish illness herself, presumably also typhus, and lost her husband suddenly a few months later. Very soon after this she began to be apprehensive, and to reproach herself with not having taken proper care of her husband. Strongly-marked delusions of sin quickly developed. She had never done anything properly, and had allowed herself to be led away by the wicked fiend. Her prayers had been no good, only she did not know that before. Her husband absolutely married the devil, and could not go to heaven, and she and her children were damned on account of her former unchristian life. Great restlessness and almost complete sleeplessness now came on. The patient lamented, shrieked, and wept persistently, her appetite quite failed, and she soon had to be brought to the hospital.

Here she was collected and clear about her surroundings, but gradually passed into a very severe state of apprehensive excitement, which found expression in monotonous and almost intolerable shrieks. She could only be interrupted for a short time by asking her questions, which she always answered. She also expressed a quantity of the most fantastic ideas. She had been the serpent in paradise, had led astray her husband, who was called Adam, and had made herself and her children accursed, and everyone unhappy. Therefore she was burning, was already in hell, and saw her fearful sins in the abyss. The firmament had fallen; there was no more water or money or food; she had ruined everything, and was guilty of the downfall of the world— "The whole world lies upon my soul." She accused herself of all these transgressions in a written document, addressed to the District Court, and begged to be taken to prison. She wrote her name on a label as "Devil."

In spite of all this, you are soon convinced that, even while she is senselessly shrieking and expressing delusionary ideas of this kind, the patient knows where she is quite well, knows the doctors, and gives broken but relevant answers to questions about the circumstances of her home. She also does sums correctly, though she returns at once to her monotonous lamentations. Sometimes it appears that she has a certain understanding of her illness. "One fancies first one thing and then another," she says. "It often seems quite different to me, as if it were not so. It often seems as if it were a dream, and often as if it were reality." As the result of sleeplessness and insufficient nourishment, she is physically quite run down, but shows no other sign of illness. She has three healthy sons,* while three of her children died in childhood. Her father is said to have been temporarily insane.

At first sight this clinical picture of disease seems different from the other and simpler forms. But it is easily shown that the variations are only a matter of degree. Both in the development of the delusions and in the strength and manifestations of the apprehension we meet with every conceivable transition, from the form first described and generally known as melancholia simplex to the present morbid condition, and to even more marked cases. Often enough the same patient presents first one and then another type of symptoms at different times. It is therefore impossible to lay down any reliable clinical line of division in these cases.

All three patients are of considerable age. This is not an accident. Melancholia, as we have described it here, sets in principally, or perhaps exclusively, at the beginning of old age in men, and in women from the period of the menopause onwards. We might regard it as a morbid expression of the feeling of growing inadequacy, usually more or less noticeable in healthy people of the same age. Those who are morbidly disposed by nature of

---

* One of them afterwards developed katatonia, and became demented.

course become melancholic most easily, as is shown by our examples, and women seem more inclined to the disease than men. Of external influences, emotional shocks, and especially the death of near relations, often figure as the exciting cause, although they cannot be regarded as the original cause, on account of their absence in other cases. The termination of the illness is generally pretty favourable.* About a third of the patients make a complete recovery. In severe and protracted cases, emotional dullness may remain, with faint traces of the apprehensive tendency. Judgment and memory may also undergo considerable deterioration. The course of the disease is always tedious, and usually continues, with many fluctuations, for from one to two years, or even longer, according to the severity of the case.

The treatment of the malady cannot, as a rule, be carried out, except in an asylum, as thoughts of suicide are almost always present. Patients who show such tendencies require the closest watching, day and night. They are kept in bed and given plenty of food, though this is often very difficult, on account of their resistance. Care is also taken to regulate their digestion, and, as far as possible, to secure them sufficient sleep by means of baths and medicines. Paraldehyde is generally to be recommended, or, under some circumstances, alcohol, or occasional doses of trional. Opium is employed to combat the apprehension, in gradually increasing doses, which are then by degrees reduced. This remedy has often done very good service with our first two patients, while with the third we have had better results from small doses of paraldehyde. Great care is needed in discharging patients. If this is done too soon, as in the case of our second patient, serious relapses may result, with attempted suicide. Visits from near relations have a bad effect up to the very end of the illness.

---

* The first of these three patients has been well for more than nine and a half years, and the second for five years. The third died of pulmonary consumption, after four and a half years' illness, while still uncured.

Kraepelin's impact upon psychiatric taxonomy is well known, so much so that it is often thought of as the beginning of modern psychiatric classification, with dementia praecox on the one hand and manic depression on the other. In spite of the continuing controversy about the taxonomic position of the atypical psychoses, and those cases which do not easily fit into the two category system, Kraepelin's classification has remained the major landmark for psychiatric nosology. How much of his system was original and how much derived from previous attempts at classification?

His ideas developed and changed over nearly three decades, and can be followed in the consecutive editions of his textbook *Psychiatrie*. The second edition was published in 1887, and the important sixth edition in 1899, containing the major revision of the concept of manic depression which is described in the first of these extracts. The eighth edition appeared in two volumes between 1909 and 1915.

Kraepelin states that manic depression includes periodic and circular insanity, simple mania, melancholia and some states of amentia. As well as these severe syndromes he also included slighter colourings of mood, both periodic and continuous, as rudiments of the more severe varieties, shading off into normality. Thus, in constructing what has been called the Kraepelinian dichotomy, he had to combine syndromes which had previously often been thought to be distinct. This was so on the manic-depression side as well as on the dementia praecox side of the divide.

The occurrence in the same individual of mania and melancholia had been documented even by the Greeks (Aretaeus), but in modern times it was the French who provided the clearest descriptions of what we would now call Affective Disorders. Pinel (1801) described his *'Manie sans delire'* as primarily an affective disturbance in the absence of intellectual, perceptual, imaginative or mnemonic decline. Esquirol (1838) concurred in the recognition of this syndrome as distinct from other forms of lunacy and dementia.

Falret (1854) described *folie circulaire* in which mania and melancholia occurred in succession, with a regularity which was the hallmark of the condition. It was at this point that periodicity entered the classification of the affective disorders and caused, over the years, considerable confusion (Lewis, 1967). Baillarger, in the same year described his *folie a double forme*: 'the succession of two regular periods, one of excitation the other of depression'. Thus it is clear from these two authorities that mania and melancholia were being thought of as one disease. Indeed, Magnan (1897) came close to Kraepelin's ideas two years before they were published, by describing *Folie Intermittente*, in which the alternating, circular and other forms of affective disorder were brought under one heading.

In the 1887 version of his textbook Kraepelin kept mania, melancholia, periodic delusional insanity and circular insanity separate. By the sixth edition, however, he defined them as the same disease. He recognized that periodicity, the criterion on which the circular forms of Falret and Baillarger had been separated from the rest, was unreliable of definition and unduly restrictive in practice. He therefore shifted the emphasis from the periodic nature of the affective disorders to the phasic; that is they could occur in two forms, mania and melancholia, at different times during the life of the victim, but strict periodicity was not necessary (Jaspers, 1965). Nevertheless periodicity had been an important observation, as it had provided theorists with evidence that some forms of affective disorder could be 'endogenous' (Lewis, 1971).

Another confusion which Kraepelin had to grapple with was that between affective disorders and psychopathic personality disorder. This came about because of the changing meaning during the 19th century of the term 'moral'. When Prichard in 1835 described 'Moral Insanity' it referred to disorders of the affective-conative functions as opposed to intellectual ones. Thus it was intended to separate out cases of affective disorder from the rest of insanity. However Prichard's clinical experience was limited and his clinical material even more so. Indeed he was forced to write asking for cases to other clinicians, such as Samuel Tuke of the Retreat. Walk, in an unpublished manuscript, pointed out that all of Prichard's seven cases began in middle age, and most suffered profound agitation, dejection, morbid depression and excitement. This appears to confirm his intent to describe affective disorders although the precision of description was lacking.

Nevertheless, throughout the 19th century writers such as Bucknill and Tuke, Maudsley, and Morison came to confound mania with psychopathy. In part this was due to the two meanings of moral, in part to the prevailing degeneracy theory of mental disorders begun by Morel, in which lack of moral sense in one generation proceeded to lunacy in the next and finally dementia in subsequent generations. In addition it may have been due to the difficulty in distinguishing the immoral acts (in the ethical and legal sense) performed during a period of hypomania from the seriously irresponsible behaviour of psychopathy.

Kraepelin, in his second edition, subscribed to the prevailing degeneracy theory, but over the course of the next four editions and ten years he developed the idea of the psychopathic personality disorder, which, along with the recognition of the unity of manic depressive disorder made the concept of moral insanity redundant (Lewis, 1974).

From the foregoing it can readily be seen that elements of the Kraepelinian synthesis were already in circulation long before the sixth edition of this textbook appeared. However, this does not detract from the impressive contribution which he made. No previous writer had had the breadth of clinical experience and ability so confidently to propose a classification of all non-organic psychoses. The care in the observation and the description of the natural history of the disorders allowed prognosis to serve as an important element of this classification. Careful follow-up would also have been necessary to see that the various forms of the disorder could occur in the same case. To some extent this was made possible by the concentration of cases in mental hospitals. Careful history taking would have been necessary to establish that all forms of manic depressive insanity could occur in the same family history.

Perhaps another element in establishing Kraepelin's reputation was the immediacy of his teaching. The lectures often begin: 'Gentlemen, you have before you today...', and so straight on into almost faultless clinical descriptions of the cases. No previous writer appears so convincingly to have been able to demonstrate the accuracy of his observations and theories by clinical demonstration.

What was Kraepelin's view of the nature of the illnesses which he was in the process of describing? Psychoanalysis was developing in Vienna, and influenced Bleuler's thinking. Kraepelin remained a sceptic. 'Empathy is a very unsure process; it plays an indispensable part in human relations and poetic creations, but as a research method it can lead to the greatest self-deception.' (Kraepelin, 1920).

He was not averse to the idea that the psychoses might be influenced by exogenous factors. But... 'The influence of external causes is probably only very general: they dictate the broad lines which the illness will follow, but the detailed symptomatology is governed by the patients own individuality'.

Thus Kraepelin rejected the notion that mental illnesses could be classified as either endogenous or exogenous; rather, all were influenced by both factors. Indeed, while disliking psychoanalytic method, he subscribed to the idea that early childhood was important, and considered the possibility that the return of repressed material may play a part in pathological states of mind. 'We must trace the phenomena of our inner life back to their roots in the psyche of the child, of primitive man, and of animals. It is also necessary to examine pathological states and try to see to what extent such forgotten stimuli are reactivated in them.' (Kraepelin, 1920).

SUBSEQUENT DEVELOPMENTS

Like all diseases, Kraepelin's two major psychoses were theories, and, once stated, were there to be tested. How have they fared so far? We have many more ways of testing disease theories today but it is clear from a perusal of current classifications that they remain, in essence, Kraepelinian.

The distinction between what is now called schizophrenia and manic depression has received some support from the differential response of the conditions to physical treatments. Antidepressants, Lithium, and ECT are all effective in manic depression, while, with the possible exception of ECT, they have no therapeutic effect in schizophrenia. On the other hand, the antipsychotic drugs are useful in calming the excitement of mania and treating the delusions which are sometimes present.

A statistical discontinuity between symptoms of schizophrenia and those of manic depression has been sought in the same way as between endogenous and reactive depression. To the extent that these methods are able to provide answers to such questions they have generally confirmed the distinction (Brockington *et al.*, 1979). However, it is acknowledged that clinically there are a large number of cases which fall at the borderline between schizophrenia and manic depression.

Biological studies in recent years have also shown different abnormalities in the two conditions, and although mixed family pedigrees are common there is a significant tendency for the two conditions to breed true.

The further subclassification of affective disorders was envisaged by Kraepelin although he thought that further divisions on the basis of symptoms alone would be unreliable. Genetic studies have lent support to the distinction between bipolar and unipolar manic depression on the basis of the presence of both affective poles in the history (Perris, 1982). The distinction between endogenous and reactive depression has also emerged as a major landmark in biological studies, but the original theory that only the reactive type would prove to be precipitated by personal trauma has not been borne out. There are numerous other subclassifications of affective disorder but none can be said to be thoroughly secure.

C. Thompson

REFERENCES

Baillarger, J. (1854). Note sur un genre de folie. *Bull. Acad. Med,* **19**, 340.
Brockington, I. F., Kendell, R. B., Wainwright, S., Hillier, V. F. and Walker, J. (1979). The distinction between the affective psychoses and schizophrenia.
Esquirol, J.-E.-D. (1838). *Des Maladies Mentales,* vols 1 and 2, J.-B. Bailliere, Paris.
Fairet, J. P. (1854). Memoire sur la folie circulaire. *Bull. Acad. Med.,* **19**, 382.
Jaspers, K. (1965). *Allgemeine Psychopathologie,* Springer, Berlin.
Kraepelin, E. (1887). *Psychiatrie,* 2nd edn, Abel, Leipzig.
Kraepelin, E. (1896). *Psychiatrie,* 5th edn.
Kraepelin, E. (1889). *Psychiatrie,* 6th edn.
Kraepelin, E. (1903–4). *Psychiatrie,* 7th edn.
Kraepelin, E. (1909–15). *Psychiatrie,* 8th edn.
Kraepelin, E. (1920). Patterns of mental disorder. *Z. ges. Neurol. Psychiat.,* **62**, 1–29.
Lewis, A. (1967). Periodicity. In *Cycles Biologiques et Psychiatrie,* O. Ajuriaguerra (Ed.), Masson, Paris.
Lewis, A. (1971). 'Endogenous' and 'exogenous'—a useful dichotomy? *Psychological Medicine,* **1**, 191–196.
Lewis, A. (1984). Psychopathic personality: a most elusive category. *Psychological Medicine,* **4**, 133–140.
Magnan, V. (1897). *Leçons Cliniques sur les Maladies Mentales,* Paris.
Perris, C. (1982). The distinction between bipolar and unipolar affective disorders. In *Handbook of Affective Disorders,* O. Paykel (Ed.), Churchill Livingstone, London.

Pinel, P. (1801). *Traite Medico-Philosophique sur L'Alienation Mentale*, Richard, Caille et Ravier, Paris.

Prichard, J. C. (1835). *A Treatise on Insanity*, Sherwood, Gilbert and Piper, London.

Walk, A. (1985). Unpublished papers on the history of psychiatry collected at his death by is wife.

13

A New Method of Shock Therapy: 'Electroconvulsive Treatment' (Summary)

U. Cerletti and L. Bini (translated by Felicity De Zulueta), 1938

First, Professor Cerletti expressed his reasons why the Cardiazol-induced convulsive treatment had become so important compared to other shock-mediated treatments used for schizophrenia and other psychoses. The reasons were essentially practical ones and, in many cases, made the above mentioned treatment preferable to insulin coma therapy; for instance, with Cardiazol-induced convulsive treatment, the doctor was left clinically responsible, fewer medical hours were required, fewer interventions were needed and it was cheaper. Having pointed out the fairly rare accidents of varying severity which had occurred after a massive and rapid injection of Cardiazol, he reminded us of a practical and fairly serious problem which was the very painful sense of annihilation which the patient experiences in the period between the injection itself and the onset of the epileptic fit. This experience makes many patients resistant to this form of treatment. Also, after the post-ictal sleeping period, the patient goes into a state of psychomotor hyperactivity due to the high dose of Cardiazol still in circulation.

For this reason, the author had looked for simpler and less toxic ways of inducing epileptic fits. For several years, in Genova, he had been involved in studies on epilepsy which consisted of inducing epileptic fits in animals, specifically in dogs using an ordinary electric current (alternating 125 volts) which was passed for a fraction of a second between two electrodes placed in the mouth and in the rectum. The technique and results on many dogs were published by a student in 1934. (Chiauzzi, *Pathologisa*, **XXVI**). The author took up the same experiments in Rome in 1935 with the assistance of Dr L. Bini, specialist in electrical techniques. The latter built a simple but practical instrument which could control both the time of passage and the voltage of an administered electric current. Another technique which had been attempted by other researchers was also adopted which involved passing an electric current through the head. Bini was able in this way to carry out many experiments on dogs.

When Cardiazol-induced convulsive therapy appeared on the scene (Sakel, Meduna), the authors thought immediately of using an electric current to achieve the same results. A great step forward in the application of this treatment was achieved through numerous experiments carried out on pigs in varying conditions, using the simple technique which is used in many slaughter houses and which makes the animals insensitive to pain by producing an electrically induced epileptic fit prior to their slaughtering. Thus, similar experiments to those done on dogs were carried out on larger animals using currents of different intensities for varying lengths of time and applying the electrodes in different sites.

In this way, it was possible to carry out experiments on humans and to determine the optimum conditions required to produce an epileptic fit. The epileptic attack thus induced in man presents as a typical epileptic fit. Once the current has passed for a fraction of a second there is an instant loss of consciousness; the patient manifests strong generalized contractions: the trunk, the legs, arms and hands take on a semi-flexed position. At first, the face reddens, then it become very pale and finally cyanosed; breathing stops. The patient has a mild tachycardia. After about 30 seconds, the face resumes its normal colouring and then becomes congested. Spastic tremors are observed in the limbs and face and then become clonic jerks of varying intensity which last for one or two minutes involving the muscles of the whole body. A gag must be placed between the teeth to prevent the patient from biting his tongue.

Occasionally he foams at the mouth, ejaculates or passes urine. There follows a phase of muscular relaxation and stertorous breathing. The patient regains consciousness little by little; his jaw muscles relax; he looks around and begins to respond to calls. After 5 minutes he can speak even though confusedly. After 8–10 minutes, he has regained full consciousness. He tends to fall asleep and, if allowed to do so, he sleeps peacefully for a few hours, waking up totally restored.

The advantages of this method of treatment observed up till now are, above all, the total lack of awareness on the part of the patient especially during the shock. When these patients are asked to give an account of their experiences, they deny any recollection other than that of having been asleep. There is not the hyperexcitability which is observed after a Cardiazol-induced fit. Following an Electroconvulsive treatment, the patient sleeps longer and wakes up in a calm and better mood than the patient who has had a Cardiazol-induced fit. The cerebrovascular system has not suffered during the shock; the only observation is of a slight rise in pulse rate in relation to the muscular contractions of the clonic phase. An important advantage is that of being able to repeat the shock without damage even a few minutes after an abortive or a complete fit.

There are not yet enough studies on the results achieved until now (which are really good) on schizophrenic patients, to be able to draw conclusions regarding the therapeutic value of Electro Convulsive Treatment, but, bearing in mind that the fit is essentially the same as that induced with Cardiazol, one can at least say that Electro Convulsive Treatment achieves the same benefits.

Bini then addressed the technical difficulties involved in measuring the intensity of the current necessary to produce a fit and he described his apparatus; this consists of a time switch to control the duration of the current in fractions of a second, and of a machine which controls and measures the alternating current. A second (provisional) circuit of continuous current is used first to gauge the resistance of the patient's head, a necessary measure to be able to estimate the required intensity and duration of the current to be applied.

He referred, in particular, to the effects of electric current on animals in a variety of experimental conditions and on the safety limits of this method. Finally, he pointed out the various effects which have been achieved up till now with patients in relation to the intensity and duration of the current administered.

In front of the Academy, once the paper had been presented, an epileptic fit was induced using Cardiazol on one patient and a similar epileptic fit was induced using an electric current on a second patient.

INTRODUCTION

In the 1930s three major physical treatments were introduced: electroconvulsive therapy, insulin hypoglycaemia and prefrontal leucotomy or lobotomy. Fifty years later, only ECT remains as a widely accepted and scientifically tested therapy. Henry Rollin (1981) has described the impact of ECT. When he started in psychiatry in the late 1930s, there was an atmosphere of therapeutic nihilism. Sedative drugs such as paraldehyde and bromides were the main treatments available. Patients with profound depression and stupor required to be force fed daily. Suicidal caution cards, which each nurse treating depressed patients had to sign, were used. Patients died of manic exhaustion and bizarre and dangerous schizophrenic behaviour was common. Rollin has no doubt that the introduction of ECT was the most important advance in psychiatric treatment so far this century. While in any league table, many psychiatrists might put Phenothiazines, antidepressants and lithium ahead of ECT there is no doubt that it has been a major advance and it has long outlived its obituarists.

CONVULSIVE THERAPY BEFORE CERLETTI

Hellebore (veractum) had been employed for thousands of years in the treatment of insanity and often caused seizures though it is not clear that ancient writers recognized the direct therapeutic effects of the seizure. Certainly Mowbray (1959) describes Paracelsus giving camphor in large doses as a cure for lunacy and by the late 18th century Auenbrugger (1722–1809) was acclaiming the use of camphor in specific types of insanity and definitely attributing the improvement to the severe and prolonged convulsions that this drug produced. Brandon (1975) quotes a number of other examples. Dr Weickhard writing in 1798 recommended epileptogenic doses of camphor in the treatment of Wahnsinn, a delusional psychotic state and Burrows in 1828 prescribed camphor in large doses, 'in a case of insanity where two scruples were exhibited, it produced a fit and a perfect cure followed'. In 1785, Dr W. Oliver, published an account of convulsive therapy in the *London Medical Journal* (Oliver, 1785). On this occasion camphor was given by mouth.

Fraser (1982) reports that in the mid-18th century Michael Shuppach 'der emmenthaler wunderdoktor' gave something resembling ECT to a Swiss farmer's wife who was diagnosed as possessed of eight devils. She was given eight consecutive daily shocks, the last one being so severe that she fell to the floor unconscious. It is not reported whether she in fact had epileptic seizures but a complete cure resulted.

The first well-recorded case of electric shock treatment was carried out by John Birch (1792), surgeon to St Thomas' Hospital. He treated a melancholic London porter, who had been depressed for about one year, with a course of six shocks which were passed through the brain, two shocks in opposite directions on each of three successive days. Birch reports that following this treatment the porter regained his spirits and remained well for seven years of follow up. Again, however, it is not clear whether any of these shocks actually produced grand mal seizures.

Working in Hungary, Ladislas Meduna had come to the conclusion that there was an antagonism between schizophrenic symptoms and epilepsy. He had observed that schizophrenic patients would temporarily lose their psychotic symptoms after a spontaneous seizure, whatever the cause of the seizure. Meduna began systematically inducing seizures in his schizophrenic patients, and the first such treatment was given on 23 January 1934, using camphor in oil by intramuscular injection (Meduna, 1935). There were considerable problems in this technique in that camphor takes 15 or 20 minutes before it produces a convulsion and during this time the patient feels extremely uncomfortable and distressed. Subsequently, Meduna replaced camphor with intravenous injection of pentylenetetrazol (metrazol) which produces an immediate convulsion. This technique of metrazol-induced convulsion was in widespread use for three years before ECT was introduced. Meduna subsequently emigrated to the United States and did no further work in convulsive therapy.

WHO WAS UGO CERLETTI?

Cerletti was born in Cornigliano, Italy, on 26 September 1877, and died in Rome on 25 July 1963. He studied medicine in Turin and Rome, and received his medical degree in Rome in 1901. He first specialized in histopathology and neuropathology, then he studied clinical psychiatry under Kraepelin and was apparently captivated by him. In 1933, he became interested in Meduna's work on schizophrenia and was subsequently an enthusiastic advocate of the hypothesis of the incompatibility of schizophrenia and epilepsy. In 1935, he was appointed as Professor of Psychiatry at the University of Rome.

Cerletti continued to work on electroconvulsive therapy until he died. According to d'Cori (1963) he formulated a theory that the humoral and hormonal changes provoked in the brain by the epileptic attack lead to the formation of substances which he called 'acroagonines'—'substances of extreme defense'. He postulated that these substances, when injected into the patient would have therapeutic effects similar to those resulting from electro-shock.

263

Frank Ayd (1963) recalled that Cerletti was in the habit of recounting the first experience of ECT regularly. On one occasion Ayd reports Cerletti as saying 'when I saw the patient's reaction, I thought to myself: this ought to be abolished! Ever since I have looked forward to the time when another treatment would replace electro-shock.'

THE DEVELOPMENT OF ELECTRO-SHOCK BY CERLETTI

This is most fully chronicled, not in the first description (given in this chapter) but in a paper by Cerletti (1950). Even at this stage it is clear that Cerletti was conscious of his place in history. Much of the introduction to the paper deals with his partnership with Bini. The paper discussed here, which was given jointly by Cerletti and Bini to the Rome Medical Academy in 1938, in fact had Bini's name first. This was the only published account available to Kalinowsky, who took it back to the United States in 1939, and used it in his bibliographies. Cerletti is at pains to point out that Dr Bini was an assistant and that his name came first on that paper because 'I also entrusted to him the task of furnishing the Academy with certain specifications about the electrical apparatus.' Cerletti was also concerned that in Russell Brayne's book *Recent Progress in Neurology and Psychiatry*, ECT is designated as a Bini-Cerletti discovery. Cerletti goes on to state 'I hasten to point out that this area is not to be ascribed to any fault on the part of Dr Bini, who has been embarrassed by the general misuse of his name in this connection. . .'

While working in Genoa, Cerletti began to experimentally provoke epileptic fits in dogs. He was interested in whether the sclerotic changes in Ammons horn found in the brains of epileptics were the result of previous injury or might be themselves consequences of repeated fits. Cerletti wanted to minimize the amount of current passing through the brain and therefore at this time was using a mouth-rectum circuit rather than one across the head. These experiments were carried out in 1933 using 125-volt AC current from the mains. With this technique some of the dogs died. Cerletti felt that this was due to the time these currents passed and he managed to abolish deaths by using stimuli from 0.1–0.5 of a second.

In 1935 Cerletti took up the Chair of Neuro-Psychiatry at Rome University and began experiments with the 'young Dr Bini'. Bini produced an apparatus which was more sophisticated with a timed stimulus and they determined that a stimulus from one tenth to one fifth of a second at 125 volts was the most reliable at producing grand mal seizures.

At this time Cerletti was using the Sakel method of treating schizophrenia with insulin coma and in 1937 they started using metrazol convulsion, as described by Meduna. Cerletti began to speculate whether electricity could be used to produce grand mal seizures in man. However, no one at the clinic took this idea seriously because deaths had been reported with voltages as low as 40 in man, and it was clear from the dog experiments that at least 125 volts was needed to produce a seizure.

In 1937 Cerletti was contacted by Professor Vanni, who told him that at the Rome slaughter house pigs were being killed by electricity. Cerletti went to see and found that the butchers took hold of the pigs by their ears with large scissor-shaped pincer electrodes. These were connected to the lighting circuit (125 volts) and current applied. Cerletti observed that the pigs did not in fact die but collapsed and began a grand mal convulsion. At this point, the butcher taking advantage of the unconscious state of the animal, cut its throat. Cerletti reports 'I at once saw that the fits were the same as those I had been producing in dogs and that these pigs were not being killed by electricity but were bled to death during their epileptic coma.'

Cerletti then began experiments at the slaughter house with the collaboration of the slaughter house director, Professor Torti. They applied currents for increasing periods of time and in various ways, across the head, neck and chest. It became clear that serious consequences, such as prolonged apnoea or death only occurred when the current was applied across the chest and that currents of up to 60 seconds could be applied across the head, on several occasions without any apparent ill effects. Cerletti concluded 'these clear proofs, certain and oft repeated, caused all my doubts to vanish, and without more ado I gave instructions in the clinic to undertake, next day, the experiment upon man. Very likely, except for this fortuitous and fortunate circumstance of pigs' pseudo-electrical butchery, electro-shock would not yet have been born.'

THE FIRST ECT MACHINE

This was constructed by Bini, together with the electrical engineers at the Rome clinic. It had two circuits, a direct one for measuring the resistance of the patient's head in ohms and an alternating current circuit to elicit the convulsion. This latter circuit included a timer which measured one-tenth of a second intervals up to one minute. It was possible to vary the voltage from 50–150 volts.

THE STORY OF THE 'FIRST' ELECTRO-SHOCK TREATMENT

This has been fully chronicled by Impastato (1960) and though the story is well known, is worth repeating here. Cerletti, Bini, Longhi, Accornero, Kalinowsky and Feischer were present. Some accounts give the impression that the first patient was found wandering in a railway goods yard in Rome, taken straight to the clinic, and because he could not speak or give an account of himself was chosen as the first subject for ECT.

On 15 April 1938 the police commissioner of Rome sent a man to the Rome clinic, with the following note: 'S.E. 39 years old. Engineer resident of Milan was arrested at the railroad station, while wandering about without a ticket on trains ready for departure. He does appear to be in full possession of his mental faculties. I am sending him to your hospital to be kept under observation. . . . The patient's condition on 18 April was as follows: lucid, well orientated. He describes, using neologisms, deliriant ideas of being telepathically influenced with related sensorial disturbances; his mimicry is correlated to the meaning of his words; mood indifferent to environment, low affective reserves; physical and neurological examination negative. A diagnosis of schizophrenic syndrome was made based on his passive behaviour, incoherence, low affective reserves, hallucinations, deliriant ideas of being influenced and neologisms.'

Cerletti decided that he was suitable as a subject for the first ECT. He writes that preparations for the experiment were carried out in 'an atmosphere of fearful silence, bordering on disapproval.' Two electrodes well wetted in a salt solution were applied by an elastic band to the patient's temples; the first stimulus was of 70 volts for 0.2 of a second. This produced a sudden jump of the patient on the bed and a short period of tensing of his muscles, before the patient immediately collapsed on the bed, but remained conscious. The patient then began to sing at the top of his voice and subsequently fell silent. Cerletti suggested a second treatment at a higher voltage and of longer duration. The staff objected, stating that if another treatment were given, the patient would probably die and they wanted further treatment postponed until the next day. The patient hearing the low toned conversation around him exclaimed clearly and in a solemn tone: 'non una seconda! Mortifera!' (Not a second! Deadly!). At this point some of the observers began to insist upon suspension of the proceedings. Cerletti's response was 'anxiety lest something that amounted to superstition should interfere with my decision urged me on to action. I had the electrodes reapplied and 110 volt discharge was sent through for 0.5 seconds.' The patient then had a typical unmodified grand mal fit and Cerletti describes how at the first deep stertorous inhalation and first clonic shudders 'the blood ran more freely in the bystanders veins as well'. At the end of the treatment, the patient sat up of his own accord, looked about him calmly with a vague smile. Cerletti asked the man: 'what has been happening to you?' He answered with no thought disorder: 'I don't know, perhaps I have been asleep.' Cerletti reports that the patient went on to have eleven complete ECTs and three incomplete ones over a period of about two months and was discharged from his clinic in complete remission.

THE FIRST ECT IN AMERICA

Dr Renato Almansi worked with Cerletti and he took an ECT machine to America in 1939, where David Impastato first did experiments on dogs and then gave the first American ECT on 6 February 1940 at Columbus Hospital, New York City.

Pulver (1961), however, reports that Dr Victor Gonda administered the first ECT. In late January 1940 at the Parkway Sanitorium, Chicago. Dr Gonda's son later reported that Gonda had tested the apparatus by placing the electrodes on his own thigh, experiencing a violent contraction of his muscles and injuring his leg, which hit the table.

DEVELOPMENTS SINCE THE INTRODUCTION OF ECT

These are described in the following figure (pp. 268–269). The most important are as follows:

1. The introduction of modified ECT.
2. The introduction of unilateral ECT.
3. The introduction of brief pulse stimuli.
4. The introduction of constant current ECT machines.

Modified ECT

Bennett (1940) did the pioneer work in this area, extracting the muscle relaxant, curare, from *Chondodendron tomentosum*, with which South American hunters paralysed the animals they wanted to capture live. Bennett originally suggested using spinal anaesthesia to prevent ECT fractures. Curare was used to prevent traumatic complications and enabled ECT to be given to patients with advanced cardiac disease, arthritic deformities and other severe physical illness. It is clear that with curare a number of unexplained deaths occurred and it was not until 1951 when succinyl choline became available that more routine muscle relaxation came into being. It was strongly criticized by Kalinowsky (1949), who felt that the side-effects of curare were more dangerous than the complications it was supposed to prevent. With the introduction of short acting relaxants the safety of the method was increased and by the mid-1950s modified ECT was being given routinely in some UK hospitals. By 1957 (Bolam versus Friern Hospital Management Committee: Bolam, 1957) it was possible for the plaintiff to allege that failure to use relaxant drugs was negligent treatment.

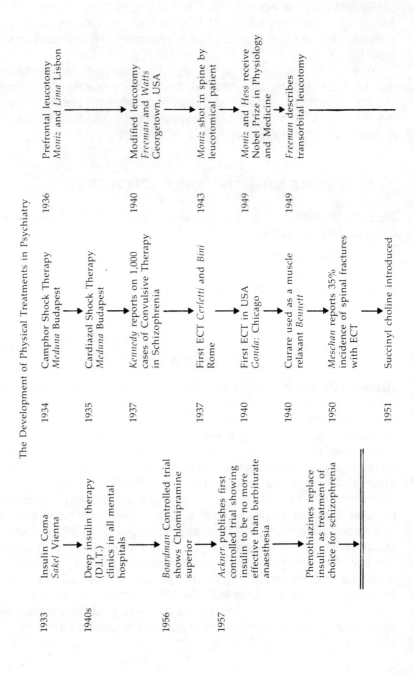

The Development of Physical Treatments in Psychiatry

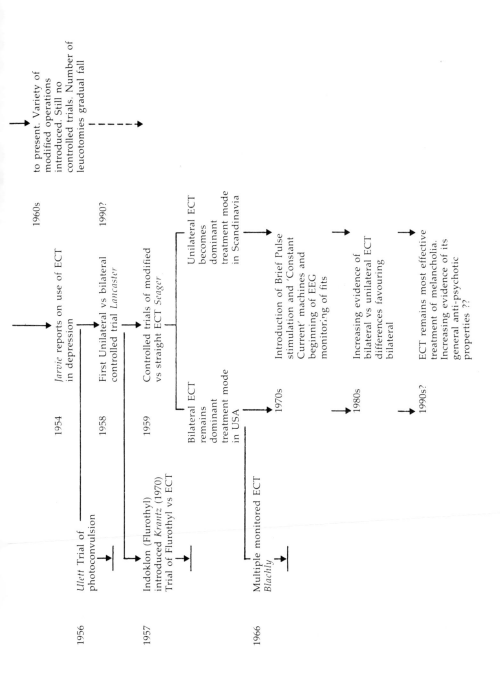

1956 *Ullett* Trial of photoconvulsion

1954 *Jarvie* reports on use of ECT in depression

1960s to present. Variety of modified operations introduced. Still no controlled trials. Number of leucotomies gradual fall

1957 Indoklon (Flurothyl) introduced *Krantz* (1970) Trial of Flurothyl vs ECT

1958 First Unilateral vs bilateral controlled trial *Lancaster*

1990?

1959 Controlled trials of modified vs straight ECT *Seager*

Bilateral ECT remains dominant treatment mode in USA

Unilateral ECT becomes dominant treatment mode in Scandinavia

1966 Multiple monitored ECT *Blachly*

1970s Introduction of Brief Pulse stimulation and 'Constant Current' machines and beginning of EEG monitoring of fits

1980s Increasing evidence of bilateral vs unilateral ECT differences favouring bilateral

1990s? ECT remains most effective treatment of melancholia. Increasing evidence of its general anti-psychotic properties ??

Unilateral ECT

Friedman and Wilcox (1942) and Wilcox (1947) first suggested the use of the unilateral electrode placement to the non-dominant hemisphere, as a way of minimizing side-effects, particularly memory impairment. It was not until 1958 that Lancaster *et al.* published the first controlled trial of unilateral versus bilateral ECT. By 1975 D'Elia and Roatma had found 29 studies where unilateral and bilateral ECT had been compared. Their clear impression was that in well-controlled clinical trials, unilateral ECT was just as effective and produced much less cognitive impairment and was therefore the treatment of choice. In scientific reports this view held sway for the next ten years, though many clinicians remained convinced that bilateral ECT was more effective, at least in some patients. The subject has recently been reviewed again (Abrams, 1986). There has been a consistent trend for published articles over the past ten years to show differential effects between unilateral and bilateral ECT, both on clinical outcome and on brain functioning. The standard conclusion that without qualification, bilateral ECT and unilateral right ECT are equal in therapeutic properties is no longer tenable.

THE CURRENT 'STATE OF ECT'

Recent developments include the introduction of constant current ECT machines and brief pulse stimulation. The former deliver a fixed dosage of electrical energy to the patient. This is important because there is wide variation in the resistance of patients' heads and without this facility patients with low head resistance may receive large amounts of energy and those with high resistance may receive insufficient to overcome the seizure threshold. All modern ECT machines give high voltage trains of brief pulse sitmuli.

In England and Wales in 1984, 125 357 ECT treatments were given to approximately 20 000 psychiatric patients. Over the past ten years the use of ECT had slowly declined but now appears to have levelled off. It remains the treatment of choice for psychotic depression and for antidepressant resistant depression. Recent studies have also indicated that it may have a role to play in the treatment of acute schizophrenia and mania. Most importantly, ECT has now secure scientific basis. There are active research programmes in many centres on both sides of the Atlantic, enquiring into the basic mechanisms and side-effects of the treatment. Its therapeutic effectiveness has been established in over ten controlled trials. Despite its critics the place of ECT in modern psychiatry appears secure.

C. P. L. Freeman

REFERENCES AND FURTHER READING

Abrams, R. (1986). Is Unilateral Electroconvulsive Therapy really the treatment of choice in endogenous depression. *Electroconvulsive Therapy*, S. Malitz and H. A. Sackheim (Eds), Annals of the New York Academy of Sciences, Vol. 462.

Ackner, B., Harris, A. and Oldham, A. J. (1957). Insulin treatment of schizophrenia: A controlled study. *Lancet, i*, 607.

Ayd, F. J. (1963). Guest Editorial: Ugo Cerletti, M.D., 1877–1963. *Psychosomatics*, **4**, A6–A7.

Bennett, A. E. (1940). Preventing traumatic complications in convulsive therapy by curare. *Journal of American Medical Association*, **114**, 322–324.

Blachly, P. H. and Gowing, D. (1966). Multiple monitored electroconvulsive therapy. *Comprehensive Psychiatry*, **7**, 100–109.

Bolam (1957). Friern Hospital Management Committee. *Times Law Report*, 24 February.

Boardman, R. H., Lomas, J. and Markowe, M. (1956). Insulin and chlorpromazine in schizophrenia: a comparative study in previously untreated cases. *Lancet, ii*, 487.

Brandon, S. (1980). The history of shock treatment, in *Electroconvulsive Therapy: An Appraisal*, R. L. Palmer (Ed.), Oxford University Press, London.

Cerletti, M. D. (1950). Old and new information about electroshock. *American Journal of Psychiatry*, **107**, 87–94.

Cerletti, V. and Bini, L. (1938). Un Nuevo metodo di shockterapie 'L'electtroshock. *Bull. Acad. Med. Roma*, **64**, 136–138.

d'Cori, F. (1963). In Memorium (Cerletti). *Journal of Neuropsychiatry*, **5**, 1–2.

D'Elia, G. and Roatma, H. (1975). Is unilateral ECT less effective than bilateral ECT? *British Journal of Psychiatry*, **126**, 83–89.

Frank, L. R. (1978). *The History of Shock Treatment*, San Francisco.

Fraser, M. (1982). *ECT: A Clinical Guide*, Wiley, Chichester.

Freeman, W. (1949). Transorbital leucotomy: the deep frontal cut. *Proceedings of the Royal Society of Medicine*, **42**, 8, suppl.

Friedman, E. and Wilcox, P. H. (1942). Electrostimulated convulsive doses in intact humans by means of unidirectional currents. *Journal of Nervous and Mental Disease*, **96**, 56–63.

Impastato, D. J. (1960). The story of the first electroshock treatment. *American Journal of Psychiatry*, **116**, 1113–1114.

Jarvie, H. F. (1954). Prognosis of depression treated by electrical convulsion therapy. *British Medical Journal*, **1**, 132–134.

Kalinowsky, L. B. (1949). The present status of electric shock therapy. *Bulletin New York Academy of Medicine*, **25**, 541–553.

Kalinowsky, L. B. (1986). History of convulsive therapy. *Annals of the New York Academy of Sciences*, **462**, 1–4.

Kennedy, A. (1937). Convulsion therapy in schizophrenia. *Journal of Mental Science*, **83**, 609–629.

Krantz, J. C. J., Truitt, E. B., Speers, L. and Ling, A. S. C. (1957). New pharmacoconvulsive agent: *Science*, **126**, 353.

Lancaster, N. P., Steinert, R. R. and Frost, I. (1958). Unilateral electroconvulsive therapy. *Journal of Mental Science*, **104**, 221–227.

Laurrell, B. (1970). Flurothyl convulsive therapy. *Acta Psychiatrica Scandinavica*, suppl. 213.

Malitz, S. and Sackheim, H. A. (1986). Electroconvulsive therapy: Clinical and basic research issues. *Annals of the New York Academy of Sciences*, **462**, 1–424.

Meduna, L. J. (1935). Versuche uber die biologische beeinflussung des abaufes der schizophrenia: camphor und cardiozolkrampfe. *Z. Ges. Neurol. Psychiatry,* **1523**, 235–262.

Meschan, I., Scruggs, J. B. and Calhoun, J. D. (1950). The impact of ECT. *Radiology,* **54**, 180.

Mowbray, R. M. (1959). Historical aspects of electric convulsant therapy. *Scottish Medical Journal,* **4**, 375.

Oliver, W. (1785). Accounts of the effects of camphor in a case of insanity. *London Medical Journal,* **120**.

Pulver, S. E. (1961). The first electroconvulsive treatment given in the United States. *American Journal of Psychiatry,* **117**, 845.

Rollin, H. R. (1980). The impact of ECT, in *Electroconvulsive Therapy: An Appraisal,* R. L. Palmer (Ed.), Oxford University Press, London.

Sakel, M. (1938). Nature and origin of the hypoglycaemic treatment of psychosis. *American Journal of Psychiatry,* **94**, suppl. 24.

Seager, C. P. (1959). Controlled trial of straight and modified electroplexy. *Journal of Mental Science,* **105**, 1022–1028.

Ulett, G. A., Smith, K. and Gleser, G. G. (1956). Evaluation of convulsive and subconvulsive therapies utilizing a control group. *American Journal of Psychiatry,* **112**, 795–802.

Wilcox, P. H. (1947). Electroshock therapy: A review of over 23 000 treatments using unidirectional current. *American Journal of Psychiatry,* **104**, 100–112.

Index

Abraham, K. 202
abreaction to psychical trauma 91–4
'acroagonines' 263
Acts of Parliament causing the increase in 'lunatics' (1845–1874) 13, 51
affective ambivalence in schizophrenia 187
affective disorders
  history of classification of 254–7
  subclassification of 257
affective insanity 11
affectivity, disturbances in, in schizophrenia 166, 178–86, 198, 205–6, 228
age
  of appearance of hereditary insanity 157–8
  of onset of melancholia 252–3
  suicide rates and 116–17
alcoholism, suicide and 120–3
alienists 162
  suicide and 134
altruism, social tendencies to 125, 129
ambivalence 187–8, 205
  affective 187
  intellectual 187
  of will ('Ambi-Tendenz') 187
amenorrhoea in anorexia nervosa 25, 28
amentia 245
anaesthesias, hysterical 88
anger in schizophrenia 182–3
Anna O, a hysterical patient 100, 101, 103
anomy, social tendencies to 125, 129, 131
anorexia, hysterical 88
anorexia nervosa 3, 25–47
  causation of 30, 34, 37–8, 43, 44–5, 46
  clinical description by Sir William Gull 25–43
  historical background to Gull's approach to 44–5
  significance of Gull's contributions on 46–7

terminology of 30, 34, 44
treatment of 27, 28–30, 31–3, 35–6, 37, 43–4
antipsychiatrists 1–2
anxiety-suicide 111
anxious (apprehensive) depression 249, 251
apepsia hysterica 30, 34, 44
apperceptive dementia, Weygandt's 229
apprehensive depression 249, 251
Aretaeus 254
arsenical chemotherapy of general paralysis of the insane 222
Aschaffenburg, G. 201
association disturbances in schizophrenia 165, 166–78, 195–6, 204, 205, 228
Associationism 202, 204
associations, loosening of 204
asthma, inheritance of 150
asylums, lunatic
  abolition of mechanical restraints in 8–10, 12
  growth in size and numbers of (1807–1877) 12–13, 49–54
Atavism 145
'attitudes passionnelles' 96
auditory sensations during epileptic seizures 60
'aura, intellectual', of Hughlings Jackson 59–83
autism 166, 190–5, 196, 206
automatic (impulsive) suicide 111–12, 134–5
automatic obedience 234
automatism, command 198

Baillarger, J. 161, 254
Balint, M. 102, 103
Bayle 218
Benommenbeit (clouded states) 200

Beyond the Pleasure Principle (Freud) 102
Bicêtre Hospital 11, 56
Bini, L. 259–70
  role in development of electroconvulsive
    therapy (ECT) by 264, 265
Binswanger, L. 202
biological psychiatry 3, 4–5
Birch, John 263
bismuth treatment of general paralysis of
    the insane 222
Bleuler, Eugen 4, 82, 165–207, 242
  biographical details 202
  concepts of schizophrenia 165–95,
    202–6
  contribution to psychiatry 201, 206–7
  differential diagnosis of schizophrenia
    195–200, 206
blocking, thought 167, 173, 176–7, 196
Bonhöffer, K. 201
bookkeeping, double-entry 190
Brain 57, 80
Breuer, J. 87–104, 204
Brill 202
Broadmoor State Criminal Asylum 52
Broca, Pierre 82
Bucknill, Charles 55, 56
Burghölzi Hospital 202, 205, 207

Calmeil 218
camphor-induced convulsive therapy 262,
    268
cardiazol-induced convulsive therapy 259,
    260, 268
catatonia 240, 241
catatonic symptoms 198
cerebral tumours, epilepsy associated with
    69, 71
Cerletti, U. 259–70
  biographical details 263–4
  description of electroconvulsive therapy
    259–61
  development of electroconvulsive therapy
    (ECT) 264–5
  the first electro-shock treatment 265–6
Chambers, R. 19
Charcot, J.-M. 82, 95–6, 99, 202
Charlesworth, E.P. 2–3
Chaslin, P. 203
chlomipramine 268
Chossat 28, 35
circular insanity 245, 254–5
clang associations 166, 174
'clouded states' 200
Clouston, T.S. 218
Collard, R. 201
command-automatism 198
community care 14
complexes in schizophrenia 204–5
'condensation' of ideas 174

confusion
  in manic depression 246
  in schizophrenia 172
congenital mental lesions, an ethnic
    classification of 15–18
Connolly, John 2–3, 7–14, 56
  growth of asylums and 12–14
  moral treatment movement and 10–12
  *Treatment of the Insane Without
    Mechanical Restraints* (1856) 2,
    7–10
conscience, double 94, 101
consciousness
  in 'dreamy state' of Hughlings Jackson
    60, 61, 63, 67, 72–3
  splitting of 94, 101–2
contractures, hysterical 88
convulsions, hysterical 88
convulsive treatment
  cardiazol-induced 259, 260
  history of 262–3, 268–9
  see also electroconvulsive therapy (ECT)
'cretin' 18
criminal behaviour in schizophrenia 184
curare in electroconvulsive therapy (ECT)
    267, 268
cycloid psychoses 242

Dämmerzustände (twilight states) 193
Darwin, Charles 4, 160
degeneracy, theory of 17–18, 19, 152–6,
    158–9, 160–2, 255
déjà vu experiences 81
  see also reminiscence
délire de persecution 240
delirium, suicide as a sort of 106–7
delusions
  in manic depression 246, 249, 251–2
  in schizophrenia 197–8, 235
  of sin 249
démence lacunaire 215
demence précoce 240, 241
dementia paranoides (paranoia) 240, 241
dementia praecox 4, 165–207, 225–37,
    241–2
  clinical description of 229–37
  general psychic clinical picture 227–9
  history of concept of 240
  prognosis of 237
  simple 241
  subdivisions of 241
  terminology of 226–7
  see also schizophrenia
depression (melancholia)
  apprehensive 249, 251
  clinical description of 248–53
  electroconvulsive therapy (ECT) in 262,
    270
  endogenous and reactive 257

in manic depression 245–7
prognosis of 253
in schizophrenia (dementia praecox)
233, 235
suicide in (melancholy suicide) 110, 112,
134, 250, 253
treatment of 253
see also manic depression
Diagnostic and Statistical Manual (DSM III)
of American Psychiatric Association
201, 242
Dictionary of Psychological Medicine
(Tuke) 54, 56
'discharging lesions' of epilepsy 60–1,
65–6, 67
'discordance' 203
dissociated thinking 172
double conscience 94, 101
double-entry bookkeeping 190
Down, J. Langdon H. 15–22
Down's syndrome 3
aetiological theories of 19–20
clinical description of 16–18
current methods of care 20–1
ethnic theory of 16, 19
prognosis of 17, 21
terminology of 21–2
'dreamy state' of Hughlings Jackson 59–81
drug treatment of psychotic disorders 262,
268–9
Durkheim, E. 2, 4, 105–38

Earlswood Asylum 16
echolalia 176, 198, 236
echopraxia 167, 176, 198, 234
ECT, *see* electroconvulsive therapy
Education Act (1981) 21
EEG (electroencephalography) 83
egoism, social currents of 125, 129, 131
die Einheitpsychose (unitary psychosis)
239–40
electroconvulsive therapy (ECT) 2, 5,
259–70
in America 267
brief pulse stimulation 270, 269
constant current machines 270, 269
current status of 268–270
the first machine 265
the first treatment 265–6
modified 267
unilateral 270
'epigastric' sensations preceding epileptic
seizures 59, 65, 67
epilepsy
haut mal 73, 77
hysterical 88
incompatibility of schizophrenia with 263
petit mal 63, 67, 73–80

temporal lobe, Jackson's description of ('a
particular variety') 3, 59–80
theory of degeneracy and 150, 161–2
see also convulsive treatment
Esquirol, J.E.D. 254
on hereditary degeneration 148, 156,
161
on suicide 105, 106
evolution, theory of, influence on psychiatry
159–61
exogenous influences on psychoses 256

Faculty Psychology 202, 203, 204
Fairbairn, W.R. D. 102, 103
Falret, J.P. 105, 201, 254
feeble-minded, *see* idiots
flexibilitas cerea (waxy flexibility) 198, 234
Flurothyl 269
folie circulaire 254
folie a double forme 254
Folie Intermittente 254
Freud, S.
Bleuler and 201, 202, 205
Hughlings Jackson and 81, 82
psychical mechanism of hysteria 87–104

Gardiner Hill, R. 2, 12
Gedankenlautwerden 197
general paralysis of the insane
aetiological theories of 211, 218–20
history of treatment of 222–3
malaria therapy in 221, 222–3
Treponema pallidum in brains of patients
with 4–5, 211–23
gout, insanity and 151
Gowers, William 80, 82
Gull, Sir William Withey 42–7
'gustatory' movements during 'dreamy state'
of epilepsy 59, 76

hallucinations in schizophrenia 197, 235
Hanwell Asylum 13
abolition of mechanical restraints in
8–10, 12
Haslam, J. 56, 57, 240
headaches, neuralgic, inheritance of 150
hebephrenia 240, 241
Hecker, E. 240
Heinroth, J.C.H. 240
Hellebore (veractum) treatment 262
hereditarianism, doctrine of 141, 142–58,
161–2
heredity of manic depression 247
Hester Adrian Centre, Manchester 20–1
Hill, R.G. 2, 12
hypnoid states 94–5, 101–2
hypnosis of hysterical patients 87, 92–3,
96–7, 99, 100
hypochondriacal ideas 249

hysteria 82
  anorexia nervosa and 30, 34, 38, 44, 46
  attacks of 88, 95–8
  curative effect of psychotherapy 99
  dispositional 95, 101–2
  psychical mechanism of 3, 87–104
  psychically acquired 95
  'traumatic' 87–94, 100
  typical course of severe 98

idiots 18, 141
  ethnic classification of 3, 15–22
  suicides by 117–19
  theory of degeneracy and 17–18, 19,
    151, 152, 154–5
imbeciles 16, 18
impulsive suicide 111–12, 134–5
incoherence of thought 172, 228
indifference in schizophrenia 178–80, 198,
  206
Indoklon 269
inner unity, loss of 227–8
insanity
  causation and prevention of 139–62
  concepts of 239–40
  facts and figures in regard to the increase
    of (1807–1877) 49–54
  moral 11, 57, 141, 255
  suicide and 105–23, 133–6
Instinctual Theory of Freud 103
insulin therapy 262, 264, 268
intellectual ambivalence 187
'intellectual aura' of Hughlings Jackson
  59–81
intermarriages, degeneracy and 153–4,
  158–9
international Classification of Diseases
  (ICD) 242
intracranial tumours, epilepsy associated
  with 59, 70–1
intrapsychic ataxia 203
irritability in schizophrenia 182–3

Jackson, Hughlings 59–83, 201
  contribution to psychiatry 80–3
  description of 'a particular variety' of
    epilepsy (temporal lobe epilepsy) 3,
    59–80
Jacob, Sarah (Welsh fasting girl) 38–9, 45
Jahnel, F. 221
Jaspers, K. 240
Journal of Mental Science 56–7, 80
Jung, C.G. 202, 203, 204, 205–6

Kahlbaum, K.L. 240
Kasanin, J. 242
Kiebedenken 175
Klein, Melanie 102
Koch 114, 119

Kraepelin, E. 4, 177, 225–57
  biographical background 239–40
  classification of psychoses 239–40,
    254–6
  clinical description of melancholy
    (depression) 248–53
  definition of manic depression 245–7,
    254–5
  dementia praecox 202, 203, 225–37
    clinical description of 229–37
    concept of 241–2
    general psychical picture 227–9
    general paralysis of the insane and
      211–12
    influence on development of psychiatry
      238, 254–7
Krafft-Ebing 219
Kränkung 91

Langfeldt, G. 242
language, importance of 103–4
Lasègue (Laseague), E.C., anorexia
  hysterica 30, 34, 44–5
laughter, affect-less 186, 198
Lejeune, Jérome 19–20
leucotomy, prefrontal 262, 268–9
Lincoln Asylum 12
lobotomy, see leucotomy, prefrontal
Lunacy Act (1845) 13, 51
Lunacy Commissioners 13, 49
  Special Report of 1897 54

Magnan, V. 201, 202, 254
malaria therapy in syphilis 221, 222–3
Malthus, Thomas Robert 160
mania
  electroconvulsive therapy (ECT) 270
  in manic depression 245–7
  simple 245
maniacal suicide 110, 134
manic depression 4, 245–57
  bipolar and unipolar 257
  clinical description by Kraepelin 248–53
  definition by Kraepelin 245–7, 254–5
  development of classification of 254–7
  inheritance of 247
  see also depression
manie sans délire 254
mannerisms 199
Mantegna, Andrea, painting of Madonna
  and Child 18, 22
Manual of Psychological Medicine (Bucknill
  and Tuke) 54, 55
marriage, consanguineous, degeneracy
  and 153–4, 158–9
Masselon, R. 189
Maudsley, Henry 4, 11, 13, 57, 80
  on causation and prevention of insanity
    139–62

on general paralysis of the insane 219
Medico-Psychological Association (MPA) 56–7, 81
Meduna, L. 263
megrims, familial predispositions to 150
melancholia, see depression
melancholy suicide 110, 112, 134
memories precipitating hysteria 91–4, 97, 101
mental disorders, concepts of 239–40
mental handicap 3, 18
  see also idiots
Mercatus, Ludovieus 145
metasyphilitic disorders 218
metrazol-induced convulsions 263, 264
Mickle, J. 218
Minkowski, E. 202
Mongolism, see Down's syndrome
monoideism 166–7, 175
monomania 240
  suicidal 106–9
Monro, James 12
mood
  changes in schizophrenia 179–81, 235
  manic depression and 245, 246
Moore, J.W. 211–17, 220
moral insanity 11, 57, 141, 255
moral treatment 10–12, 57–8
  of anorexia nervosa 37, 43
Moreau (de Tours), J.J. 105–6, 161, 201, 240
Morel, B. 200
  degeneracy theory 153, 162, 255
  démence précoce 226, 240
Morselli 117, 118, 119
Mott, F. 219–20, 221
Mourning and Melancholia (Freud) 102
mouth movements during 'dreamy state' of epilepsy 76
muscle relaxants used in electroconvulsive therapy (ECT) 267, 268–9

'naming' 167, 175
negativism 198–9
neologisms 196–7
neuralgias, hysterical 88
neuralgic headaches, familial predispositions to 150
neurasthenia, suicide and 113–19, 124, 135, 137
neurology in relation to psychiatry 80, 81–2, 83
neuropsychiatry 83
neuroses
  familial predispositions to 150
  traumatic 88, 89, 100
Noguchi, Hideyo
  biographical details 220–1

demonstration of Treponema pallidum in brain of patients with general paralysis 211–17, 220
Nonne, M. 211
noopsyche, Stransky's 228
Normansfield Hospital 18

Obsessive suicide 111, 134
onanism, dementia praecox and 233
optic neuritis, epilepsy associated with 59, 69–71
organic brain disease, epilepsy associated with 59, 70–2
Osler, W. 218–19

paralyses, hysterical 88
paralysis of the insane, general, see general paralysis of the insane
paramimia 186
paranoia (dementia paranoides) 240, 241
parasyphilitic disorders 218
parathymia in schizophrenics 185–6
penicillin 223
pentylenetetrazol (metrazol)-induced convulsions 263, 264
periodic insanity 245, 254–5
perplexity in manic depression 246
perserveration 175
personalities, multiple 196
personality, splitting of 196
  see also temperament
phenothiazines 268
phthisis, insanity and 151–3
Pick, A. 226, 240
Pinel, P. 11, 56, 201, 240, 254
Poor Law Act (1834) 12–13
Popper, Karl 4
prefrontal leucotomy 262, 268–9
pressure of thoughts 167
Prichard, J.C. 11, 12, 255
psychoanalysis 3–4, 100, 205, 256
psychopathic personality disorders 255
psychoses, concepts of 239–40
puberty, appearance of hereditary insanity at 157–8

reality, detachment from (autism) 166, 190–5, 196, 206
reflex reactions to psychical trauma 91
religion, suicide rates and 115–16
reminiscence (recollection)
  by hysterics 91
  in 'intellectual aura' of Hughlings Jackson 59, 62–3, 64, 72, 74, 77, 78
repression 101, 102–3
restraints, mechanical, treatment of insane without 7–14
The Retreat, York 11, 12, 53, 56, 255

retrograde metamorphosis (retrogression) 18, 154–5, 161
   see also degeneracy, theory of

St. Luke's Hospital 49–50
Salpêtrière Hospital 11
Savage, George 81, 82
schizo-affective psychosis 242
schizophrenia 3, 165–207
  accessory symptoms 165, 188–90, 203–4
  affectivity in 178–86, 198, 205–6
  ambivalence in 186–8, 205
  association disturbances 165, 166–78, 195–6, 205, 206, 228
  autism in 190–5
  Bleuler's concepts of 165–95, 202–6
  current diagnostic criteria 242
  differential diagnosis, significance of individual symptoms in 195–200, 206
  differentiation from manic depression 256–7
  electroconvulsive therapy (ECT) in 261, 263, 270
  fundamental symptoms 165, 166, 203–4, 205–6
  latent 166
  terminology of 202, 226–7, 241
  see also dementia praecox
schizophreniform psychosis 242
Schneider, K. 200, 204, 242
scrofula, insanity and 151–2
Séguin 19
sejunction, Wernicke's theory of 203
sex differences in suicide rates 114–15
sex of parents, inheritance of insanity and 156–7
Shuttleworth, G.E. 19
sleeping sickness, similarity to syphilis 219–20
smell, sensations of, during epileptic seizures 59, 65, 67
social causes of suicide 113, 123–33, 136–8
sociology, role of Emile Durkheim in 133
Spaltung (splitting) of mental functions 203, 206
  see also splitting
spasmodic movements, familial predispositions to 150
Spencer, Herbert 82, 160
spirochaetes (Treponema pallidum) in brain of patients with general paralysis 4–5, 211–20
splitting
  of consciousness 94, 101–2
  of mental functions 203, 206
  of personality 196

stereotype 166, 173, 174–5, 199
Stransky, E. 203, 227–8
stupor
  differential diagnosis of 199–200
  in schizophrenia 194
suggestion, unconscious 90
suicide 105–38
  anxiety- 111
  in depression (melancholy) 110, 112, 134, 250, 253
  impulsive or automatic 111–12, 134–5
  maniacal 110, 134
  obsessive 111, 134
  problems of statistical analysis 137–8
  psychopathic states (insanity) and 105–23, 133–6
  social element of 113, 123–33, 136–8
super-ego 102
suppression 93, 102
symbolization 89
syphilis
  history of treatment of 221, 222–3
  intracranial (cerebral) 70, 212
  see also general paralysis of the insane

taste, sensations of, during epileptic seizures 59
temperament
  phthisical 152
  suicide and 124
thought
  autistic 194–5
  blocking 167, 173, 176–7, 196
  deprivation (withdrawal) 177
  dissociated 172
  incoherence of 172, 228
  Klebedenken 175
  pressure of 167
thought disorders in schizophrenia 166–78, 195, 204, 205, 228
Thurnam, John 55
thymopsyche, Stransky's 228
tics 199
  hysterical 88–9
  inheritance of 150
transference 100
transitivism 196
trauma, psychical
  abreaction to 91–2, 93
  precipitating hysteria 87–94, 100
traumatic neuroses 88, 89
Trélat, U. 161
Treponema pallidum in brain of patients with general paralysis 4–5, 211–20
trypanosomiasis, similarity to syphilis 219–20
tryparsamide treatment of general paralysis of the insane 222

tuberculosis
  latent, anorexia nervosa and   25, 27, 42
  theory of degeneracy and   17, 19, 151–3
Tuke, D. Hack   3, 49–58
  biographical details   55–7
  humane management of the insane and
    56
  on the increase in insanity from 1807 to
    1877   49–54
Tuke, Samuel   11, 53, 255
Tuke, Williams   11, 53
twilight states   193

the unconscious   100, 103
unconscious suggestion   90
unitary psychosis (die Einheitpsychose)
  239–40
unity, inner, loss of   227–8

veractum (Hellebore) treatment   262

verbigeration   199
visual disturbances
  hysterical   88
  preceding epileptic seizures   60, 66
vomiting, hysterical   88
Vorbeidenken   170

Wagner-Jauregg, J.   222–3
Wallace, A.R.   159
Warnock Report (1978)   21
Wassermann Test   219
waxy flexibility (flexibilitas cerea)   198, 234
Welsh fasting girl (Sarah Jacob)   38–9, 45
Wernicke, C.   203
Weygandt, W.   229
word associations   204
word-blindness after epileptic seizures
    66–7
word-deafness after epileptic seizures   6–7